Esthetic Dentistry and
Ceramic Restorations

D 340 TOU

Esthetic Dentistry and Ceramic Restorations

Bernard Touati DDS DSO
Past-President, European Academy of Esthetic Dentistry
Institut Dentaire
33 rue de Prony
75017 Paris
France

Paul Miara DDS
Scientific President, Société Française de Dentisterie Esthétique
Private Practice
24 rue de Rocher
75008 Paris
France

Dan Nathanson DMD MSD
Professor and Chairman
Department of Restorative Sciences and Biomaterials
Goldman School of Dental Medicine
Boston University, Boston MA, USA

With a special contribution by

Russell Giordano DMD DMSc
Boston University, Boston MA, USA

MARTIN DUNITZ

© Martin Dunitz Ltd 1999

First published in the United Kingdom in
1999 by Martin Dunitz Ltd, The Livery House, 7–9 Pratt Street
London NW1 0AE

A CIP catalogue record for this book is available from the British Library

ISBN 1-85317-159-X

Distributed in the United States and Canada by:
Thieme New York
333 7th Avenue
New York, NY 10001
USA
Tel. 212 760 0888, ext 110

Composition by Scribe Design, Gillingham, Kent
Printed and bound in Singapore by Imago

Contents

Forewords

John W McLean

The advancement of standards in esthetic dentistry has now become a worldwide effort, and no country can claim a monopoly of expertise in this every-expanding area. It is therefore a pleasure to see the type of international cooperation that is evident in this Atlas, embracing both sides of the Atlantic. The subjects selected reflect the distinct changes that our profession is now making in deciding whether to use conventional metal–ceramic crowns or to adopt the more conservative approach of the bonded ceramic laminate veneer or inlay. Even our approach to the treatment of early caries is moving towards minimal preparation in order to conserve human enamel, which is still our best restorative material.

I have, over the years, become familiar with Dr Bernard Touati's contribution to the advancement of esthetic dentistry, and, in particular, his porcelain inlay technique, which is respected and much admired internationally. The work presented in this Atlas by Bernard, Paul Miara and Dan Nathanson continues this tradition of excellence.

It is a credit to the authors that they have found time in their busy practices to record their work. Color photography and printing have reached such a high quality that today's practitioner is given a unique opportunity to share the exacting standards that the authors set. They have, over the years, been able to assess many new materials and techniques, and I have greatly valued their clinical judgement. Today, the clinician is faced with a constant stream of new ceramics and dentin bonding agents, and manufacturer's claims often fail to meet expectations. Postgraduate education based on good science and clinical expertise is the only way to unravel the mysteries of the advertisements, and the authors have made significant contributions in this area by their teaching. This new book is a further step in sharing knowledge that has taken many years to accumulate and then refine into a critical reappraisal of many of our current practices.

John W McLean OBE
Consulting Professor in Fixed Prosthodontics and Biomaterials,
Louisiana State University, New Orleans LA, USA
Formerly Clinical Consultant to the Laboratory
of the Government Chemist

Peter Schärer

Esthetic dentistry, a term that originated in the USA, has been generally accepted all over the world and has become one of the main areas of interest in clinical dentistry. More and more practitioners have become involved in this area over the past 10 years.

To the extent that periodontology and gnathology as basic factors in restorative dentistry have become accepted, and methods suitable to general practitioners as well as for specialists have been developed and refined, the esthetic aspects of dentistry have become increasingly interesting to all those colleagues who consider themselves to be pioneers seeking a better restorative dentistry.

The increasing interest in esthetics has been accompanied by developments in new tooth-colored materials, with ever-improving clinical properties. Today these factors contribute to the high level of satisfaction felt by even the most critical patients.

It has been one of the major contributions of Drs Bernard Touati and Paul Miara to promote high quality esthetic dentistry, first in France, and because of their competence in the English language, all over the world. Dr Dan Nathanson, a renowned expert in biomaterials, has brought the essential fundamentals to the understanding and practice of modern esthetic dentistry.

The quality of the pictures and drawings in this Atlas, the wide range of techniques discussed in this book, and the multitude of restorative methods presented will provide the readers with a complete overview of esthetic possibilities. It is by the continuous efforts of such authors as these three that esthetic dentistry in Europe, the USA and all over the world did not turn into a passing phase. Rather, it has made a genuine contribution to the profession, and has improved the quality of our work.

I congratulate them on their efforts in esthetics, and look forward to even further advancements in this exciting area of restorative dentistry.

Peter Schärer
Professor and Chairman,
Department of Biomaterials and Prosthodontics,
University of Zurich Dental School, Zurich, Switzerland

Preface

Many studies have already been published on esthetic techniques in specialized areas of dentistry.

The steady advance in the development of materials and, in particular, in the understanding of certain principles underlying ceramic bonding, reinforcement and light transmission, has served to promote further evolution of esthetic dentistry. Throughout the 1980s, restorative dentistry has been based on the four following basic principles: biocompatibility of materials, reduced tissue damage, longevity, and esthetic considerations.

This text aims to present basic principles as well as clinical and laboratory procedures, providing both the practitioner and the technician with an overview of the opportunities and limitations that innovative esthetic treatments can offer.

It is not our intention to produce an encyclopedia on esthetic dentistry or a textbook on one specific subject; instead, we intend this text to be a practitioner's guide and introduction to esthetic techniques for improving, restoring, or rebuilding single teeth with various ceramic systems.

If we have succeeded in our aim, this book could be followed by a sequel on more invasive dentistry (as occasionally required), necessitating the use of bridges or implants.

The text classifies the different types of ceramics now available, describing their main characteristics and indications. It also traces the history and development of bonding, listing the main principles and providing an overview of this rapidly developing field.

A special chapter is devoted to basic data on color and the effects of light transmission – certainly one of the key elements to cosmetic success.

Observations on the color of natural teeth and deviations that may occur throughout life are also fully discussed. Several chapters cover in detail treatment methodology – from chemical techniques, such as bleaching or microabrasion, to prosthetic techniques, for various indications.

Ceramic laminate veneers, jacket crowns, inlays and onlays are also fully documented, and the basics of dental photography, transfer of esthetic information and various laboratory techniques are discussed.

We hope that this book will provide dental practitioners with all the information needed to understand and implement up-to-date esthetic procedures, as part of their daily everyday practice. The text should also aid in developing the skills of critical observation, analysis and decision-making before embarking on a programme of treatment.

BT
PM
DN

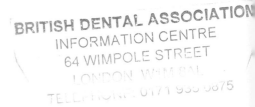

Acknowledgements

We would like to thank our families for their patience and understanding during our many absences while we were working on this book: our wives – Liliane Touati, Monique Miara and Sinaia Nathanson; and our children – Vanessa, Elisa and Laurine Touati, Alexandre Miara, and Natalie and Doria Nathanson. We also thank our dental assistants for their support: Angélique Gouget, Anne-Marie Delhoume and Sylvie Piot.

Books often draw on suggestions and collaboration from friends and colleagues, and we would particularly like to thank the following for their contributions and their inspiration: Drs Sylvain Altglas, Nitzan Bichacho, Claude Cohen-Coudar, Robert Eskenazi, Didier Fillion, Youssef Haikel, Gilles Laborde, Pierre Machtou, John McLean, Jaoa Pimenta, Michel Rogé, Rafi Romano, Peter Schärer and Jean-Claude Senoussi; and our laboratory technicians: Marc Cristou, Jacques Diligeart, Jean-Marc Etienne, Willi Geller, Jean-Paul Jourdain, Laboratoire GH, Jean-Pierre Levot, Harry Levy, Gilbert Moricet, Serge Tissier and Gérald Ubassy.

We gratefully acknowledge assistance from: Marylène Scagni of *L'Information Dentaire* for the graphics; Gérard Bouhot for advice and help with the chapter on photography; Fred Picavet (Bisico, France); Ulrich Schmidt (Ivoclar Vivadent, France); Yves Scialom (Cédia, France); Herfried Eder (Komet, France); Philippe Gruat (Kerr); Zermack; GC International; Dentsply-DeTrey; Ducera.

Finally, we owe a considerable debt to the following: Dr Stephen Dunne (King's College Dental School, London), for his general help and advice, and for reviewing the text through its various stages; Dr Russell Giordano (Goldman School of Dental Medicine, Boston University) for his valuable contribution to the text; Stephen Sweeney (Montage Media), for scanning the majority of the slides and for the excellent quality of the reproduction; and Alison Campbell (Martin Dunitz Publishers), for her collaboration and careful co-ordination of the project.

CHAPTER 1

Introduction to Bonded Ceramic Restorations

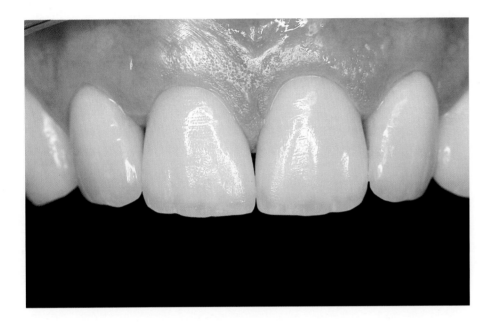

Restorative dentistry has witnessed some major discoveries during the past two decades, to the extent that many routine procedures in modern dental practice vary considerably from the way in which they were practised for over half a century.

The conventional ground rules for restorative dentistry still taught in most modern dental schools include two objectives: debridement of carious tissue and establishment of a cavity preparation with specific form. The form and dimensions of cavity preparations are designed to contribute to resistance against functional stresses as well as to counteract displacement of restorative material from the tooth (retention). Another traditional feature in cavity design, 'extension for prevention', has become less popular in recent years, but still finds its use in many applications.

Traditionally, the retention of the restorative material would be provided by mechanical undercuts in the cavity preparation. This arrangement, still the basis for retention of silver amalgam and other restorations, does not provide perfect microscopic alignment of the restorative material with the cavity walls; in fact, a gap may exist between the tooth structure and the restorative material. This gap may be large enough to allow saliva, salivary ions and bacteria to enter the space, causing microleakage. Silver amalgam restorations survived through a process of formation of self-sealing corrosion layers at the tooth–restoration interface. Indirect restorations (e.g. gold inlays) functioned because of the use of cements for sealing and retention. But resinous tooth-colored material is a poor candidate for restoration by mechanical retention. Polymerization shrinkage and the lack of a seal are distinct disadvantages.

Adhesive dentistry

With the advent of enamel etching (Buonocore, 1955) as a means of retention, new restorative possibilities with resin materials have become available. Consequently, cavity preparation guidelines were changed to accommodate this new form of retention. Because resin penetration into microscopic irregularities of the etched enamel produces such reliable retention (Dogon et al, 1980; Jordan, 1980), it is no longer necessary to rely on undercutting and mechanical retention for restoration survival. A new era of 'adhesive dentistry' has emerged that relates to restorative procedures based on filled resins aided by acid-etched retention. The 'bond' to enamel proves to be strong, consistent, reliable and durable, providing excellent sealing in addition to retention (Figure 1.1). A side-benefit to this development is the opportunity for tissue conservation by reduced cutting for mechanical purposes, as well as an increased ability to produce esthetic restorations that integrate well with the remaining tooth structure.

Dentin adhesion

The reported successes with 'bonding' to enamel has caused researchers to expand their trials to include dentin. However, early attempts with dentin bonding were unsuccessful. The etching of dentin with phosphoric acid did not produce any retention with several resin restorative materials tested. Furthermore, studies by various researchers demonstrated potential pulpal damage due to the application of acid to cut dentin (see Chapter 2). For a while, it seemed that bonding to dentin was a hopeless fantasy. However, in

the early 1980s new adhesive systems were introduced with measurable adhesion to dentin. These materials, containing esters of phosphates or phosphonates, relied on ionic attraction with calcium molecules to provide the adhesion effect on the dentinal surface.

The use of dentin-bonding agents of the so-called 'first generation' was somewhat limited by the low level of bond strengths attained, but adhesive dentistry has changed further to rely even less on mechanical undercutting. The problem with early dentin adhesives was that bond strength values (in laboratory testing) were in the range of only 3.5–7.0 MPa. Polymerization shrinkage forces reach magnitudes of 10 MPa and more, and thus distort and disrupt dentinal adhesion.

'New generation' dentin adhesives

Further development of dentin adhesives led to the introduction in the late 1980s of systems capable of producing bonds of 15 MPa and above, often surpassing those reported with enamel systems. The 'new generation' dentin adhesives rely on a more sophisticated retention mechanism than previously utilized. By partial alteration or total removal of the smear layer followed by treatment of the dentin surface with 'bonding promoters', better wetting of the dentin surface by modified BIS–GMA resin is accomplished. The bonding resin finds its way into the dentinal tubules and attains intimate contact with the cleansed and at times partially decalcified dentin surface. The excellent wetting coupled with tubular penetration creates a combined micromechanical and adhesive bond, leading to relatively high resistance against separation (see Chapter 2).

By forming a layer at the dentin level (hybridization) (Nakabayashi et al, 1982), these far more ecologically sound bonding techniques seal off the tubules, which blocks the entry of bacteria, thus limiting inflammation of the pulp and ensuing postoperative sensitivity.

These developments have further changed the nature of preferred cavity preparation for the use of resinous restoratives. A new degree of reliability in terms of retention and sealing has been introduced which makes the preparation process so conservative that often mechanical cutting is totally obviated and the restorative material is held by adhesive retention only.

The quality and magnitude of bonding both to enamel and dentin enabled the development of the concept of bonded ceramic restorations (see Chapter 2). Ceramics, which are still the materials of choice for

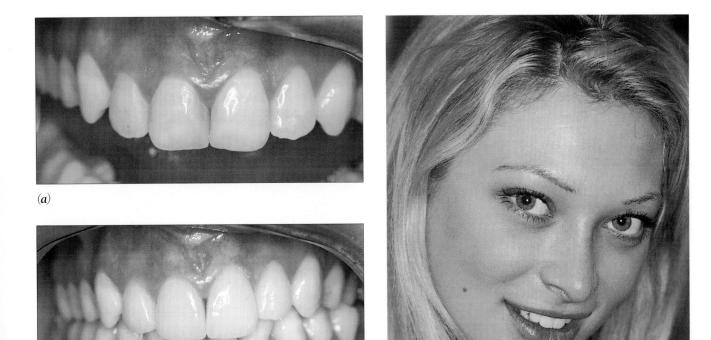

(a)

(b)

(c)

Figure 1.1 (a) *Central and lateral incisors restored by extensive composite fillings have an unesthetic appearance.* (b) *Four ceramic laminate veneers have been bonded onto the vital teeth, after conservative preparations have been performed.* (c) *The smile of the young patient.*

offering unequalled esthetics and resemblance to tooth structure, are somewhat restricted in use because of limitations in their mechanical properties. Previous experience with jacket crowns has shown that the brittle nature of ceramics and their inability to handle tensile stresses results in inevitable failures (McLean and Hughes, 1965). However, the ability to microetch the inner surfaces of ceramic restorations and the use of resins as intermediary materials between tooth and ceramic, have produced yet another new kind of restoration, namely, the bonded ceramic.

Bonded ceramic restorations

Bonded ceramic restorations were an exciting new entity of the 1980s, and are now accepted as a valid treatment modality. They offer the benefits of excellent esthetics, conservative tissue management, resistance to degradation and discoloration, and a lower potential for marginal caries. Since the technique involves no alloy, there is virtually no risk of corrosion or galvanic reactions (Figure 1.2).

With bonded ceramics, restorations can be more easily 'integrated' with tooth structure, since the new bonding mechanism can virtually establish a continuity from tooth structure to restoration. There is no other material that can emulate tooth structure in terms of color and texture as closely as ceramics. Through the input of a skilled dental technician and with appropriate clinical procedures, a dentist can achieve excellent esthetic results with bonded ceramics.

The longevity of these restorations still has to be determined. Because they have been introduced

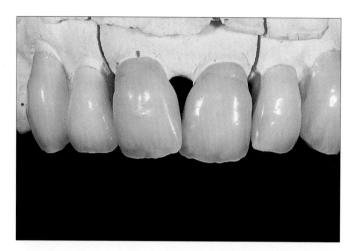

Figure 1.2 Most ceramic restorations can be fabricated on refractory investment, such as these laminate veneers, which greatly simplifies laboratory procedures.

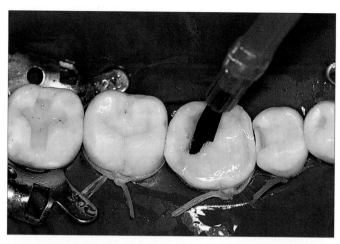

Figure 1.3 The quadrant has to be restored by four esthetic inlays. Single-component dentin adhesive is applied to the conditioned dentin surface, dried and light-cured.

relatively recently, long-term (15–20 years) clinical data do not exist. However, early observations demonstrating virtually no wear of the ceramic, only limited discoloration, and a good overall record over the initial few years of service lead to the conclusion that longevity may surpass that of other 'direct' restorative methods.

Esthetic dentistry

Composite cements, with a capacity for light transmission similar to that of natural teeth and great scope for variations in chroma, endow restorations with exceptional vitality.

There is now a movement, at least in the case of single teeth, away from metal alloy reinforcements, which remain esthetically detrimental, even after opaquing, acting as screens serving to direct light rays into dental and gingival tissues.

Use of fluoride and the development of dental care and prophylaxis in the West has led to a reduction in the number of extractions, and to detection of caries often before the pulp is involved. At the same time, patients' life expectancy has increased. This situation is conducive to conservative esthetic dentistry relying on restorations devoid of metal. Ceramics offer the benefits of proven biocompatibility and reduced propensity for retaining bacterial plaque. In contrast to composite

resins, ceramics offer the potential for long-term functionality. In common with composite resins, after bonding, the tooth is reinforced (Figures 1.3–1.5).

Economic circumstances do not favor short-lived materials requiring frequent repair. Moreover, the advantage of conservation of tooth tissue is lost if frequent repairs are required. It appears likely that advances in the chemistry of synthetic resins will lead to an improvement in the structure and longevity of these materials, but for the time being only ceramics can offer long-term esthetics as well as biocompatibility.

It is for these reasons that we have elected to introduce innovative aspects of these bonded materials in this book. Few reference works have been devoted to this subject, a fact that further aroused our enthusiasm. We shall be stressing the importance of preparation, the extent of which has diminished in recent years and often involves intra-enamel reduction, such as the veneer preparation.

We shall also stress the clinical benefits offered by ceramic laminate veneers, jacket crowns, and inlays and onlays, while detailing the precise indications for each procedure.

After 10 years' experience with these restorations, we can report clear and accurate results. In contrast to the prevailing view during the 1980s, under the influence of conservative clinicians, the failure rate of these prostheses has not exceeded that of conventional metal–ceramic structures when used appropriately.

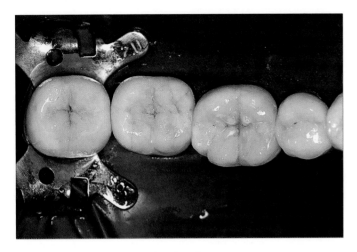

Figure 1.4 *The inlays are luted with a composite cement.*

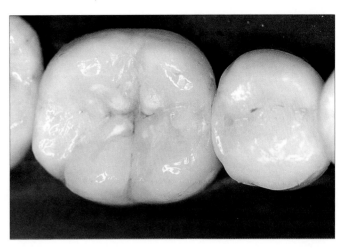

Figure 1.5 *A higher magnification view of the inlays shows that the margins are hardly visible.*

However, this does not mean that these techniques have no shortcomings. In particular, as with any other bonding technique, failure to attend to even minor details can bring about clinical failure. This reliance on technique requires knowledge and familiarity with the materials used, which is not easy to achieve considering the number of new products steadily flowing on to the market and the varying procedures they require.

Not all setbacks arise from ignorance of the materials used or errors in clinical technique: poor analysis of the clinical case can often be responsible. We aim to help the clinician in this consideration.

This book, then, is the fruit of 25 years' clinical experience, wide reading, and our teaching activities amongst both students and practitioners. We should have liked to have cited all those shaping our knowledge, but consideration of this would have detracted from our objective to provide a synthesized clinical atlas. The best tribute we can pay to our mentors is to present case histories in which patients' teeth are not just treated, but are restored to a sound, healthy and esthetic state.

Knowing that the good is the enemy of the best, we have approached this task with humility as well as determination. We have attempted to make strides towards genuinely esthetic dentistry, while realizing that the successes achieved are only relative, and that much more progress needs to be made.

It should also be stressed that successful esthetic dentistry implies teamwork, with the laboratory technician playing a major role. Success may be measured in terms of the technician's powers of observation, artistry and technological discipline.

Bruce Clark commented in a 1931 edition of *Dental Digest* that most writers in the field of dental ceramics and esthetic dentistry mention the many difficulties encountered in reproducing tooth color in ceramics, and that nearly all ceramic laboratory technicians believe that most of their troubles would be over once the color problem had been solved.

Solving the color problem in ceramics is still our main concern today (see Chapter 5). Despite our improved regulation of clinical preparation, fashioning in the laboratory and bonding procedures, we come up against the same problems of establishing color shades and communicating these to the laboratory (Ubassy, 1993). Far from simplifying matters, dispensing with metal substructures in the anterior region tends to complicate the cosmetic success of our prostheses, since the final color shade will be dictated not only by the ceramic material but also by the bonding substance and the underlying tooth structure (Preston, 1983).

This book also aims to impart a basic knowledge of color and visual aspects of the natural tooth (see Chapter 4). Our approach to the study of ceramic

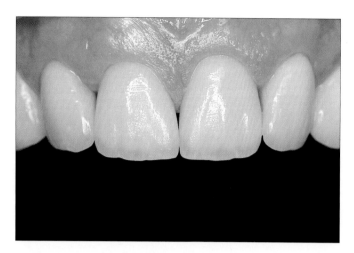

Figure 1.6 Empress (Ivoclar) ceramic laminate veneers (stratification technique) require less invasive preparations than jacket crowns, and yet provide appealing esthetic results thanks to their texture and opalescence.

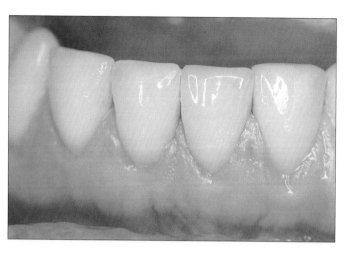

Figure 1.7 Bonded jacket crowns on lower incisors: the soft tissue looks pink and natural, and the teeth are pleasingly translucent owing to the absence of any metallic substructure.

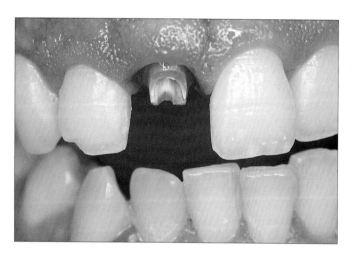

Figure 1.8 A fractured devitalized central incisor on a young patient.

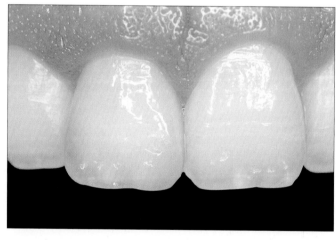

Figure 1.9 Bonded, low-fusing ceramic crown (Duceram-LFC, Ducera) reproducing the natural appearance of the adjacent teeth.

restoration will therefore consist of assessing the effects of light and light transmission through the prosthesis at all the different clinical and laboratory stages. In this way we shall attempt to explain how preparations, for example, for laminate veneers or jacket crowns, can exert an influence on such transmission (Figures 1.6 and 1.7; see also Chapters 9 and 10).

If our preference now tends toward restorations devoid of metal substructures in the anterior region, this is due to our belief that they hamper natural light transmission.

The potential for transparency and opacity of different ceramic powders and composite cements allows us to reproduce the visual qualities of dental tissue. In this way, we can produce restorations with luminous or translucent appearance, as required (Figures 1.8 and 1.9).

The task of reproducing a tooth in ceramic goes well beyond making the right choice of shape or colour.

In view of the importance of light transmission, we shall explain

- the laws governing light transmission;
- color mechanisms and the principles underlying visual perception;
- the 'language of color' and contemporary methods of communication using it;

- the color of the natural tooth in its various forms.

The chapters detailing these subjects will aim to provide all the information required to improve the natural aspect of our prostheses (see Chapters 4–6).

Finally, thanks are always due to our patients for their forbearance, encouragement and the financial sacrifices to which they consent – even those who sometimes expect too much of us! This study is dedicated to the patients themselves, since it is they who reap the benefits of our refinements.

References

Buonocore MG, A simple method of increasing the adhesion of acrylic filling materials to enamel surfaces. *J Dent Res* 1955; **34**: 849–53.

Dogon IL, Nathanson D, Van Leeuwen MJ, A long term clinical evaluation of Class IV acid etched composite resin restorations. *Compend Contin Educ Dent* 1980; **6**: 385.

McLean JW, Hughes TH, The reinforcement of dental porcelain with ceramic oxides. *Br Dent J* 1965; **119**: 251–67.

Nakabayashi N, Kojima K, Masuhara E, The promotion of adhesion by the infiltration of monomers into tooth substrates. *J Biomed Mater Res* 1982; **16**: 265–73.

Preston JD, The elements of esthetics – application of color science. In: *Dental Ceramics: Proceedings of the First International Symposium on Ceramics.* Chicago: Quintessence, 1983: 491–520.

Ubassy G, *Shape and Color: The Key to Successful Ceramic Restorations.* Berlin: Quintessence, 1993.

CHAPTER 2

Development and Mechanism of Dental Adhesive Procedures

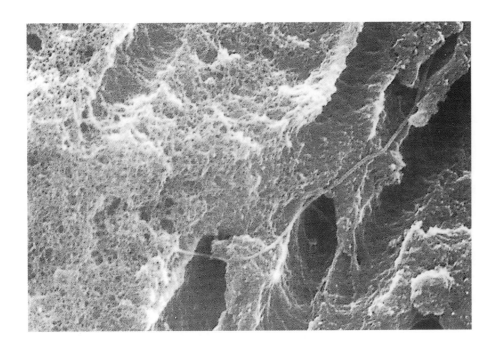

Dental restorative procedures require the securing of restorative materials to tooth structure. The use of adhesion and adhesive materials makes much sense in achieving retention in the oral cavity. Nevertheless, adhesives are a newcomer to dentistry.

Adhesion requires certain conditions that are not easily found within the oral environment. For instance, adhesion is optimal with relatively smooth, dry, clean homogeneous surfaces. Tooth structure is heterogeneous, normally moist, covered with various organic films, and is constantly bathed in saliva.

In generic terms, adhesion is the joining of two solids. It usually occurs through an adhesive medium – normally in a liquid state – that is capable of wetting the two solid surfaces and then solidifying, thus providing a joint between the two solids. The mechanism keeping the adhesive in close contact and permanently connected to the solid surface can be chemical, mechanical or a combination of both. Chemical adhesion occurs when the adhesive reacts chemically with the solid surface or achieves extremely close molecular contact with it. Mechanical adhesion derives from incorporation of the liquid adhesive into irregularities and mechanical undercuts of the solid surface. This phenomenon is sometimes referred to as micromechanical interlocking.

Good wetting of the adherent surfaces by the adhesive is imperative for good adhesion, and therefore the adhesive–adherent compatibility is of great importance. Good wetting usually occurs with solids that exhibit high surface energies. Adhesives in general should have low viscosities or low surface tension to increase their wetting capabilities.

The enamel surface, relatively smooth with no provision for micromechanical attachment, is also wet and has a relatively low surface energy, making it a poor substrate to adhere to. In addition, enamel is usually covered with a pellicule which may also interfere with adhesion. Paradoxically, removal of the pellicule by polishing also reduces the surface energy, making the enamel even more resistant to the flow of liquids and wetting. In fact, the polishing of enamel with fluoride-containing prophylaxis paste as a dental hygiene procedure is believed to have the benefit of preventing or reducing the adherence and accumulation of dental plaque (Glantz, 1969).

Acid etching of the enamel surface, as originally proposed by Buonocore (1955), induces a microscopic roughness to the surface that affects adhesion in several ways: It increases the surface area available for adhesion, increases the surface energy of the enamel and produces microscopic irregularities suitable for mechanical interlocking. When such a surface is covered with a dental adhesive (e.g. a diluted BIS–GMA resin), excellent wetting occurs. The adhesive then sets by polymerization over the surface and in the microscopic undercuts, achieving the desired micromechanical interlocking. This adhesion phenomenon with etched enamel, routinely referred to as 'bonding', is the basis of most adhesive procedures now practised in the various disciplines of dentistry.

From the initial experiments of Buonocore, who used citric acid for etching and poly(methyl methacrylate) as the adhesive resin, the technique has evolved to the use of highly specialized adhesive systems and new etching agents. Various laboratory studies have been reported in which the micromechanical bond to etched enamel was tested and found to produce bond strengths in excess of 16 MPa. In clinical studies the bonding process produced reliable restorations repeatedly, with high rates of success over long follow-ups.

Initial enamel-bonding procedures involved the use of phosphoric acid solutions in concentrations ranging from 37% to 50% in strength. The routine application procedure called for repeated wetting of the enamel surface for at least 60 seconds and up to 120 seconds.

Gwinnett (1971) and Silverstone et al (1975), observing the microscopic patterns of the etched enamel surface, reported three main formations. The type 1 etching pattern exhibited a honeycomb formation where the cores of the enamel prisms were removed. This was assumed to be the most common pattern. The type 2 etching pattern was described as the reverse of type 1, with the enamel cores protruding and the peripheries removed. The type 3 etching pattern is less organized, with a more amorphous pattern that gives no hint to the enamel prism formation. Nathanson et al (1982) quantified the three etching pattern formations and showed that the type 3 pattern was actually the most prevalent and the type 1 pattern the least prevalent – only about 15% of the surfaces exhibited this formation.

Enamel etching provides excellent retention for composite restorations (Dogon et al, 1980) that are bonded to enamel. Another significant benefit is the sealing effect achieved with margins that are enamel-bonded, and a significant decrease in microleakage (Crim and Shay, 1987). Bonding to enamel can also create the effect of cusp strengthening in posterior teeth (Share et al, 1982; Morin et al, 1984) as compared with non-bonded restorations (e.g. amalgam), which contribute little to tooth strength.

In the mid-1970s phosphoric acid gels became popular. These gels, in concentrations of 40% or less, required single applications for 60 seconds and were then washed off with water. Glasspoole and Erickson (1986) tested the effects of different etching times on enamel and found that 15 seconds of etching produced as reliable a retention as one-minute treatments. This finding prompted a new etching regimen requiring only 15 seconds of acid application for all routine enamel-bonding procedures.

More recently, a new enamel etching procedure, utilizing 10% maleic acid, has been introduced in conjunction with a dentin adhesive system (Scotchbond Multipurpose, 3M, Minneapolis/St Paul, MN, USA). Although microscopically the enamel etched with such

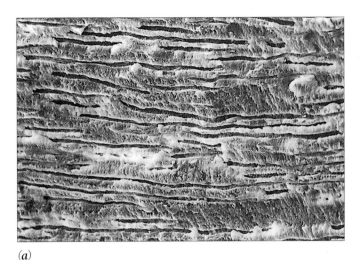
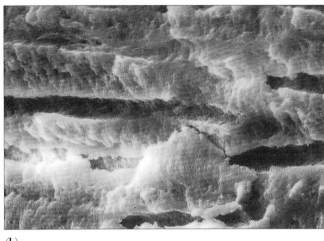

(a)   (b)

Figure 2.1 (*a*) *This split section of tooth shows the tubular structure of dentin (SEM, ×1000);* (*b*) *magnification (SEM, ×5000) of section from* (*a*), *exhibiting the microstructure of tubular dentin – note the interconnecting tubules.*

conditioner shows a somewhat less pronounced etching pattern, the bond strength is claimed not to change substantially. This finding has been challenged by some researchers (Swift and Cloe, 1993).

Adhesion to dentin

Adhesion to dentin surfaces has been a more difficult and challenging task than bonding to enamel. Researchers have tried bonding methods similar to those used for enamel, namely, acid-etching the dentin surface and application of low-viscosity resins. However, the results in terms of bond strength have been disappointing. Also, the direct application of acids to dentin has raised concern about the potential adverse effects on the pulp (Retief et al, 1974; Stanley et al, 1975).

The complexity of adhesion to dentin derives from the fact that dentin is more heterogeneous than enamel, has a lower level of calcified structure and has a much higher water content. Compared with the highly calcified enamel, dentin is composed of a collagen–hydroxyapatite–water combination that is only 45% inorganic. Dentin is a tubular tissue, with dentinal tubules radiating from the pulp toward the dentinoenamel junction

(Figure 2.1). In the deeper section, towards the pulp, each tubule houses an odontoblastic process that extends from the pulp (Yamada et al, 1991). The tubules of vital dentin are filled with fluid that is under slight pressure. Tubule diameter changes from an average of 2.5 μm close to the pulp to 0.8 μm at the enamel side. The tubule density also varies with the depth of the dentin: on average 30 000 tubules/mm² at the dentino-enamel junction to 45 000/mm² at the pulp (Heymann et al, 1988; Paul and Schärer, 1993) (Figures 2.2–2.4).

Simply opening the tubules by acid etching and dissolving the smear layer followed by the application of a conventional bonding resin did not produce any substantial bond strengths. Hydrophobic conventional bonding agents could not fill and attach themselves to the tubules in the presence of the tubular fluid. This aspect of incompatibility was enhanced by the pressure of the tubular fluid in the direction opposite to the flow of the resin.

With the introduction of the so-called 'first-generation' dentin-bonding agents, some chemistry was utilized to achieve better adhesion. These materials were based on phosphate esters that exhibited an ionic attraction to the positively charged calcium ions found in the smear layer and dentin surface. Because they were supposed to react

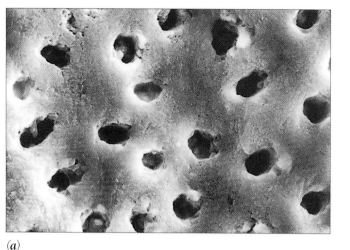

(a)

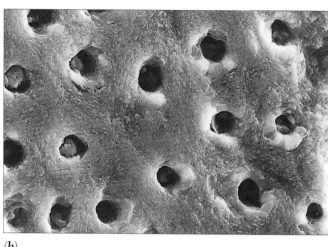

(b)

Figure 2.2 *Dentin surface after (**a**) treatment with 10% phosphoric acid for 15 seconds – note removal of smear layer and open tubules (SEM, ×5000); (**b**) after treatment with 10% phosphoric acid for 60 seconds – this decalcified surface exposes collagen fibers and has a characteristic appearance (SEM, ×5000).*

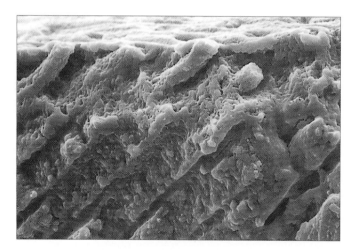

Figure 2.3 *Split section of dentin (SEM, ×3000), showing smear layer on top with some smear layer plugs blocking the tubule openings.*

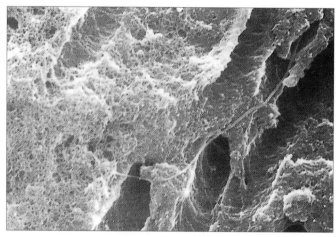

Figure 2.4 *Tubular dentin (SEM, ×5000) after acid conditioning, revealing decalcified surface.*

with the smear layer, its removal through dentin conditioning was not recommended. In fact, the deliberate creation of a smear layer (e.g. via surface roughening) was a commonly recommended procedure.

Although measured bond strengths ranging up to 7 MPa were reported, bonding the dentin with these early products remained unsatisfactory. Not only was

the limited bond strength too weak to support many dental applications, but it was also often counteracted by the forces of polymerization shrinkage acting in the opposite direction (Davidson et al, 1984; Munksgaard et al, 1985). Another concern was the potential hydrolysis of phosphonate esters over time in the presence of water (Eliades and Vougiouklakis, 1989).

Materials in the second generation of adhesives included Scotchbond (3M, Minneapolis/St Paul, MN, USA), J & J Dentin Bonding Agent (Johnson & Johnson, East Windsor, NJ, USA), Creation Bond (Den-Mat, Santa Maria, CA, USA), Bondlite (Kerr, Glendora, CA, USA), and Dentin Adhesit (Ivoclar Vivadent, Schaan, Liechtenstein). One of these early dentin adhesive systems utilized a different monomer, isocyanate, to produce a bond to dentinal tissue. Clearfil Liner Bond (Kuraray, Osaka, Japan), combining a phenyl phosphate ester and HEMA (hydroxyethyl methacrylate), was shown to produce some bond strength to etched dentin (Fusayama et al, 1979). In general, in vitro testing of these products produced only modest bond strengths, hinting at their limited bonding potential, or required application techniques that were difficult to follow (Solomon and Beech, 1983).

Clinical performance of phosphate esters as reported in the dental literature was relatively poor (Ziemecki et al, 1987; Heymann et al, 1988; Tyas, 1991). Additional retention from enamel etching was a prerequisite for any predictable results. Mechanical undercutting to enhance retention was also often recommended. Apparently the mechanism of bonding the smear layer was flawed and could not produce consistent and reliable bonds.

'Third-generation' dentin bonding systems included products such as Scotchbond 2 (3M), GLUMA (Bayer), Tenure (Den-Mat), Prisma Universal Bond 3 (Dentsply-Caulk), X–R Bond (Kerr) and Syntac (Ivoclar Vivadent). Bond strengths for these systems were reported to be substantially higher than those obtained with the 'second-generation' adhesives, and at times approached those of etched enamel-bonding values (Barkmeier et al, 1986; Barkmeier and Cooley, 1989a,b; Chappell et al, 1991; Retief, 1991). Also, bonds obtained in vitro did not differ significantly from those tested in vivo (Gray and Burgess, 1991).

Third-generation dentin adhesives used various chemistries to obtain a bond to dentin. GLUMA (Bayer) was a three-component system that used EDTA at a pH between 6.5 and 7.0 to clean the smear layer and condition the dentinal surface (Asmussen and Munksgaard, 1984). The conditioned surface would then be treated with a resin-containing HEMA and glutaraldehyde. HEMA would provide the hydrophilic action and glutaraldehyde the affinity to collagen at the conditioned dentin surface. A third application of an unfilled resin containing BIS–GMA would follow, to which the restorative resin would ultimately be bonded.

Scotchbond 2 (3M) used an aqueous solution of maleic acid and HEMA as a dentin conditioner that would dissolve the smear layer and remain attached to the slightly demineralized surface. An application of a resin adhesive containing HEMA and BIS–GMA would follow, to polymerize over the conditioned surface.

'Oxalate bonding', introduced by Bowen (1965), utilized an oxalate solution for conditioning of the dentin surface. The solution, containing some nitric acid, would also remove the smear layer and expose the dentin surface and tubules. To enhance dentin bonding, the procedure required the subsequent application of the materials NTG–GMA (N-(p-tolyl)glycine and glycidyl methacrylate) and PMDM (polymellitic dianhydride and 2-hydroxyethyl methacrylate). These materials are dissolved in acetone, rendering the solution very hydrophilic. A separate application of BIS–GMA would follow before the placement of the restorative composite.

The first commercial product based on 'oxalate bonding' was Tenure (Den-Mat). Other products utilizing similar bonding technology include Mirage Bond (Myron Labs), and Dentastic (Pulpdent). All Bond (Bisco) was a modification of the Bowen technique that used BPDM (bisphenol dimethacrylate) instead of PMDM, and was reported to achieve excellent bond strengths in both dry and wet environments.

In addition to achieving better bond strengths with dentin, these newer bonding agents were also shown to have better sealing properties than the former generation of adhesives (Barkmeier and Cooley, 1989b). Sealing of the dentinal margins and reduction of microleakage around restorations, particularly in posterior teeth, is extremely important for elimination of sensitivity and recurrent caries. This could only be accomplished at enamel margins with the acid-etched bond, but not with early dentin adhesives. The 'third-generation' adhesives for the first time offered dentinal sealing that seemed to have a significant reduction, although not complete elimination, of marginal leakage (Swift and Hansen, 1989).

Dentin etching

Fusayama et al (1979) introduced the concept of 'total etching', advocating the treatment of both enamel and dentin with phosphoric acid prior to bonding. This technique has become relatively popular in Japan, but initially met with resistance in the USA. Early animal studies indicated that etching the dentin may be harmful to the pulp (Retief et al, 1974; Stanley et al, 1975; Macko et al, 1978). But clinical experience in humans hardly supports these observations, and it is unlikely that acid etching actually causes irreversible

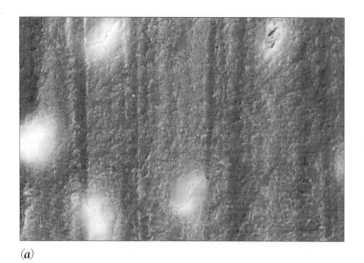

(a)

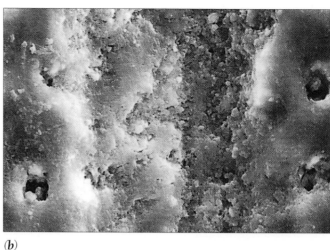

(b)

Figure 2.5 (*a*) *Surface of dentin after cutting and polishing is covered by amorphous smear layer. Tubules are blocked, and streaks are caused by polishing in one direction (SEM, ×5000).* (*b*) *Another area of dentin surface covered with smear layer exhibiting incomplete blockage of dentin tubules (SEM, ×5000).*

pulpal damage (Lee et al, 1973). Furthermore, the realization that new dentin adhesive technology may require the dissolving of the smear layer and some demineralizing of superficial dentin has made total etching a more widely accepted treatment methodology in the USA (Kanca, 1989, 1992).

Proponents of the 'total etching' method would point out that all dentin adhesives of the third generation include a dentin conditioner that is acidic, so etching of dentin would occur with any of the systems. Some researchers, however, pointed out that there was a

Table 2.1 Relative acidity of various dentin primers

Product	Manufacturer	pH
Scotchbond II Primer	3M	2.3
Universal Bond II Primer	Dentsply-Caulk	2.6
X-R Primer	Kerr	2.8
Gluma Cleanser	Columbus	6.4
Mirage Bond Primer	Myron Labs	2.1
Tenure Dentin Primer	Den-Mat	2.2
37% phosphoric acid enamel etchant		1.0

From: White RC, College Park, TX, personal communication

substantial difference both in pH and the effect of various conditioners on the dentin surface (Table 2.1; Nathanson et al, 1992a).

A comparison of scanning electron micrographs of dentin surfaces before (Figure 2.5) and after conditioning (see Figures 2.2–2.4) shows the effect of various conditioners. Some produce total removal of the smear layer, while others create a less visible effect of dissolving it and increasing its penetrability.

Testing the chemical make-up of surface dentin before and after conditioning via surface element analysis in a scanning electron microscope (EDAX) reveals indirectly the 'depth' of the conditioning effect and the degree of demineralization. It is evident that most dedicated dentin conditioners maintain a surface that is rich in calcium and phosphorus even if the smear layer is totally dissolved. In contrast, etching the dentin with 37% phosphoric acid for 30 seconds or more results in total demineralization of the dentinal surface. These surfaces under surface element analysis appear to be rich in carbon (from the organic collagen) but lack any calcium or phosphorus. These findings suggest that dentin is very susceptible to decalcification by phosphoric acid as compared with milder or organic acids. When phosphoric acid is used to condition the dentin before bonding, one must be careful with the 'strength' of the acid as well as the duration of contact. Longer exposure to the inorganic acid can induce significant surface demineralization and reduced bonds with certain systems (Nathanson et al, 1992b).

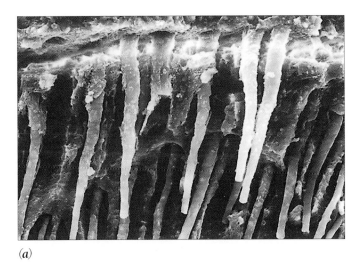

(a)

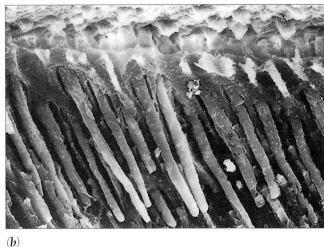

(b)

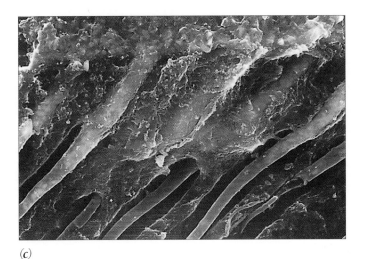

(c)

Figure 2.6 (a, b) Resin tag formation of dentin adhesive after application (SEM, ×2000). Sample surface was decalcified subsequently to reveal tag formation. Note 2 μm-thick hybridization layer on top with different configuration; (c) Magnified (×2500) area from (b), showing resin tags through the area of hybridization.

Current dentin adhesives ('fourth' and 'fifth' generations) rely both on some conditioning of the dentin surface and on the utilization of bifunctional monomers that have a chemical affinity to different constituents of dentin. In addition, these monomers can be combined with hydrophilic resins to achieve better wetting of the moist dentin surface.

The various products now available as dentin adhesive systems utilize two main approaches in relation to pretreatment of the dentin surface prior to the application of adhesive. One approach favors only minimal or no change in the smear layer prior to bonding. The other approach requires total removal of the smear layer before the application of the bonding resin. This is usually accomplished by acidic conditioners or primers. Either way, the adhesive resins have been shown to

enter the dentin tubules and to set against the dentin. This dentinal tubule penetration was considered to be a mechanism that is at least partially responsible for bond strength. With more complete removal of the smear layer or with use of stronger acid conditioners, decalcification of the surface dentin occurs to a depth of from 0.5 to 10–15 μm. The adhesive resin can penetrate this decalcified layer and set among the collagen fibrils, in effect incorporating itself in this portion of dentin. This layer was first identified by Nakabayashi et al (1982), who called it the hybrid zone. Other researchers referred to it as the resin-impregnated layer or the resin inter-diffusion zone (Van Meerbeek et al, 1992, 1993a,b).

Further microscopic analysis of the conditioned dentin and the relationship between the adhesive monomers and the tooth structure give more details on the possible

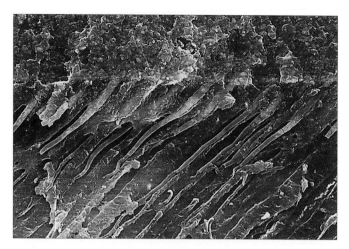

Figure 2.7 Cross section through dentin treated with dentin adhesive. Adhesive layer, seen on top, forms a hybrid connection with dentin to a depth of about 10 µm. Beyond this point resin tags are more defined and seem to lose contact with tubular walls (SEM, ×1000).

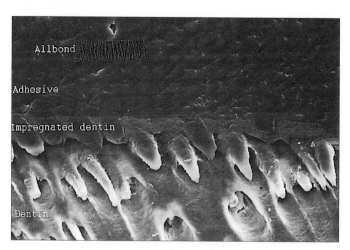

Figure 2.8 Section of dentin after application of adhesive (All Bond 2) shows a layer approximately 2 µm wide where resin has impregnated the decalcified surface dentin, and resin tag formation into tubules (SEM, ×3000).

mechanisms of adhesion to these surfaces (Erickson, 1992; Van Meerbeek et al, 1992, 1993a,b; Eick et al, 1993). Scanning electron microscopy shows evidence of the formation of a zone that differs from both the bonding resin and the underlying dentin (Figures 2.6–2.8). Transmission electron microscopy used to analyze this layer shows further evidence of collagen fibrils and resin-adhesive impregnated within it (Thomas and Carella, 1984; Van Meerbeek et al, 1993b). There is no evidence that the bond is chemical or covalent, and most researchers feel that the nature of the 'bond' is secondary or micromechanical (Erickson, 1992; Van Meerbeek et al, 1992). There is some substantiation of this theory of a mechanical bond through infrared photoacoustic work (Spencer et al, 1992). Others feel that there exists a potential for a covalent bond to collagen (Lee et al, 1973; Asmussen and Bowen, 1987). Munksgaard et al (1985) investigated the possibility of chemical adhesion to the collagen matrix. They classified this adhesion as follows:

(1) adhesion based on ionic polymers;
(2) adhesion by coupling agents;
(3) adhesion by grafting reactions.

Regardless of the exact nature of the bond, virtually all new adhesive resins include a hydrophilic group that is 'attracted' to the conditioned dentin surface. Resins containing this group wet the surface well and penetrate the collagen network, sometimes making it recover

almost to its original level before the decalcification. This resin–collagen interface is assumed by many researchers to be the primary mechanism for adhesion. A study by Gwinnett (1993) demonstrates that a significant portion of the bond also derives from penetration of the dentinal tubules. One in vitro study of new dentin-bonding agents found a correlation between the presence of resin tags (into tubules) and bond strength (Kraivixien et al, 1993), confirming the validity of this mechanism. For resin tags extending into the dentinal tubules to be effective for retention, the resin must adhere to the tubule walls, through much the same mechanism as used for resin adhesion to the intertubular dentin.

The most recent generation of dentin adhesive systems have been presented by their manufacturers as materials that can be used over acid-etched dentin. These systems include All Bond 2 (Bisco), Clearfil Liner Bond (Kuraray/Morita), Scotchbond Multipurpose Plus (3M), OptiBond (Kerr), Imperva Bond (Shofu) and Dentastic (Pulpdent). Several dentin-etching systems may be utilized, such as 10% phosphoric acid, 32% phosphoric acid, 10% maleic acid, etc.

Because the depth of decalcification of the dentin surface may vary according to the strength of the conditioner/acid used as well as the duration of the application, the practitioner must be aware of this effect and compensate for deep etching by allowing sufficient resin diffusion into the demineralized zone. Scanning and transmission electron microscope observations show that at times the demineralized layer is much wider than the area impregnated by the resin (Van Meerbeek et al, 1993b). This is of concern because the uninfiltrated collagen may be subjected to collapse and degradation over time. One method to ensure good penetration of the decalcified layer of dentin is to keep the surface wet during the bonding procedure. Because virtually all dentin adhesive resins are hydrophilic, they are attracted to water, and the procedure of wet bonding includes a phase where water is being replaced by the resin.

Wet bonding has been primarily advocated for use with the All Bond 2 system (Kanca, 1992). The procedure calls for etching the dentin with either 10% or 32% phosphoric acid. The etched dentin is rinsed but allowed to stay wet for the bonding process. The primer, containing a combination of NTG–GMA and BPDM, both dissolved in acetone, is applied to the wet surface repeatedly, for five or more coats, without drying the surface between applications. This method allows the acetone to combine with water and gradually replace it. In this procedure the primer is carried by the acetone into the demineralized zone of the surface dentin. This step is followed by the application of a more conventional BIS–GMA-based unfilled resin that is attracted to the primer and can copolymerize with it.

Wet bonding is primarily suited for systems in which the primer is dissolved in acetone. Such systems include Tenure (Den-Mat), All Bond 2 (Bisco), ProBond (Dentsply-Caulk) and Dentastic (Pulpdent). In testing All Bond 2 under various conditions, Gwinnett found out that drying the dentin significantly reduced the bond strength, but acid conditioning did not seem to have an important effect. Also, removal of the collagen fibrils in the decalcified zone by use of sodium hypochlorite did not have an effect on bond strength, suggesting that the outer demineralized zone may not be responsible for the bonding mechanism. HEMA-based systems are also capable of bonding to wet dentin, but there may not be as strong an effect as with acetone-based systems. Swift and Triolo (1992) reported bond strengths for a HEMA-based system (Scotchbond Multipurpose, 3M) that were slightly higher on wet dentin (21.8 MPa) than on dry dentin (17.8 MPa).

Clinical uses for dentin bonding

Dentin bonding is used as a primary form of retention for some direct restorations, namely class V cavities where there is minimal enamel. This use was almost unthinkable in the 1970s and 1980s, when mechanical retention was still required. At present, dentin adhesives are sufficiently reliable to offer retention based on bonding and without undercutting the tooth.

But there are many other applications where dentin bonding has become an integral part of the procedure. The potential sealing and cuspal reinforcement properties have made dentin adhesive a natural amalgam-bonding material. The adhesive bonds to the dentinal cavity wall, and the amalgam is condensed over it to form a micromechanical union via surface irregularities.

The amalgam simply intermixes with the wet layer on the surface of the resin. When both materials achieve final setting, they are interlocked, forming a strong union. Using dentin bonding in conjunction with amalgam restorations produces better retention. This can be used in lieu of other retentive methods, thus employing a more conservative process. Some undercutting and potential weakening of the tooth can be avoided. Still, a study by Lo et al (1994) shows that retention of amalgam by pins is on average six times stronger than retention with amalgam bonding alone.

Cuspal reinforcement is another important potential benefit. Alone, amalgam offers minimal cuspal protection, but with dentin bonding there may be a significant strengthening of the cusps. Also, amalgams, particularly of new formulations, are subjected to marginal leakage during the initial weeks after placement. Dentin bonding counteracts leakage by providing a continuous marginal seal.

Another important use is with indirect restorations, that is, composite inlays, ceramic inlays/onlays and ceramic crowns. Beyond retention and sealing, current dentin-bonding systems can improve the strength of all-ceramic systems by providing a better foundation and more continuous union with tooth structure (Figure 2.9).

Adhesion techniques have become an integral part of retaining ceramic restorations to tooth structure. With the improvement of adhesive systems, bonding to etched ceramics has also been enhanced. Most current dental adhesives are designed to achieve good union with etched ceramic surfaces. Although etching the surface with the appropriate ceramic etchant (usually hydrofluoric acid or a derivative) is the most important factor in producing retention with a composite cement, bonding can be enhanced by utilizing the various universal bonding systems that are available. Special bonding enhancers, usually silane formulations, are used to

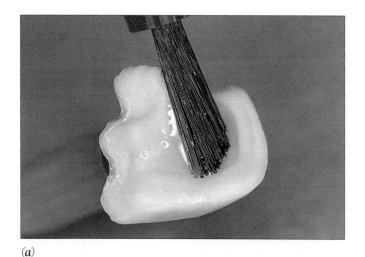

(a)

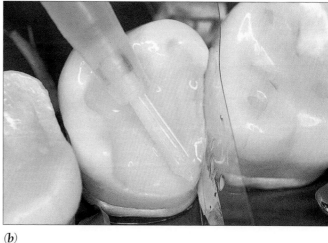

(b)

(c)

Figure 2.9 (a) *A single-component dentin adhesive is brushed onto the internal surface of the onlay, prior to gentle drying and light polymerization.* (b) *Adhesive is applied to the preparation surfaces, left in place for a few minutes, and then gently dried.* (c) *The adhesive is light-cured, and the onlay is ready to be bonded with a resin cement.*

enhance the bond. Dentin adhesives can also improve the bond via better surface wetting and some ionic affinity with components of the ceramic material (Stangel et al, 1987). In one study of machineable ceramics the most important factor in achieving optimal bond strength was the application of a bonding resin before using the resin cement (Nathanson and Kraivixien, 1992).

The potential for tooth strengthening via bonded ceramic and composite restorations has been reported (Frydman et al, 1993; Nathanson et al, 1992b) and confirms early observations that bonded direct composites make a significantly greater contribution to cuspal reinforcement than amalgam restorations (Share et al, 1982). Hence the new dentin adhesive systems are a factor in stress resistance of restored teeth. Further

research is needed to determine the clinical significance of this finding.

Current trends

In comparing bonding to dentin with bonding to enamel, several differences become evident.

- The application of conditioners and adhesive to enamel is generally simpler and involves fewer steps.

- For enamel bonding, the technique is less demanding. Dentin bonding may necessitate multiple steps, and they have to be carried out in a precise fashion.

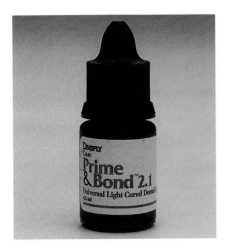

Figure 2.10 Prime & Bond 2.1 (Dentsply-Caulk).

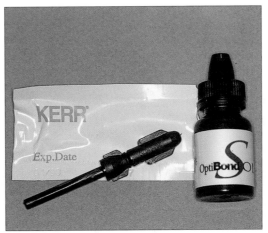

Figure 2.11 OptiBond Solo (Kerr).

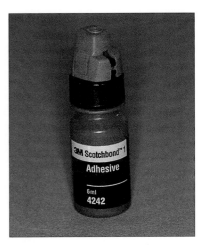

Figure 2.12 Scotchbond 1 (3M).

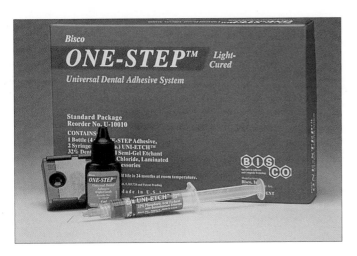

Figure 2.13 One-Step (Bisco).

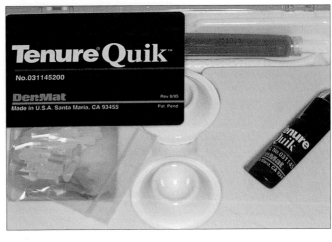

Figure 2.14 Tenure Quik (Den-Mat).

Another way to express this is that dentin bonding is 'technique-sensitive', and deviations from the appropriate application methodology can cause significantly reduced bond strengths.

- Data reported from clinical studies involving dentin bonding show a wide variance in results among researchers. Enamel bonding varies less among studies, and within studies. Standard deviations from mean bond strength are generally less for enamel bonding than for dentin bonding.

- As a substrate for bonding to, enamel shows less variance than dentin. With dentin, the depth of the restoration, the region of dentin in the tooth, the age of the patient and other factors may have an impact on bond strength.

In summary, bonding to dentin is a much more involved procedure than bonding to enamel, and the potential for not achieving an optimal bond strength – or even minimal adhesion – is much higher than with enamel. Dental manufacturers are trying to make new

---

Table 2.2 Composition of One-Step (Bisco) adhesive system

Monomers
    BPDM   (hydrophilic resin)
    HEMA   (hydrophilic resin)
    BIS–GMA (hydrophobic resin)

Photo-initiator
    Tertiary amine
    Camphoroquinone

Solvent
    Acetone/ethyl alcohol (60–65%)

Table 2.3 Composition of Tenure Quik (Den-Mat) adhesive system

Resins
    BIS–GMA (hydrophobic)
    HEMA   (hydrophilic)
    NTGGMA (hydrophilic)

Water

Photo-initiator

Acetone (46%)

Table 2.4 Composition of Prime & Bond (Dentsply-Caulk) adhesive system

Resins
    Resin (R-5-62-1)   (elastomeric urethane resin)
    UDMA   (urethane dimethacrylate)
    BPA–DMA   (phenol A dimethacrylate)

Penta   (adhesion promoter by
                               wetting, cross-linking)

Photo-initiator

Acetone (75–80%)

Table 2.5 Composition of Syntac Single-Component (Ivoclar Vivadent) adhesive system

	Weight %
Methacrylate-modified polyacrylic acid	6.0
Hydroxyethyl methacrylate	43.6
Water (deionized)	46.0
Maleic acid	3.0
Fluoride compound	0.1
Catalysts and stabilizers	1.3

---

adhesive procedures easy to follow, and the systems easy to use, in order to make dentin bonding less complex and time-consuming while increasing the likelihood of a strong bond.

A clear current trend is to reduce the bonding steps as well as the number of components in the adhesive kit. 'Single-component' dentin adhesives have been introduced that include only one bottle of material. These products, such as Prime & Bond (Dentsply-Caulk), One-Step (Bisco), Scotchbond 1 (3M) and OptiBond Solo (Kerr) combine the primer and adhesive in the same liquid (Figures 2.10–2.14). They may require more

than one application, but there is an advantage in the fact that there is no mixing and no risk of applying the incorrect material.

Single-component dentin adhesion

General 'single-component' ('fifth-generation') dentin adhesives are based on combinations of conventional hydrophobic resins such as BIS–GMA, together with hydrophilic resins and solvents. Hydroxyethyl methacrylate (HEMA) is often used as a hydrophilic monomer.

Table 2.6 Composition of OptiBond (Kerr) adhesive system

Primer
    HEMA   (hydroxyethyl methacrylate)
    GPDM   (glycerylphosphate dimethacrylate)
    PAMM   (phthalic acid monoethyl
                      methacrylate)
    CQ   (camphorquinone)
    Ethanol
    Water

Adhesive
    Resin
        BIS–GMA   (bisphenol glycidyl methacrylate)
        HEMA   (hydroxyethyl methacrylate)
        GDM   (glyceryl dimethacrylate)

    Filler
        Barium–aluminum–borosilicate glass (average
        particle 0.6 μm)
        Fumed silica
        Disodium hexafluorosilicate

    Photo–initiator
        CQ   (camphorquinone)

Acetone, alcohol or a combination of both can be used as hydrophilic solvents. Several systems include water in various quantities to make the compound as an aqueous solution. The composition of four single-component dentin adhesive systems – Prime & Bond (Dentsply-Caulk), One-Step (Bisco), Tenure Quik (Den-Mat) and Syntac Single-Component (Ivoclar Vivadent) – are presented in Tables 2.2–2.5.

What makes single-component adhesive systems effective is the strong hydrophilic action derived from their constituents. These hydrophilic parts relate well to the dentin tissue with its high water content. Hydrophilic monomers as well as solvents are attracted to water and are able to penetrate into the dentin, carrying the hydrophobic resins along with them. For effective hydrophilic action some products must rely on high amounts of acetone or alcohol, in the range of 60–80% of the material's composition. With such formulations dentin bonding is particularly effective on wet substrates. In fact, wet dentin may be a prerequisite for obtaining optimal adhesion values. It has been suggested that drying the dentin surface by blowing air from the air syringe before the application of high-acetone content adhesives may create an 'under-wet' syndrome, resulting in significantly lower bond strengths.

Two factors that may further enhance bond strengths with systems that are based on a high content of acetone or alcohol are (a) multiple applications and (b) allowing the solvent to evaporate thoroughly. It should also be noted that single-component dentin adhesives are light-curable only. Autopolymerization does not occur. For certain applications in which the light may not reach the dentin adhesive layer (e.g. cementing a cast metal crown with resin cement), a dual-cure bonding system may be more appropriate.

Another new trend in dentin adhesive technology is to provide an intermediate layer between the cavity wall and the restorative material. This layer assumes the role of a liner with a lower modulus of elasticity, which can compensate for various stresses that may occur around the restoration. Practically all restorative resins exhibit a significant amount of shrinkage during polymerization. With current formulations this shrinkage is inevitable and can lead to significant stresses both inside the restoration and along the restoration-wall interface. The use of the lower-modulus liner-adhesive can relieve the stresses by the adhesive resin acting as an elastic buffer between the dentin wall and the shrinking restorative resin.

In addition to stresses generated from polymerization shrinkage, teeth are subjected to various other stresses that are intermittent. A major source for the dynamic stressing of restorations can be the direct functional occlusal forces of chewing and clenching, as well as the indirect stresses due to the flexing of teeth under occlusal loading. Tooth flexure is considered to be a factor in the etiology of cervical erosion lesions, and can also influence class V restorations adversely. The relatively high elastic modulus of modern hybrid dental composites does not allow them to flex with restored teeth, particularly in the cervical area. This inflexibility may cause loss of retention and restorative failure. It is believed that the use of a dentin adhesive that can form a flexible intermediary layer between the restoration and tooth structure would contribute to better retention and marginal integrity of class V restorations.

One dentin adhesive system that functions both as a bonding agent and an elastic liner is OptiBond (Kerr). This system contains a glass-filled (48%)

adhesive resin that maintains an average thickness of 75 μm compared with the approximately 5–10 μm thickness of conventional unfilled dentin adhesives. The OptiBond adhesive is designed to act as a low-modulus, flexible 'shock absorber' that can compensate for composite shrinkage during polymerization. It should also relieve functional flexure stresses during mastication. The composition of OptiBond is shown in Table 2.6.

Another novel approach to providing a liner-adhesive layer utilizes the combination of a modified glass-ionomer and a resin adhesive. The material (Fuji Bond LC, GC) is provided as a powder and liquid, which need to be mixed before application. The powder contains the fluoro-aluminosilicate reaction glass. The liquid contains the polyalkenoic acid as well as the light-curable components. The material sets via the conventional glass-ionomer acid–base reaction as well as by visible-light photoinitiation. In addition to low modulus liner qualities, the product offers high fluoride output, which is thought to be advantageous in preventing marginal caries. The material is compatible with virtually all composites and other resin restoratives.

Summary

Modern dental adhesives have changed the nature of restorative dentistry dramatically. The decades of performing dental restorations with mechanical retention and reliance on non-adhesive cements have given way to an era that enables the dentist to use esthetic tooth-like materials to rebuild teeth in a more conservative way. The advantages to patients are enormous – less-invasive procedures, conservative tooth preparations, less discomfort, more esthetic restorations and stronger teeth. This trend continues with the ongoing research and development of even newer materials that make the application and treatment easier, yet ensure optimal results. However, both continuous education and clinical research will be necessary in order to incorporate the full potential of these developments into clinical practice.

References

Asmussen E, Munksgaard EC, Formaldehyde as a bonding agent between dentin and restorative resins. *Scan J Dent Res* 1984; **92**: 480–83.

Asmussen E, Bowen RL, Effect of acidic pretreatment on adhesion to dentin mediated by Gluma. *J Dent Res* 1987; **66**: 1386–88.

Barkmeier WW, Shaffer SE, Gwinnett AJ, Effects of 15 vs. 60 second enamel acid conditioning on adhsion and morphology. *Oper Dent* 1986; **11**: 111–16.

Barkmeier WW, Cooley RL, Shear bond strength of the Tenure Solution dentin bonding system. *Am J Dent* 1989a; **2**: 263–65.

Barkmeier WW, Cooley RL, Resin adhesive sytems. In vitro evaluation of dentin bond strength and marginal microleakage. *J Esthet Dent* 1989b; **1**: 67–72.

Bowen RL, Adhesive bonding of various materials to hard tooth tissues. II. Bonding to dentin promoted by a surface-active comonomer. *J Dent Res* 1965; **44**: 895–902.

Buonocore MG, A simple method of increasing the adhesion of acrylic filling materials to enamel surfaces. *J Dent Res* 1955; **34**: 849–53.

Chappell RP, Eick JD, Theisen FC, Carracho AJL, Shear bond strength and scanning electron microscope observation of current dentinal adhesives. *Quintessence Int* 1991; **22**: 831–39.

Crim GA, Shay JS, Effect of etchant time on microleakage. *J Dent Child* 1987; **54**: 339–40.

Davidson CL, de Gee AJ, Feilzer A, The competition between the composite–dentin bond strength and the polymerization contraction stress. *J Dent Res* 1984; **63**: 1396–99.

Dogon IL, Nathanson D, Van Leeuwen MJ, A long term clinical evaluation of Class IV acid etched composite resin restorations. *Compend Contin Educ Dent* 1980; **6**: 385.

Eick JD, Robinson SJ, Cobb CM et al, The detinal surface: its influence on dentinal adhesion. Part III. *Quintessence Int* 1993; **24**: 571–82.

Eliades GC, Vougiouklakis GJ, 31P-NMR study of P–based dental adhesives and electron probe microanalysis of simulated interfaces with dentin. *Dent Mater* 1989; **5**: 101–8.

Erickson RL, Surface interactions of dentin adhesive materials. *Oper Dent* 1992; **17(Suppl 5)**: 81–94.

Frydman L, Riis D, L'Herault R, Nathanson D, In vitro resistance to fracture of computerized ceramics vs. indirect composite restorations. *J Dent Res* 1993; **72**: 186 (abstract 743).

Fusayama T, Nakamura M, Kurosaki N, Iwaku M, Non-pressure adhesion of a new adhesive restorative resin. *J Dent Res* 1979; **58**: 1364–70.

Glantz P, On wettability and adhesiveness. *Odont Rev* 1969; **20**(Suppl 17): 1.

Glasspoole EA, Erickson RL, Effect of acid etching and rinsing times on composite to enamel bond strength. *J Dent Res* 1986; **65**: 285 (abstract).

Gray SE, Burgess JO, An in vivo and in vitro comparison of two dentin bonding agents. *Dent Mater* 1991; **7**: 161–65.

Gwinnett AJ, Histologic changes in human enamel following treatment with acidic adhesive conditioning agents. *Arch Oral Biol* 1971; **16**: 731–8.

Gwinnett AJ, Quantitative contribution of resin infiltration/hybridization to dentin bonding. *Am J Dent* 1993; **6**: 7–9.

Heymann HO, Sturdevant JR, Brunson WD et al, Twelve-month clinical study of dentinal adhesives in Class V cervical lesions. *J Am Dent Assoc* 1988; **116**: 179–83.

Kanca J, Bonding to tooth structure: a rational rationale for a clinical protocol. *J Esthet Dent* 1989; **1**: 135–8.

Kanca J, Resin bonding to wet substrate. I. Bonding to dentin. *Quintessence Int* 1992; **23**: 39–41.

Kraivixien R, Jaochakarasiri P, Nathanson D, Effect of ageing on bond strength of dentin adhesives in vitro. *J Dent Res* 1993; **72**: 282 (abstract).

Lee HL, Orlowski JA, Scheidt GC, Lee JR, Effects of acid etchants on dentin. *J Dent Res* 1973; **52**: 1228–33.

Lo CS, Millstein PL, Nathanson D, In vitro shear strength of pin-retained vs. resin–bonded amalgam. *J Dent Res* 1994; **73**: 2285 (abstract).

Macko DJ, Rutberg M, Langeland K, Pulpal response to the application of phosphoric acid to dentin. *Oral Surg Oral Med Oral Pathol* 1978; **45**: 930–46.

Morin D, DeLong R, Douglas WH, Cusp reinforcement by the acid–etch technique. *J Dent Res* 1984; **63**: 1075–79.

Munksgaard EC, Irie M, Asmussen E, Dentin–polymer bond promoted by Gluma and various resins. *J Dent Res* 1985; **64**: 1409–11.

Nakabayashi N, Kojima K, Masuhara E, The promotion of adhesion by the infiltration of monomers into tooth substrates. *J Biomed Mater Res* 1982; **16**: 265–73.

Nathanson D, Kraivixien R, Resin cement adherence to machined ceramic restorations. *J Dent Res* 1992; **72** (Special issue): 516.

Nathanson D, Bodkin J, Evans J, SEM of etching patterns in surface and subsurface enamel. *J Pedodontics* 1982; **7**: 11.

Nathanson D, L'Herault RJ, Frankl SN, Dentin etching vs. priming: surface element analysis. *J Dent Res* 1992a; **71**: 1193 (abstract).

Nathanson D, Amin F, Ashayeri N, Dentin etching vs. priming: effect of bond strengths in vitro. *J Dent Res* 1992b; **1**: 1188 (abstract).

Nathanson D, Vongphantuset R, L'Herault RJ, Bond strengths of luting resins to etched glass ceramic in vitro. *J Dent Res* 1992c; **71**: 1186 (abstract).

Paul SJ, Schärer P, Factors in dentin bonding: A review of the morphology and physiology of human dentin. *J Esthet Dent* 1993; **15**: 5–8.

Retief DH, Adhesion to dentin. *J Esthet Dent* 1991; **3**: 106–13.

Retief DH, Austin JC, Fatti LP, Pulpal response to phosphoric acid. *J Oral Pathol* 1974; **3**: 114–22.

Share J, Mishell Y, Nathanson D, Effect of restorative material on resistance to fracture on tooth structure in vitro. *J Dent Res* 1982; **61**: 237.

Silverstone LM, Saxton CA, Dogon IL, Fejerskov O, Variations in the pattern of acid etching of human dentin enamel examined by scanning electron microscopy. *Caries Res* 1975; **9**: 373–87.

Solomon A, Beech DR, Bond strengths of composite to dentin using primers. *J Dent Res* 1983; **62**: 677 (abstract).

Spencer P, Byerley TJ, Eick JD, Chemical characterization of the dentin/adhesive interface by Fourier transform infrared photoelastic spectroscopy. *Dent Mater* 1992; **8**: 10–15.

Stangel I, Nathanson D, Hsu CH, Shear strength of composite bond to etched porcelain. *J Dent Res* 1987; **66**: 9: 1460 (abstract).

Stanley HR, Going RE, Chauncey HH, Human pulp response to acid pretreatment of dentin and to composite restoration. *J Am Dent Assoc* 1975; **91**: 817–25.

Swift EJ, Cloe BC, Shear bond strengths of new enamel etchants. *Am J Dent* 1993; **6**: 162–4.

Swift EJ, Hansen SE, Effect of new bonding systems on microleakage. *Am J Dent* 1989; **2**: 77–80.

Swift EJ, Triolo PT, Bond strengths of Scotchbond Multi–purpose to moist dentin and enamel. *Am J Dent* 1992; **5**: 318–20.

Thomas HF, Carella P, Correlation of scanning and transmission electron microscopy of human dentinal tubules. *Arch Oral Biol* 1984; **29**: 641–6.

Tyas MJ, Three year clinical evaluation of dentine bonding agents. *Aust Dent J* 1991; **36**: 298–301.

Van Meerbeek B, Inokoshi S, Braem M et al, Morphological aspects of the resin–dentin interdiffusion zone with different dentin adhesive systems. *J Dent Res* 1992; **71**: 1530–40.

Van Meerbeek B, Mohrbacher H, Celis JP et al, Chemical characterization of the resin–dentin interface by micro–Raman spectroscopy. *J Dent Res* 1993a; **10**: 1423–28.

Van Meerbeek B, Dhem A, Goret–Nicaise M et al, Comparative SEM and TEM examination of the ultrastructure of the resin–dentin interdiffusion zone. *J Dent Res* 1993b; **72**: 495–501.

Yamada T, Nakamura K, Iwaki M, Fusayama T, The extent of the odontoblastic process in normal and carious human dentin. *J Dent Res* 1991; **62**: 798–802.

Ziemecki TL, Dennison JB, Charbeneau GT, Clinical evaluation of cervical composite resin restorations placed without retention. *Oper Dent* 1987; **12**: 27–33.

CHAPTER 3

Current Ceramic Systems

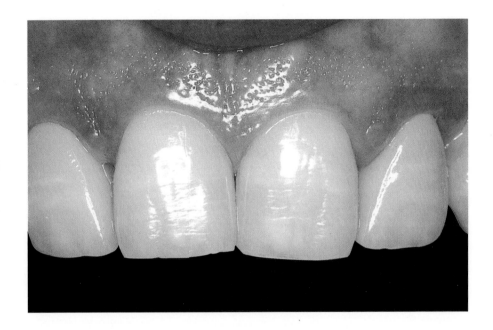

Ceramics originally referred to the art of fabrication of pottery. The term derives from the Greek *keramos*, which means 'a potter or a pottery'. It is believed that this word is related to a Sanskrit term meaning 'burned earth', since the basic components were clays from the earth, which were heated to form pottery (Frieman, 1991).

Ceramics are nonmetallic, inorganic materials. The term 'ceramic' applies to a wide variety of materials, including metal oxides, borides, carbides, nitrides, and complex mixtures of these materials. In general, ceramics are said to demonstrate 'long-range' order due to their periodic crystalline structure, and they may exhibit ionic or covalent bonding. Ceramics may also be broadly classified according to their composition and defined as traditional ceramics or advanced engineering ceramics.

Traditional ceramics typically use clay as one of their main components, along with other metal oxides such as alumina (Al_2O_3), feldspar ($K_2O.Al_2O_3.6SiO_2$), potash (K_2O), and soda (Na_2O). Stoneware (tiles), porcelain (tableware and china), earthenware (pottery), bricks, and sanitary ware are all items characterized as traditional ceramics (Kingery et al, 1976).

Advanced ceramics used in electronics, automotive engines, lasers, and other areas may be composed of oxide or nonoxide materials. Electronic

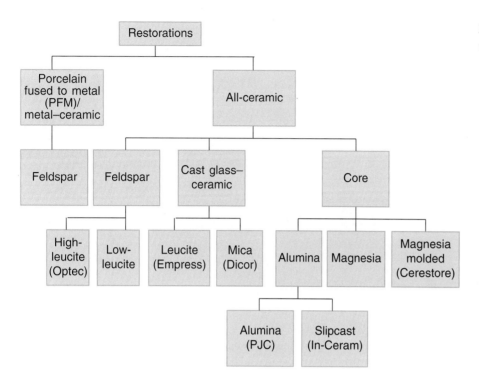

Figure 3.1 Classification of dental ceramic restorative materials.

devices often rely on aluminum nitride (AlN) or boron nitride (BN) as the substrate material. Silicon carbide (SiC) is used as a semiconducting ceramic as well as for special mirrors required in outer-space applications. Certain lasers rely on optical ceramic crystals such as YAG (yttrium aluminum garnet) for production of the laser beam. Automotive and machine components that are in frequent motion are coated with titanium nitride (TiN) or titanium carbide (TiC) to improve the wear resistance of the parts.

Dental ceramics are composed primarily of metal oxides and other 'traditional' ceramic materials. However, with increasing interest in improving the esthetic quality of restorations, a wide variety of ceramic materials and processes have been developed. Dental ceramics may be classified by composition, firing temperature, or process of fabrication. Figure 3.1 illustrates the wide variety of ceramic systems available to the dentist. Ceramics in this diagram are classified by composition and fabrication technique. The majority of ceramics are feldspar-based, and are used for metal–ceramic restorations. However, the possible esthetic advantages of all-ceramic restorations has led to the development of a number of systems such as In-Ceram, Empress and Dicor.

Feldspar ceramics may be further classified by fusing temperature. High-fusing feldspar ceramics are used primarily for denture teeth, and are fired in the temperature range 1260–1400°C. Medium-fusing feldspar ceramics are employed in porcelain jacket restorations, and are fired between 1080 and 1260°C. Low-fusing ceramics made up the bulk of the material for producing metal–ceramic restorations. These are commonly fired at temperatures ranging from 900 to 1080°C. With recent developments in ceramics, it is necessary to add a fourth category, ultra-low-fusing ceramics, which are fired in the range 650–850°C (McLean, 1982).

Dental porcelain

Of all materials used in dentistry to restore the natural dentition, ceramics have by far the best optical properties to mimic tooth structure in appearance and color. Processing ceramics requires the expertise of a skilled technician, and is a form of art as much as it is a vocation. In the hands of those who can use them properly, ceramics can provide restorations that are so similar to natural teeth in shape, texture, color reflectance, and translucency that distinguishing them from natural teeth could be impossible.

The physical properties of ceramics are very suitable for materials to be used as dental restoratives. Their optical, thermal, solubility, and corrosion properties enable the processing of restorations that can provide good appearance and tolerance to the oral environment. The mechanical properties of ceramics, however, are only partially suitable for making dental restorations. Therefore they must be manipulated, designed, and used in such a way as to compensate for the deficiencies.

Uses of dental porcelain

Ceramic materials are used for a variety of dental restorations. These include the fabrication of denture teeth, single crowns, and fixed partial dentures. More recently, the use of ceramics has been expanded to include labial veneers, and inlays and onlays in posterior teeth.

Composition

Porcelain is particularly suitable as a restorative dental material because of its glass-like properties and its optical resemblance to tooth enamel. It is different from glass in the fact that all constituents in regular glass (primarily potash and silica) fuse to form a single-phase transparent material. Porcelains contain ingredients that are infusible at the porcelain firing temperature. They remain as crystals surrounded by the fusible ingredients, forming a translucent (but not transparent) material that is multiphasic, i.e. with a dispersed (or crystalline) phase and a continuous amorphous phase.

In principle, dental ceramics are based on constituents that are similar to those used in household and ornamental ceramics. These compounds include feldspar, silica, and kaolin (also refined as clay). The main difference in composition between porcelain used in dentistry and that used for other products (i.e. dishes and china) is in the proportions of the main ingredients: clay is the main constituent in these other porcelains, whereas dental porcelain is based primarily on feldspar.

Feldspar is a gray, crystalline material that is found in rocks in certain geographical locations. The chemical composition of common feldspar is $K_2O.Al_2O_3.6SiO_2$, or potassium aluminum silicate. Other ingredients found in feldspar rocks are iron and mica. Iron is an impurity that is removed mechanically by splitting the feldspar rocks and examining the thin splinters visually for the presence of the impurity (which appears more opaque than the pure feldspar). The pure feldspar pieces are selected and subjected to further grinding and milling to make the material into a powder. The remaining iron impurities are removed at this stage using strong magnets.

The main source of silica (SiO_2) is quartz crystals. Quartz is heated then quenched in cold water so that it cracks. It is then ground and milled to a fine powder. Iron impurities are removed magnetically as described for feldspar. The quartz powder makes up roughly 15% of dental porcelain. It remains unchanged during the firing of the porcelain, and forms the crystalline layer that contributes to the optical properties (translucency) and limits shrinkage during firing.

Kaolin, a form of clay found in river beds and river banks, occurs naturally: feldspathic rocks are washed out continuously by water, which dissolves the potassium away and produces a hydrated aluminum silicate ($Al_2O_3.2SiO_2.2H_2O$) – kaolin. To prepare a pure form of kaolin, the clay has to be washed, dried, and screened, resulting in a fine white powder. Kaolin is used in dental porcelain in small quantities (i.e. 4%). Its main function is that of a particle binder: mixed with water, kaolin becomes sticky and helps keep the wet porcelain particles together. This allows manipulation of the powder–liquid mass by the technician to obtain various forms. In firing the porcelain, the kaolin coats the nonfusible particles and does not contribute much to the porcelain volume.

To allow the fabrication of porcelain restorations in tooth colors, small quantities of coloring agents are added to porcelain powders. These pigments (also called 'color frits') are derived from metallic oxides that are ground and mixed with feldspar powder. This mixture is then fired and fused to a glass. The pigmented glass is then reground to a powder. Commonly used oxides include tin oxide for opaquing, iron oxide for brown shading, copper oxide for green shading, titanium oxide for yellows, cobalt oxide for blue, nickel oxide for brown, and manganese oxide for purple. Rare-earth elements are added in small quantities to provide fluorescence and make the porcelain reflect ultraviolet light in a similar manner to natural teeth.

Porcelain fusion – fabrication of porcelain crowns

All-porcelain restorations can be fabricated either on refractory dies that are produced by replicating the master models, or by utilizing platinum foils (0.025 mm

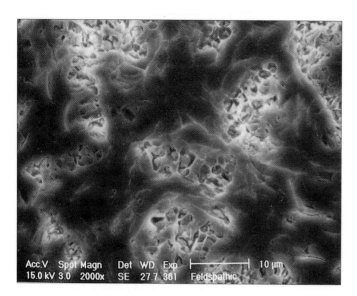

Figure 3.2 Etched feldspathic porcelain – note the leucite crystals.

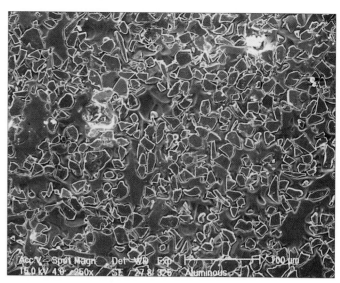

Figure 3.3 Etched aluminous porcelain – alumina crystals in a glass matrix.

thick) that are swaged onto the dies to assume their exact shape. Both the refractory dies and the platinum foil retain the mixed porcelain powder in the porcelain firing oven and keep its shape during the firing process.

The porcelain powder of adequate shade is mixed by the technician with distilled water and applied to the refractory die or platinum foil with a fine brush. First the 'dentin layer' is applied. Mild vibration accomplished with hand instruments is required in order to condense the wet porcelain particles and obtain a dense mass. Blotting with absorbent tissue paper helps to reduce excess water. The dentin porcelain is applied to an oversize shape to compensate for the significant shrinkage that occurs during the porcelain fusion. Repetitive firings are normally used to achieve the layer effect and to correct for shrinkage. In this manner, the enamel layer is added (usually a more translucent shade). After cooling, the restoration can be adjusted by mechanical means to assume the correct shape, contour, size, and fit.

A final firing can then be employed in which the porcelain completes its fusion. Shrinkage is minimal at this stage, since it mostly occurs during the initial firing (the bisque stage). By controlling the final firing temperature, time and firing in air (without vacuum), a 'self-glaze' layer can be produced over the outer surface of the restoration. Alternately, a low-fusing glaze can be applied to the surface and fired separately. Firing needs to be performed with a controlled temperature rise in the oven (i.e. 100°C/min) because porcelain is a poor thermal conductor. Raising the heat too rapidly may overfire the outer layer before giving the inner layer a chance to fuse properly.

Both condensation of the particles and the firing regimen influence the properties of porcelain greatly and hence the final quality of the porcelain restoration (Vergano et al, 1967).

Porcelain properties

Porcelain is a brittle material with little plastic behavior. It has a compressive strength of about 170 MPa, a flexural strength of 50–75 MPa, and a tensile strength of about 25 MPa. Values of other physical properties include an elastic modulus of 69–70 GPa (enamel 46 GPa), a linear coefficient of thermal expansion of $(12-14) \times 10^{-6}/°C$ similar to that of tooth structure, and a surface hardness of 460 KHN (versus 340 KHN for enamel) (Figure 3.2).

Porcelain strengthening

Because porcelain is a brittle material with relatively poor tensile properties, it may be prone to failure when used in stress-bearing restorations. Traditionally, jacket crowns were known to fail after several years of service. Failure mechanisms related to microcracks that would be evident in the porcelain crown internal surface. These would occur during the firing and cooling process, and are subjected to continuous stressing in the oral cavity. The inner porcelain surface would be subjected to tensile forces, making these microcracks open and propagate further. With propagation continuing toward the surface, by the time the outer surface is reached, the crown exhibits complete failure and breakdown.

Different mechanisms have been devised and employed to reduce the potential of ceramic crown failure due to repeated stressing. They involve strengthening or supporting the porcelain internally (the layer closest to tooth structure) with materials of adequate strength.

One of the most effective strengthening methods is the use of a metallic substructure (i.e. metal coping) onto which the porcelain is added and fired. This method (metal–ceramic, or PFM) seems to be by far the most successful in producing restorations that are resistant to occlusal stresses.

Metallic substructures, however, tend to be problematic in terms of esthetics. The metallic shade needs to be blocked and eliminated from view, and this is difficult in margin areas as well as areas of thin porcelain. Also, the translucency of the restoration is greatly reduced by the metal substructure. In recent years, a technique has been presented that combines a metallic substructure with porcelain margins. The technician 'cuts back' the metal coping, thus allowing space for full porcelain margins. For accuracy, special margin–porcelain preparations are used. Products are now available that couple porcelain powder with a wax pattern and allow waxing-up of the margins in preparation for firing and finishing the crowns.

Another approach is to eliminate the metallic coping altogether and use a reinforced porcelain core material. McLean and Hughes (1965) developed aluminous porcelain jacket crowns in 1965. A high-strength ceramic containing 50 wt% fused alumina crystals forms the core onto which a matched (thermal expansion) veneer porcelain is applied. The labial surface is made with a reduced thickness (approximately 0.5 mm) to allow room for the application of regular porcelain for esthetic appearance. This so-called 'aluminous porcelain jacket crown' is said to be twice as resistant to fracture as the unreinforced porcelain jacket crown. This was an improvement; however, light transmission is limited because of the alumina crystals, and the

strength is still insufficient for use in the posterior region (Figure 3.3) (McLean, 1983).

In-Ceram

A more recent development by Sadoun in 1985 makes use of aluminous cores that are infiltrated with a glass to achieve high-strength substructures that can support crowns and bridges.

In-Ceram belongs to a class of materials known as interpenetrating-phase composites. These materials consist of at least two phases that are intertwined and extend continuously from the internal to the external surface. These materials may possess improved mechanical and physical properties compared with the individual components. They may have improved strength and fracture resistance due to the fact that a crack must pass through alternating layers of both components no matter what direction the crack takes. Materials such as ceramics and metals or ceramics and resins may be combined to produce novel materials with improved strength and flexibility (Budiansky et al, 1988; Faber and Evans, 1983; Clarke, 1992; Taya et al, 1990).

An all-ceramic restorative system, In-Ceram, is based on the slip casting of an alumina core with its subsequent glass infusion. An impression of the mastercast preparations is made with an elastomeric impression material. A special gypsum supplied with In-Ceram is then poured into the impression to produce the die onto which the In-Ceram alumina is applied.

Alumina powder (38 g) is mixed with 5 ml of deionized water supplied in a premeasured container. One drop of a dispersing agent is added to help create a homogenous mixture of alumina in the water. One-half of the alumina is added to a beaker containing the water/dispersant and then sonicated for 3 minutes in a Vitasonic. This initiates the dispersion process. A second quantity of powder equal to one-half of the remaining amount is then added to the beaker and sonicated again for 3 minutes. The remaining powder may be added and sonicated for 7 minutes; during the last minute, a vacuum is applied to remove air bubbles. This solution of alumina is referred to as 'slip', which is then 'painted' onto the gypsum die with a brush. The alumina is built up to form the underlying core for the ceramic tooth. The water is removed via capillary action of the porous gypsum, which packs the particles into a rigid network.

The alumina core is then placed in the Inceramat (Vita Corporation) furnace and sintered using program 1. This cycle involves a slow heating of approximately 2°C/min to 120°C to remove water and the binding agent. A rapid temperature rise would boil off remaining water and binder, producing cracks in the framework. The second stage of the sintering involves a temperature rise of approximately 20°C/min to 1120°C for 2 hours to produce approximation of the particles with minimal compaction and minimal shrinkage of the alumina. Shrinkage is only about 0.2%; thus an interconnected porous network is created, connecting pores on the outer surface with those on the inner surface.

A lanthanum aluminosilicate ($LaAl_2O_3SiO_2$) glass is used to fill the pores in the alumina. The glass is mixed with water and placed on a platinum–gold alloy sheet. The external surface of the core is placed on the glass. The core is then heated in the Inceramat to 1100°C for 4–6 hours. The glass becomes molten and flows into the pores by capillary diffusion. A 4-hour infusion time is recommended for single units, while 6 hours should be used for bridges. The excess glass is removed by sand blasting with alumina particles (Figure 3.4) (Pelletier et al, 1992; Pober et al, 1992).

The index of refraction of the infusion glass is closely matched to the alumina, resulting in a translucent core. The interpenetrating network also aids in producing an extremely strong all-ceramic core. The last step in the fabrication of the restoration involves the application of an aluminous porcelain (Vitadur Alpha, Vita) to the core to produce the final form of the restoration. The In-Ceram core material is apparently one of the strongest all-ceramic materials available for restorative procedures. Flexural strength values for the core range up to 600 MPa, but may decline as the veneer porcelain is added or the core thickness decreases. The In-Ceram system is discussed further in Chapter 12, 'Dental Ceramics and Laboratory Procedures'.

In-Ceram Spinell

A second generation material, In-Ceram Spinell, based on the In-Ceram technique, has recently been introduced. The techniques of fabrication are essentially the same as the original system. The primary difference is a change in composition to produce a more translucent core. The porous core is fabricated from a magnesium–alumina powder to form a porous network after sintering. This type of material has a specific crystalline structure referred to as a 'spinel' (magnesium aluminate, $MgAl_2O_4$). The porous spinel is secondarily infused with

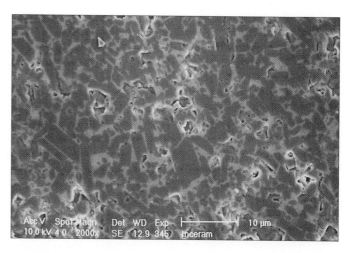

Figure 3.4 *Glass-infused In-Ceram: alumina crystals (dark) surrounded by a lanthanum aluminosilicate glass matrix.*

a glass, which produces a more translucent substructure upon which the Vitadur Alpha is placed to form the final restoration. The In-Ceram spinal core material is not as strong as the original system, but flexural strength values of up to 350 MPa have been reported (Giordano et al, 1995; Seghi et al, 1990a,b).

Glass–ceramics

In recent years, new ceramic systems that allow fabrication of crowns by casting or injection molding have been adapted for dental use. One of the main differences between feldspathic porcelain and castable glass–ceramic is the fact that castable glass–ceramics are cast as noncrystalline materials and are later made into crystalline structures by heat treatment (Shand, 1958).

Glass–ceramic materials may be ideally suited for use as dental restorative materials. This class of materials consists of a glass matrix surrounding a second phase of individual crystals. Glass–ceramics generally have improved mechanical and physical properties, such as increased fracture resistance, improved thermal shock resistance, and erosion resistance. The exact properties depend upon the crystal size and density and the interaction between the crystals and matrix. The crystals help to slow crack propagation, and may even pin cracks by a combination of dispersion strengthening and compressive stress generated around each crystal as it grows.

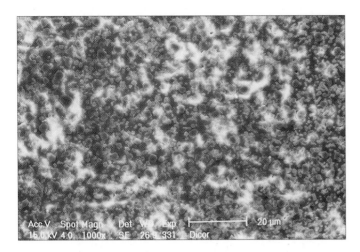

Figure 3.5 Etched Dicor castable ceramic: fluoromica crystals in a glass matrix.

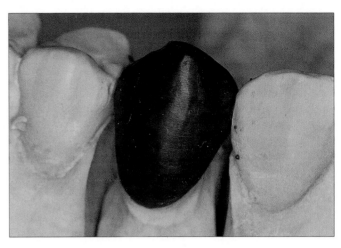

Figure 3.6 Master cast with wax pattern prepared for Empress crown fabrication.

Glass–ceramics are in widespread use for cookware, missile nose cones, and even heat shields on space vehicles. They may be opaque or translucent, depending upon their chemical composition.

Dicor, a castable glass–ceramic, was developed by Grossman (1973) at Corning Glass Works. Dicor consists of SiO_2, K_2O, MgO, and small amounts of Al_2O_3 and ZnO_2. The crystalline phase of Dicor is composed of tetrasilicic fluoromica ($K_2Mg_5Si_8O_{20}F_4$), which provides fracture resistance and strength (Hoekstra, 1986). It is one of the most translucent of the all-ceramic systems. However, color must be developed using several coats of surface glaze, or the Dicor must be veneered with an aluminous porcelain. During sintering, micaceous crystals form, which reportedly give the Dicor material improved strength and machining qualities due to the generation of compressive stress around the crystals (Figure 3.5).

Dicor also presents a unique problem. When cast and ceramed, one surface – called the 'ceram layer' – is significantly different in composition from the rest of the glass–ceramic material. Removal of the external ceram layer has been reported to affect fracture strength, increasing the strength from 93 to 154 MPa or decreasing it from 149 to 143 MPa. The ceram layer contains large micaceous crystal 'whiskers' as well as greater porosity with respect to the rest of the material.

A primary advantage of this system is the option of casting (or injection molding) the material into a special

mold produced by the lost-wax technique. This technique simplifies the process of making all-ceramic crowns, and has resulted in good accuracy and fit (Malament and Grossman, 1992).

Casting is accomplished in a special centrifugal casting machine driven by an electric motor. The glass ingot is heated to about 1300°C in a special carbon crucible. The mold, made of a phosphate-bonded investment, is heated in several stages and finally held at around 900°C for casting. The cast restoration is divested; at this stage it is clear and transparent. It requires further heat treatment for the ceraming and external coloration to give it the appearance of a tooth. Prior to ceraming (crystal development), the sprues are removed and the restoration again invested and heat-treated in a predetermined heat regimen for several hours. This process produces crystals of a mica ceramic in the glass. The ceramed restoration is again divested and coated with a staining glaze that is fired at a lower temperature.

Injection molding

IPS Empress (Ivoclar, Schaan, Liechtenstein) recently introduced an injection molding system that uses a leucite (40–50%) reinforced feldspathic porcelain. The leucite crystals may improve the strength and fracture resistance of the feldspathic glass matrix in a manner similar to that which occurs in glass–ceramics like Dicor

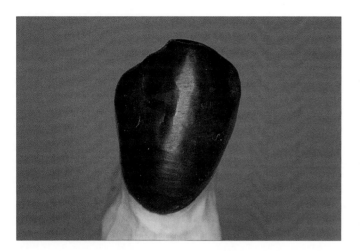

Figure 3.7 Completed wax pattern on master die.

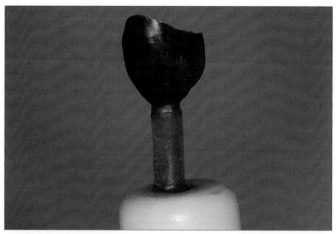

Figure 3.8 Wax pattern for Empress coping, mounted on sprue former, ready for investing.

or in dispersion-strengthened aluminous porcelains (Lehner and Schärer, 1992; Mackert and Evans, 1991; Mackert and Russell, 1995).

A conventional lost-wax technique is employed, except for the use of a special investment and a prolonged burnout cycle. The wax patterns are placed in a furnace along with the Empress ingots, and are slowly heated to approximately 1200°C. The investment mold is then placed in the bottom of the Empress injection molding system at a temperature of about 1150°C, and the selected glass ingot is placed in the upper chamber for molding under a pressure of about 0.4 MPa (Figures 3.6–3.19).

The ingots are supplied in several shades, and two techniques may be employed to fabricate the restoration. The restoration may be cast to its final contours and subsequently stained and glazed to provide an esthetic match. Alternatively, a coping may be molded upon which porcelain is added to achieve the final shape and shade of the restoration. Empress restorations are very translucent, and have reported flexural strengths of up to 160–180 MPa (Figure 3.20).

Low-fusing ceramics

Low-fusing ceramics have been developed primarily for use with titanium frameworks. Titanium is now being

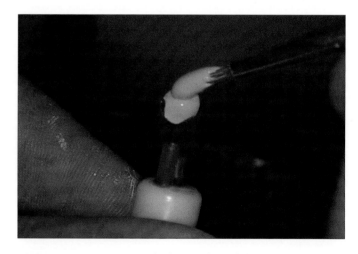

Figure 3.9 Investment applied to surface of the wax pattern.

used for metal–ceramic restorations because of its biocompatibility and corrosion resistance. Low-fusing porcelains are required to adequately match the thermal expansion coefficient of titanium to reduce residual stress, which may result in failure of the overlying ceramic. The fusing temperature of these materials may range from about 650°C to 850°C. Lower fusing temperatures may also preserve the microstructure of the ceramic, in contrast to higher-fusing materials, which

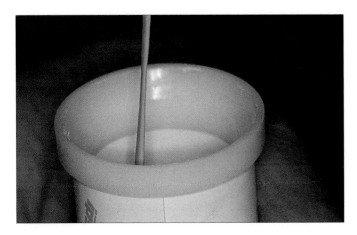

Figure 3.10 *Wax pattern and sprue former are attached to the ring former – the ring former is now filled with investment material*

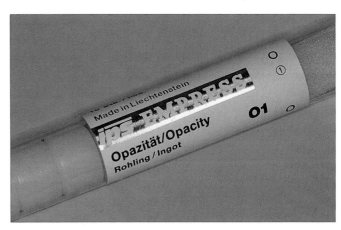

Figure 3.11 *Empress ceramic ingots.*

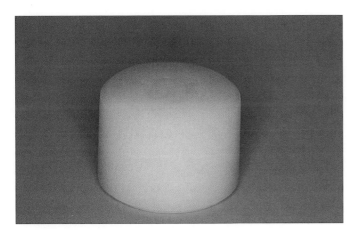

Figure 3.12 *Ingot, type O1, selected for casting.*

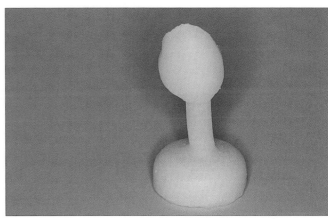

Figure 3.13 *Cast Empress crown attached to the ceramic ingot button.*

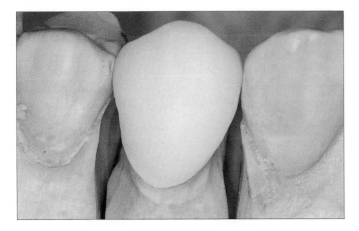

Figure 3.14 *Empress crown seated on master die: contours, contact points, and fit may be adjusted with diamond burs.*

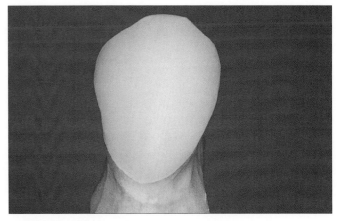

Figure 3.15 *Empress crown with external stains applied to adjust shade and characterize the restoration.*

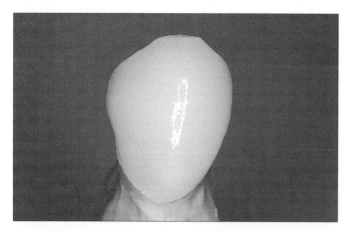

Figure 3.16 Empress crown glazed after stain application: initial application of veneering porcelain.

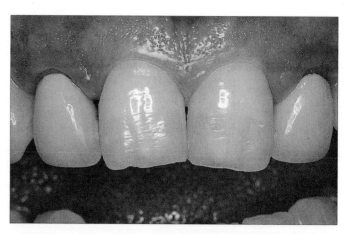

Figure 3.17 Lateral incisors have old metal–ceramic restorations which are to be replaced with Empress crowns.

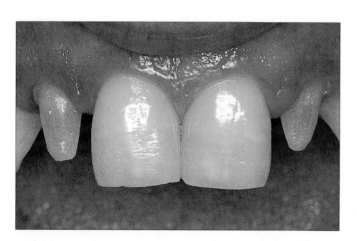

Figure 3.18 The metal–ceramic crowns are removed, and the preparations refined for fabrication of Empress crowns.

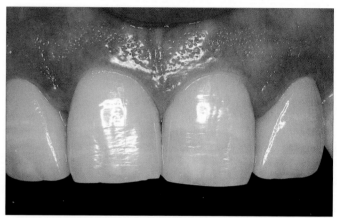

Figure 3.19 Empress crowns cemented in place – the esthetics may be enhanced due to the increased translucency of the all-ceramic restoration.

may suffer from dissolution of the crystalline component. These lower temperatures can result in a more natural, lifelike appearance of the porcelain. Flexural strengths are similar to that of conventional feldspathic porcelain (Hoffman and Casellini, 1988).

Ducera presently makes a low-fusing ceramic, Ducera LFC, which can be fired at 660°C. This ceramic can be used directly to fabricate all-ceramic inlays, onlays, and veneers. Additionally, repair and correction of porcelain or metal–ceramic margins may be accomplished with this ceramic.

Ceramic machining systems

CAD–CAM (computer-assisted design–computer-assisted manufacture) systems have also recently been introduced to the dental profession. Development of CAD–CAM systems for the dental profession began in the 1970s with Duret in France, Altschuler in the USA, and Mormann and Brandestini in Switzerland (Rekow, 1987; Rekow et al, 1992, 1993; Rice and Mecholsky, 1977). Mormann's work led to the development of Siemens' CEREC CAD–CAM system. This system allows

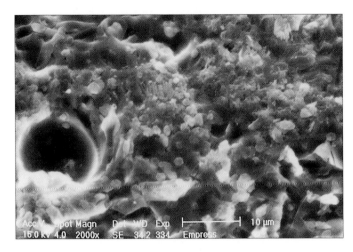

Figure 3.20 Etched Empress ingot: numerous fine leucite crystals are surrounded by a feldspathic glass matrix.

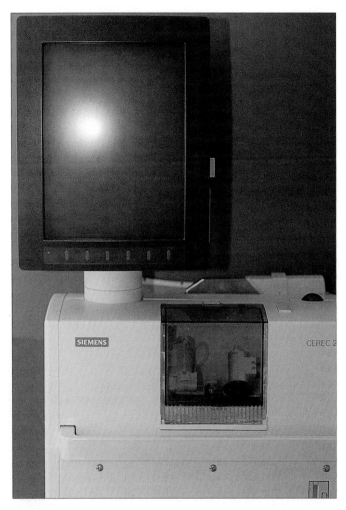

Figure 3.21 The Siemens CEREC II CAD-CAM system.

the dentist to make an 'optical' impression of the tooth preparation and, with the aid of a computer, design the restoration. The restoration is then milled from a block of ceramic material using a diamond wheel; the restoration is 'custom-fitted' to the patient's occlusion using diamond burs. The restoration produced by the CEREC I system must be ground and polished to develop the proper occlusal contacts and anatomy. The new CEREC II system also mills the occlusal surface of the restoration, and may be used to fabricate crowns in addition to inlays, onlays, and veneers (Figure 3.21). The ceramic material used for this system is either a glass–ceramic (Dicor MGC) or a feldspar-based ceramic (Vitabloc MKII). Dicor MGC is also a fluoromica glass–ceramic, but reportedly has a higher concentration of crystals and higher strength than the castable Dicor material (Mormann et al, 1986; Shearer et al, 1993).

Another system that machines ceramic inlays, onlays, crowns, and bridges is the CELAY system (Figure 3.22) (Siervo et al, 1994). This is a precision copy milling machine that uses similar types of ceramic materials, but is not computer-driven. A light-cured composite replica of the restoration is fabricated directly in the patient's mouth or on a master cast. The replica is mounted on one side of the CELAY system (the scanning side), and a ceramic block is mounted on the milling side. Scanning tools are used to trace the surface of the restoration while a corresponding milling tool removes the ceramic. The system uses a sequential milling procedure proceeding from coarse to fine milling burs, and

can mill a typical restoration in about 15–20 minutes. The internal and occlusal surfaces are fully formed with this technique. Vitablocs similar to CEREC Vitablocs may be used in this system. However, In-Ceram alumina blocks can also be used to fabricate single- and multiple-unit In-Ceram cores for production of all-ceramic crowns and bridges. The In-Ceram porous alumina is milled with the CELAY system and subsequently infused with glass before application of the overlying porcelain (Figure 3.23).

All-ceramic restorations

There are several criteria by which dentists may judge restorative systems. These include esthetics, strength,

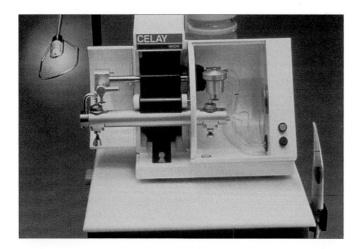

Figure 3.22 The Mikrona CELAY system.

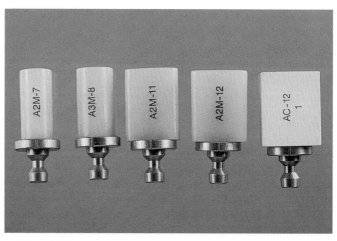

Figure 3.23 Vitabloc MKII and In-Ceram blocks for use with CELAY and CEREC II.

marginal fit, cost, and ease of fabrication. The Dicor, Empress, In-Ceram, and In-Ceram Spinell materials all fulfill these criteria to varying degrees. The esthetics of each system varies primarily with respect to the degree of translucency. Dicor is generally considered to be the most translucent of all the ceramic systems. However, the strength of this material is not as high as that of Empress or In-Ceram, and in some cases it is too translucent. Empress and In-Ceram Spinell follow, in order of degree of translucency. The strength of Empress is somewhere between those of Dicor and In-Ceram Spinell. Empress and In-Ceram Spinell are both excellent materials for use in cases where the natural dentition is fairly translucent and strength is of intermediate concern. In-Ceram is the strongest all-ceramic core material available (Figure 3.24). In cases where strength is the overriding concern, this system may be considered the material of choice. Even though its translucency is not as high as the other materials, the core does have some translucency, and excellent esthetics can be achieved.

The fit of these all-ceramic systems has been shown to range from 25 to 75 μm. Generally, the fit is clinically adequate for all of these systems. Ease of fabrication varies greatly for each material. The casting procedures for Dicor and the heat-cycle/injection-molding procedures for Empress must be followed carefully to achieve proper fit, strength, and esthetics. The critical step in the fabrication of In-Ceram restorations is the dispersion of the alumina/spinel and the application of this 'slip' to the gypsum die. The appli-

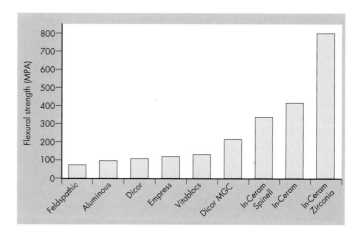

Figure 3.24 Mean flexural strength values for restorative ceramic materials.

cation and carving of the structure must be done properly so as not to introduce defects at this stage, since these may later result in premature failure of the restoration. Overall, any of these systems can provide well-fitting, natural-looking restorations as long as care is taken during the preparation and fabrication procedures (Rosenstiel et al, 1989; Morena et al, 1986; Mould, 1959; Probster, 1992; Giordano et al, 1995; Seghi et al, 1990a,b).

References

Budiansky B, Amazigo JC, Evans AG, Small scale crack bridging and the fracture toughness of particulate reinforced ceramics. *J Mech Phys Solids* 1988; **36**:167–87.

Clarke DR, Interpenetrating phase composites. *J Am Ceram Soc* 1992; **74**:739–59.

Faber KT, Evans AG, Crack deflection processes: 1. *Theory Acta Metall* 1983; **31**:565–76.

Frieman S, Introduction to ceramics and glasses. In: *ASM Engineering Materials Handbook, Vol 4: Ceramics and Glasses*. Philadelphia: ASM International, 1991: 1–40.

Giordano R, Campbell S, Pelletier L, Pober R, Flexural strength of an infused ceramic, glass ceramic, and feldspathic porcelain. *J Prosthet Dent* 1995; **73**:411–18.

Grossman DG, Tetrasilicic mica glass–ceramic material, 1973. US Patent No. 3732087.

Hoekstra KE, Dicor research facts. In: *Proceedings of the International Symposium on Alternatives to the Use of Conventional Porcelains*. Amsterdam, The Netherlands, 1986: 49–77.

Hoffman HR, Casellini RC, New low fusing synthetic porcelain: a solution to ceramo-metal problems. *Trends & Techniques in the Contemporary Dental Laboratory* 1988; **5**:44–7.

Kingery WD, Bowen HK, Uhlmann DR, *Introduction to Ceramics, 2nd edn*. New York: John Wiley, 1976.

Lehner CR, Schärer P, All-ceramic crowns. *Curr Opin Dent* 1992; **2**:45–52.

Mackert JR Jr, Evans AL, Effect of cooling rate on leucite volume fraction in dental porcelain. *J Dent Res* 1991; **70**:137–9.

Mackert JR Jr, Russell CM, Leucite crystallization during Empress processing. *J Dent Res* 1995; **74**:166 (Abstract 1236).

Malament KA, Grossman DG, Bonded vs non-bonded Dicor crowns. *J Dent Res* 1992;**71**:321 (Abstract 1720).

McLean JW, *The Science and Art of Dental Ceramics. Volume 2: Bridge Design and Laboratory Procedures in Dental Ceramics*. Chicago: Quintessence, 1982: 28–31.

McLean JW, The future of dental porcelain. In: *Dental Ceramics: Proceedings of the First International Symposium on Ceramics*. Chicago: Quintessence, 1983.

McLean JW, Hughes TH, The reinforcement of dental porcelain with ceramic oxides. *Br Dent J* 1965; **119**: 251.

Morena R, Lockwood PE, Fairhurst CW, Fracture toughness of commercial dental porcelains. *Dent Mater* 1986, **2**:58–62.

Mormann W, Jans H, Brandestini M, Ferru A, Lutz F, Computer machined adhesive procelain inlays: Margin adaptation after fatigue stress. *J Dent Res* 1986; **65** (special issue):72.

Mould RE, The strength and static fatigue of glass. *Glastech Ber* 1959, **32K**:18–28.

Pelletier L, Giordano R, Campbell S, Pober R, Dimensional and compositional analysis of In-Ceram alumina and die material. *J Dent Res* 1992;**71**(special issue): 253.

Pober R, Giordano R, Campbell S, Pelletier L, Compositional analysis of In-Ceram infusion glass. *J Dent Res* 1992; **71** (special issue): 253.

Probster L, Compressive strength of two modern all-ceramic crowns. *Int J Prosthodont* 1992; **5**:409–14.

Rekow ED, Computer aided design and manufacturing in dentistry: A review of the state of the art. *J Prosthet Dent* 1987; **58**:512–16.

Rekow ED, Thompson VP, Slater ELD, Musolf W, CAD/CAM restoration surface finish as a function of tool wear. *J Dent Res* 1992; **71** (special issue): Abstract 1399.

Rekow ED, Thompson VP, Jahanimir S, Lloyd L, Anand D, Factorial design technique to investigate the effect of machine tool parameters and machining environment on surface finish. *J Dent Res* 1993; **72** (special issue): Abstract 570.

Rice RW, Mecholsky JJ, The science of ceramic machining and surface finishing: III. *Natn Bur Stand Soc Publ* 1977; No.562:351.

Rosenstiel S, Balker M, Johnston W, A comparison of glazed and polished dental porcelain. *Int J Prosthodont* 1989; **6**:524–9.

Seghi RR, Daher T, Caputo A, Relative flexural strength of dental restorative ceramics. *Dent Mater* 1990a; **6**:181–4.

Seghi RR, Sorensen JA, Engelman MJ, Roumanas E, Torres TJ, Flexural strength of new ceramic materials. *J Dent Res* 1990b; **69** (special issue): Abstract 1521.

Shand EB, *Glass Engineering Handbook, 2nd edn*, New York: McGraw-Hill, 1958: 50–1.

Shearer AC, Heymann HO, Wilson NH, Two ceramic materials compared for the production of CEREC inlays. *J Dent* 1993: **21**:302–4.

Siervo S, Bandettini B, Siervo P, Falleni A, Siervo R, The CELAY system: a comparison of the fit of direct and indirect fabrication techniques. *Int J Prosthodont* 1994; **7**:434–9.

Taya M, Hayashi S, Kobayashi A, Yoon HS, Toughening of a particulate reinforced ceramic matrix composite by thermal residual stress. *J Am Ceram Soc* 1990; **5**: 1382–91.

Vergano PJ, Hill DC, Uhlmann DR, Thermal expansion of feldspar glasses. *J Am Ceram Soc* 1967; **50**:59–60.

CHAPTER 4

Color and Light Transmission

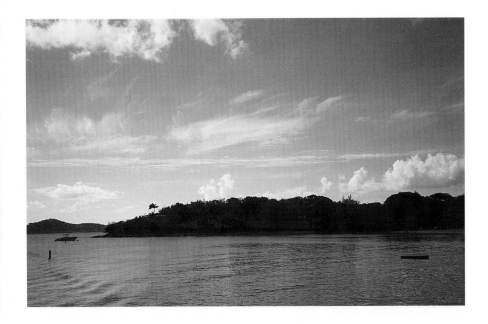

Visual impressions pervade our daily lives. These visual experiences can occasionally change into emotion, depending on our mood or state of mind. There are hundreds of different ways of seeing things; seeing is an art in itself. Whereas a superficial look at things imparts commonplace, everyday information, a closer look yields a wealth of detail and all the information essential for the understanding, transmission and reproduction of shape and colors.

For the majority of painters, sculptors, craftsmen and architects, creation and invention are processes always accompanied by much questioning on the three-dimensional aspects of the shape and color of their subjects, and, above all, of how they are perceived. Esthetics is sometimes defined as the 'art of perception' (Ancient Greece).

In dentistry, one must apply the same principles if successful ceramic coloring is to be attained. One must learn to see and try to understand the laws of physics, physiology, and psychology governing the perception of the shapes and colors seen in natural teeth, which one normally aspires to reproduce as closely as possible.

It is impossible to cover such a vast subject thoroughly in just a few pages, bordering, as it does, on such complex fields as physics, biology, histology, psychology, mineralogy, medicine and esthetics. Similarly, the merit of a 'shade' in ceramics goes far beyond mere color, since a decisive role in

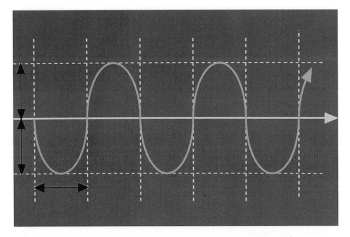

Figure 4.1 Electromagnetic waves. The wavelength is the distance between successive peaks (or successive troughs). The amplitude is the wave height with relation to the directional axis of the wave.

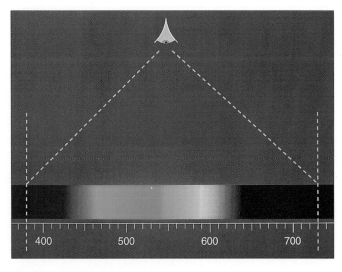

Figure 4.2 Spectrum of light that is visible to the human eye (wavelengths are in nanometers).

determining the success of the esthetic effect is played by shape, surface texture, surrounding tissue, spatial arrangement, ceramic build-up techniques, bonding cements, and the quality of the substrate and of integration. This subject has been dealt with in numerous books, articles and lectures, and some of these, such as the first publication of Dr Bruce Clark in 1931, were already laying the basic foundations of color measurement. Other authors, such as Sproull (1973a,b), Billmeyer and Saltzman (1967), Munsel (1961), Preston and Bergen (1980), Nakagawa et al (1975) and Yamamoto (1972), subsequently improved our grasp of the complexity of light transmission through transparent and, especially, translucent objects.

Knowledge of these different theoretical, clinical and practical analyses is essential for understanding the mechanisms underlying color perception and for applying this understanding to our everyday clinical activities.

Understanding the language of colors

Without becoming too involved in the complex mechanisms underlying color perception, it should be remembered that sight cannot exist without light and that tooth shape and color can only be perceived if the tooth reflects or emits light rays reaching the eye, producing signals that pass to the brain, where they trigger a visual perception process.

In attempting to understand the basic relationship between light and visual perception, it should be pointed out that light is a form of energy, which propagates according to the laws of physics. This energy spreads in the form of waves characterized by two different parameters: wavelength and amplitude (Figure 4.1).

Light is the form of electromagnetic energy visible to the human eye. Color perception depends on both objective and subjective phenomena, and occurs as a result of vision, or, in other words, the pattern of optical and cerebral response over a very narrow band of the electromagnetic spectrum. The 380–760 nm electromagnetic wave range can be discerned perfectly well by the naked eye (Figure 4.2). The human eye can distinguish violet, blue, green, yellow, orange and red, but finds it difficult to establish clear boundaries between different hues.

The fact that every color has its own matching wavelength is of interest: short wavelengths of 400 nm correspond to blue hues for example, medium wavelengths of 540 nm to greens, and long wavelengths of 700 nm to reds.

So color is nothing more than an energy wave of a specific wavelength; it is visual perception of a given

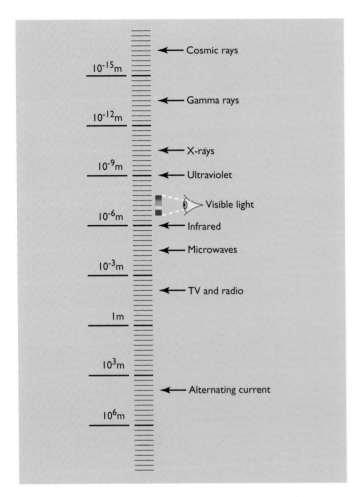

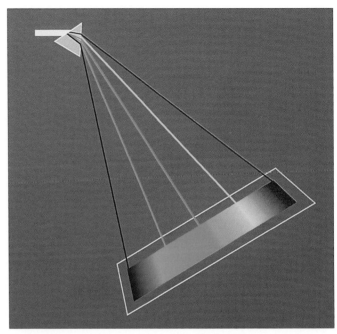

Figure 4.4 Splitting of white light as it passes through a prism. Different wavelengths are perceived by the human eye as colors.

Figure 4.3 The electromagnetic spectrum by wavelength. Note the narrow range of wavelengths for visible light.

wavelength that determines the color of what the eye has seen.

The electromagnetic spectrum ranges from 10^{-14} m (gamma rays) to 10^6 m (radio waves) (Figure 4.3). It is only rays within the 380–760 nm range that, through their action on specialized cells, elicit photochemical reactions from the retina, responsible for triggering visual perception of shapes and colors within the brain. This is why we cannot distinguish either ultraviolet or infrared rays (with wavelengths of less than 380 nm or more than 760 nm respectively).

There are three main natural sources of light – the sun, the moon and fire – and three principal artificial sources – incandescent light, fluorescent tubes and photographic flash. Each of these light sources is defined either by its light spectrum or its corresponding temperature. A particular source is often defined by its 'color temperature' rather than its spectrum. The color temperature is measured in degrees kelvin (K). The kelvin scale starts at 0 K, corresponding to a temperature of –273°C.

Natural light typically ranges between 5000 K and 5500 K . An object will take on different colors when seen under different types of light. It is important for us, as dentists, who rarely work under a consistent light, to bear this in mind.

Concept of color and colorimetry

Color

Color is a purely subjective impression, formed in a specific portion of the brain, owing to the specialization of certain cells, rods and cones, distributed over the retina.

Light produced by the sun is made up of different wavelengths, which can be revealed using a simple prism (Figure 4.4). The prism splits up the light into components of different wavelengths, each of which is perceived by the eye as a different color; the shortest and longest wavelengths visible to the eye are violet and red respectively.

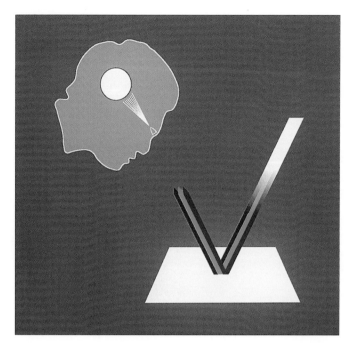

Figure 4.5 *A surface appears white when it reflects all light rays.*

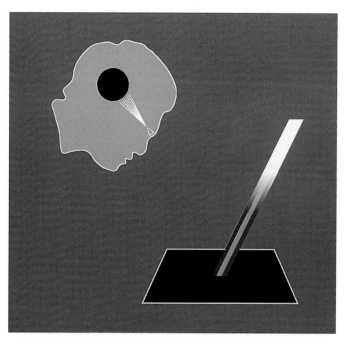

Figure 4.6 *A surface appears black when it absorbs all light rays.*

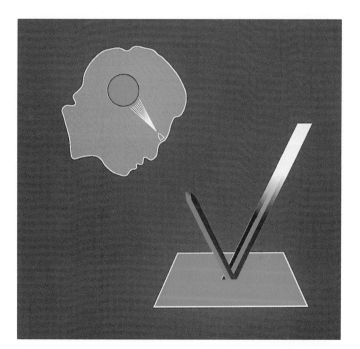

Figure 4.7 *A surface appears blue when it reflects short and medium waves but absorbs long waves.*

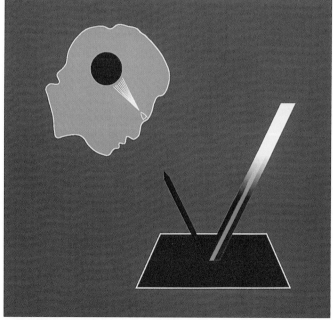

Figure 4.8 *A surface appears red when it reflects long waves but absorbs short and medium waves.*

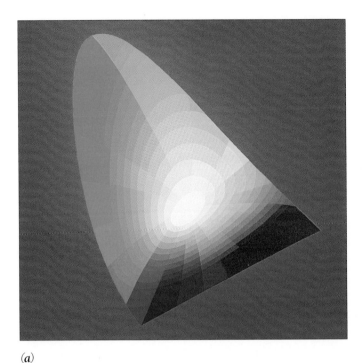

(a)

New colors may be synthesized by adding or subtracting others. The principle of subtraction of certain light constituents serves to explain why a lemon is yellow or a tomato red.

A surface or an object may appear red, for example, when it reflects long waves but absorbs short and medium waves (Figure 4.5). More specifically, the proportion of the light absorbed always complements that of the light reflected.

In the above example, the red surface reflects red light, but absorbs light of the complementary color, blue. The reverse also applies: a surface appears blue when it reflects short and medium waves but absorbs long waves (Figure 4.6).

When a neutral light (the sun) strikes a surface reflecting all its rays, the eye sees the surface as white (Figure 4.7). A surface appears gray when all the wavelengths of neutral light are reflected and absorbed in equal measure, and a surface appears black when the light is totally absorbed and no reflected ray can stimulate the retinal cells (Figure 4.8).

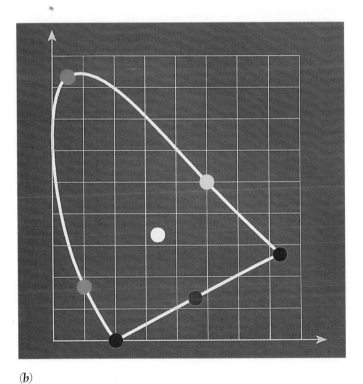

(b)

Figure 4.9 (a) The standard CIE rating system is a theoretical model based on the ranking of colors. (b) White occupies the central position and each color has a set position according to its degree of chroma.

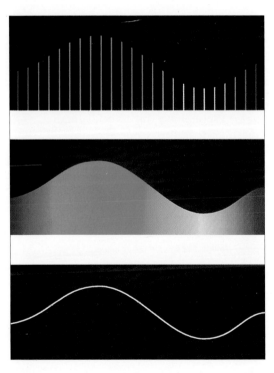

Figure 4.10 An emission curve is obtained by measuring the light intensity of each wavelength once every 10 or 20 nm. This curve, which may be augmented by colors of the spectrum, enables the intensity of a certain color or of different light rays to be determined.

Colorimetry

The intensity of a light source may be established by the energy it gives off.

Reflectivity is a measure of the capacity of a given surface or substance to reflect light. A white surface, for example, has 100% reflectivity. A black surface, where all rays are absorbed, has 0% reflectivity. A certain number of light rays do, in fact, strike the retina, but without producing sufficient energy for the cells to react. All these energy levels equate to photometric levels measurable by photometers as adopted by the CIE (Commission Internationale d'Eclairage) (Figure 4.9).

Colorimetry is a precise technique that aims to specify color by taking accurate measurements expressed either quantitatively or, better still, graphically. In fact, transmission or reflection of light produced by any light source can be analyzed according to its spectral composition (Figure 4.10). Light or color playing an important role in various applications, whether scientific, industrial or technical, can be accurately measured by means of spectral analysis. It is spectral analysis that enables the exact color of a painting or textile to be reproduced. Within our own field, this technique enables us to analyze the color of natural teeth, shade guides and ceramic materials, and even to test the true effect of chemical bleaching agents, for example. Although widely used for the manufacture of shade guides and ceramic powders, spectral analysis still remains at the experimental stage for establishing the color of natural teeth.

Although Ronchi (1970) stated that it should be remembered that light is a mental phenomenon and cannot possibly be measured in the same way as physical phenomena, we do need to have some physical points of reference.

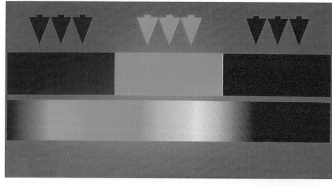

(a)

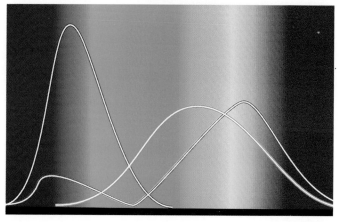

(b)

Figure 4.11 (a) The retina has three types of cone cell, sensitive to radiation of short (blue), medium (green) and long (red) wavelengths respectively. Color perception is governed by the laws of additive and subtractive synthesis. (b) These curves illustrate the sensitivity spectrum of the three categories of cone cells, which react with various intensities depending on the type of lighting, to produce the sensation of color within the brain.

Color perception

Numerous hypotheses on the mechanism of color perception have been put forward. Aristotle maintained that white light was of greater intensity than colored light, and perception of color resulted from differing degrees of mixing between light and shade. These concepts became more scientific with the advent of Hooke's theory, followed by that of Newton, who established the composition of white light. Finally, in 1801, Thomas Young attributed the diversity of colors to combinations between the three fundamental qualities of the retina: 'Three types of nerve fiber appear to exist within the eye; excitation of these produces red, green and blue respectively'.

This theory, according to which the eye can pick out the three primary colors by means of specialized cells, was taken up again 60 years later by Helmholtz. The existence within the eye of three types of cell, photosensitive to short, medium and long wavelengths corresponding to the three primary colors, is now generally accepted (Figure 4.11). Any light containing either part of the spectrum only, or having some constituents of higher intensity than others, is therefore perceived as colored by the eye.

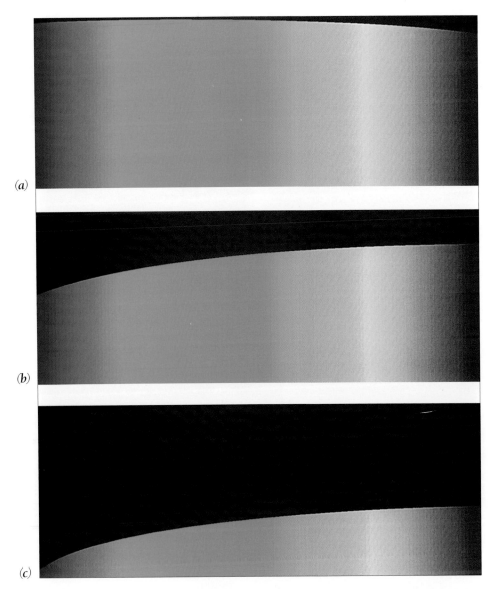

(a)

(b)

(c)

Figure 4.12 *Emission curves of three types of light:* (**a**) *Light of colour temperature 5000 K; the proportions of different parts of the visible spectrum are roughly identical.* (**b**) *Light of 2000 K ; the proportions of red and green wavelengths is high.* (**c**) *Light of 1000 K ; the proportion of red and green wavelengths is still higher.*

Turning to artificial light, we can discriminate

- incandescent light, invented by Edison in 1878;

- fluorescent light emitted from lamps or tubes.

In incandescent light, the rays emitted by heated filaments produce a reddish-yellow light, and it is appar-ent from the emitted spectrum that this type of light is of greatest intensity in the long-wave band (color temperature 3000 K–4000 K) but does contain all parts of the spectrum (Figure 4.12).

Fluorescent lamps usually operate using a mixture of several fluorescent powders. Lights giving off different shades of white light can be produced in this way. Three standard types exist, each giving out a specific type of light according to the kelvin scale:

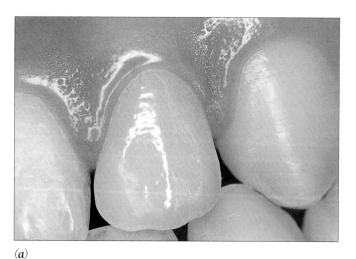

(a)

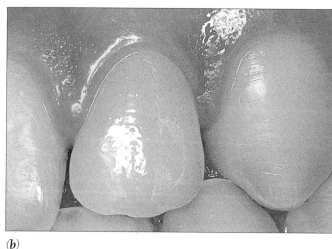

(b)

Figure 4.13 A ceramic laminate veneer on the maxillary lateral incisor: note how the shade is a good match under one lighting condition (a), but shows a mismatch under different lighting conditions (b).

- warm white (3000 K)

- standard white (4000 K)

- daylight (6000 K)

A 5000 K light may be considered neutral compared with the sun's surface, at 6500 K (pure white). An international daylight standard of 5500 K has been adopted. Spectral graphs indicate that a 5000 K light is the best balanced (see Figure 4.12a). Many authors, e.g. Winter (1993), consider that a 5500 K light is too bright to appraise color. They favor a 5000 K light, combining 6000 K neon tubes with 3000 K incandescent light. As explained in Chapter 5, 'Color of Natural Teeth', a 5000 K light will be used to select hue and chroma and a much fainter light to choose value.

Any alteration in the intensity of light will also alter the color of anything illuminated by it; a few examples will now be given to illustrate this point. Yellow and blue will appear as orange and indigo respectively under an incandescent (reddish-yellow) light. When lighting matches the color of the object illuminated, it becomes more heavily saturated. A red surface appears more heavily saturated under a red light, for instance – a color reinforcement phenomenon. Lighting complementary to the color it illuminates inhibits the latter, and the color verges on gray. Under a bluish neon light, bright pink

becomes more gray. As far as neutral, white and gray shades are concerned, white shades are seen to turn orange-yellow under incandescent light, but appear blue-gray when illuminated by a fluorescent tube.

Light sources can also affect color value; certain colors remain unchanged, whereas others will appear darker or lighter (Figure 4.13).

Metamerism is another phenomenon that has a strong impact on color perception. Metamerism is a phenomenon whereby two colored objects look the same under source of one light and different under another light. Two colors or objects with the same spectral curves cannot be described as metameric, while two colors or objects with different spectral curves can manifest varying degrees of metamerism (Figure 4.14). Metamerism is discussed further on page 59.

Photoluminescence: fluorescence and phosphorescence

Substances giving off a certain type of light when struck by invisible ultraviolet rays are described as photoluminescent. Such substances can be divided into two groups:

- phosphorescent substances, which continue to emit visible light after ultraviolet rays have struck them;

- fluorescent substances, which emit visible light only as the ultraviolet rays are striking them.

This phenomenon may be explained by the fact that these substances are able to transform invisible short-wave ultraviolet rays into longer, visible waves.

Such substances are widely used as optical brighteners in detergents, creating the impression of 'whiter than white'. These brighteners do not really make white any whiter, but simply make it look more luminous. Whites actually look brighter with a slight bluish overtone, thus reflecting more rays of shorter wavelengths. An optical brightener, employing a fluorescent substance, in effect turns invisible ultraviolet rays, by reflection, into rays with higher wavelengths within the spectrum of vision of between 400 and 500 nm, that is, into a blue shade.

It should be remembered that teeth and tooth enamel in particular, are fluorescent substances. Not all dental ceramics are fluorescent, however, and this has to be borne in mind when assessing the value of natural teeth (Figure 4.15).

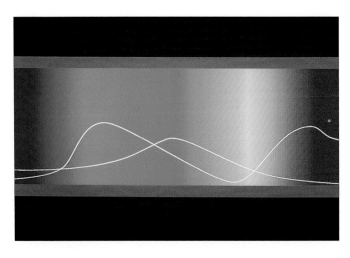

Figure 4.14 Reflectance curves of two metameric colors: the spectral compositions of the two colors are completely different; they can produce either the same or a different sensation of color, depending on light conditions. The emission and transmission curves of colors resembling each other can be superimposed.

Aspects of color measurement

When studying a colored surface, numerous difficulties arise in defining its color. Sproull (1973a) rightly remarked that this sensory perception involves three separate phenomena, and these are:

- a physical phenomenon existing outside the body, namely light;

- a psychophysical phenomenon, namely the eye's response to stimulation by light;

- a psychosensory phenomenon, namely the cerebral response to coded messages transmitted by retinal receptor cells.

Color can thus be defined in three different ways.

- From the standpoint of physics, color is defined by three parameters: intensity of energy emitted, wavelength and spectral composition. This aspect therefore involves radiant energy only.
- From a psychophysical standpoint, color is defined by another three parameters: luminance, dominant wavelength and colorimetric value. This aspect is involved only with light energy caught by the eye.

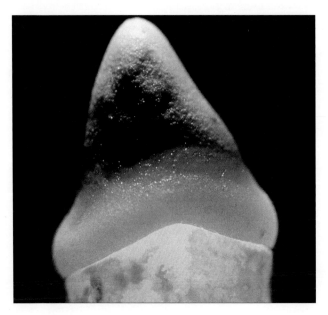

Figure 4.15 Excellent fluorescence at the margins obtained with Margin (Creation) ceramic material. (Courtesy of Jean-Marc Etienne.)

- Finally, from the psychosensory standpoint, color is again defined by three parameters: hue, value and chroma. This aspect relates to the way that the brain interprets color, and this is the concept that interests us for the purposes of quantifying color in our day-to-day clinical activities.

Just as the three measurements of height, length and width enable us to describe an object, color too is traditionally defined by the three measurements of hue, value and chroma – terms known to many among us. Unfortunately, few of us understand exactly what these terms imply and, more specifically, what scales of measurement are used to evaluate them. Despite this, they must be used to convey color information to dental laboratories.

As far as opaque objects are concerned, the eye discriminates colors with respect to the three measurements of hue, value and chroma. In the case of teeth, as we shall see, a fourth measurement should be added, namely that of translucency.

Spatial classification of colors

The three dimensions of hue, value and chroma are those used in the spatial classification of color. Numerous color classification systems exist, but Munsel's (1961) system is that which best serves to rank tooth color, since it views differences between neighboring colors as regular intervals. Hue, value and chroma are very well represented on Munsel's color scale.

To give a clearer picture of the arrangement of colors in Munsel's color system (Figure 4.16) they are basically represented as a sphere. It should be noted that the various colors (hues) are represented by the leaves that surround the axis. The axis of the system corresponds to

the value scale, which Munsel takes, arbitrarily, as ranging from 1 to 9, thus distinguishing nine value scales, with 0 representing black and 9 representing full white. The radii of the different discs represent chroma, starting with 'pure' color at the outer edge and becoming progressively less saturated towards the central axis.

The three dimensions can easily be associated to define a color by a notation such as 5.R 5/4. The first figure stands for degree of value, R for the red hue and the third, expressed as a fraction, to the degree of chroma.

This system makes it possible to quantify, convey and reproduce a color very accurately, and has the added advantage of international acceptance. Unfortunately, the system was intended for evaluation of opaque surfaces and therefore is not fully applicable for teeth, whose surfaces are translucent. Therefore a fourth dimension, that of translucency, has to be added to make this system effective for dentists. The four dimensions of color – hue, value, chroma and translucency – should be quantified as clearly and accurately as possible in defining natural tooth or ceramic color. These four parameters can be considered our basic color language for day-to-day practice; dental practitioners must take every opportunity to become acquainted with these four dimensions and accustomed to their use. Such aids as spectrophotometry, colorimetry and photography are essential for determining these values, although shade guides remain the most modern technique for use in dental offices or prosthetic laboratories.

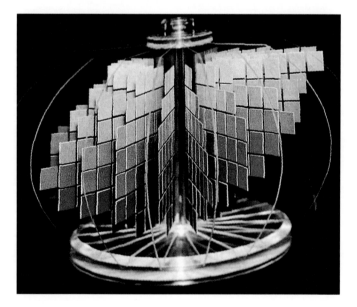

Figure 4.16 *Munsel's color system.*

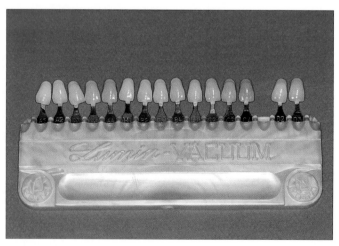

Figure 4.17 *The Vita shade guide.*

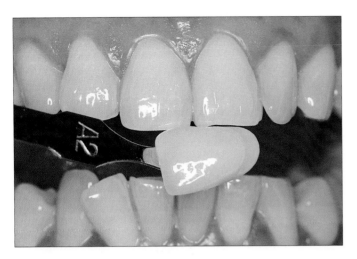

Figure 4.18 *The Vita shade guide comprises four color 'families'. Before defining tooth color, the 'family' to which it belongs must be established.*

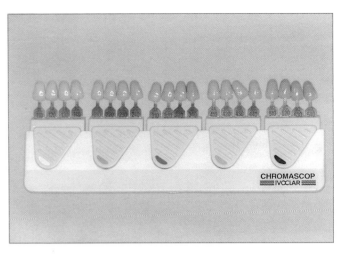

Figure 4.19 *The Chromascop (Ivoclar) shade guide. Differences in value can best be grasped by means of a black and white photograph.*

Shade guides

There is no such thing as an ideal shade guide, although some can be very comprehensive, such as that introduced by Hayashi (1967) or Clark's 'tooth color indicator' (1933), with 125 and 60 shades respectively. Unfortunately, most widely used shade guides – those that serve as a standard for most ceramic materials – only include 15 shades, and therefore cannot cover the entire range of natural tooth color, or the common method of shade arrangement (Figure 4.17).

Hue

Hue is the easiest scale to define. According to Munsel, it is this quality that distinguishes one color family from another. Thus, in describing an object as green, blue or red, one is defining its hue. This always corresponds to the wavelength of the light reflected by the teeth.

The Vita shade guide comprises four hues: A (reddish-brown), B (orange-yellow) C (greenish-gray) and D (pinkish-gray). Accordingly, it is possible to define the hue of a tooth by stating that the tooth belongs to group A, B, C or D (Figure 4.18).

It should be remembered that the hue must always be selected under appropriate light (5000 K).

Value

This is the factor distinguishing light from dark colors. Each shade guide may, in fact, display a different degree of value, as shown with Munsel's color scale and its nine value scales ranging from black to white.

A good illustration of the separation of value from color can be obtained by suppressing the color facility on one's television set: the 'brightness' facility then determines the value of the pictures. Two football teams playing in differently colored shirts, such as red and blue, but of the same value, appear to be wearing identical shirts. High- and low-value colors then appear light and dark respectively.

Value is by far the most important factor in color determination.

Light intensity has already been seen to exercise a decisive influence on the apparent value of a tooth. Hence it is always preferable to confirm tooth value by referring to a standard shade guide under average or even dim light, which will optimize contrast. We have become accustomed to assessing value at the following four different light intensities during shade selection:

- by average natural light (5000 K)

- by dim natural light (3000 K)

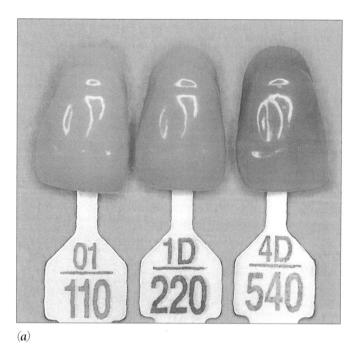

(a)

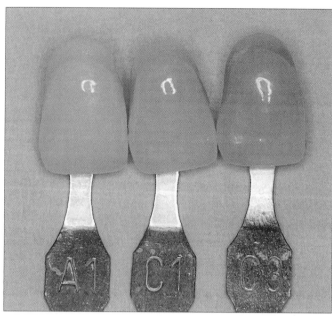

(b)

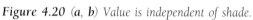

Figure 4.20 (a, b) Value is independent of shade.

- by average artificial light (5000 K)

- by dim artificial light (3000 K)

What appears to be the best value should always be chosen. If in doubt, values obtained under dim light are preferred.

Another way of assessing value consists in taking black and white photographs of the teeth and shade guides, using either conventional photography or, more simply, Polaroid instant photography (Figures 4.19–4.21). This testing method may identify a difference in value for two teeth with identical hues. Similarly, two teeth with different hues may exhibit the same value. It has been suggested by some clinicians that the Vita shade guide could be rearranged according to increasing value rather than by hue sets.

Chroma

Chroma is the portion of a hue that is pigmented. It can also be defined in relation to the amount of pigment contained in a hue shade. In the case of blue, for example, a pure, bright blue may be imagined as representing high chroma, followed by several less saturated blue shades, tending towards increasingly light blues, with less chroma.

In the standard Vita shade guide, four different chroma levels will be found for the same reddish-brown hue, with, for instance, A1 being less saturated than A4. It can thus be seen that value and chroma are at least connected, if not actually mingled, in this type of color guide (Figure 4.22). Chroma rises with increasing value. It can be seen that value and chroma are also connected in the case of natural teeth – although much less closely.

The concept of color desaturation seen in layered ceramic build-up has been particularly well researched by Yamamoto (1992) and Ubassy (1993). The latter recommends the use of a neutral ceramic powder to desaturate a color shade, to be mixed with the basic powder in varying amounts according to the degree of desaturation desired. In fact, the higher the degree of desaturation, the less pigment will the mixture contain. Most major ceramic brands now offer a range of more or less saturated ready-to-use dentin powders.

On reaching the shade selection stage, one may well choose an A3 shade of varying degrees of chroma. One

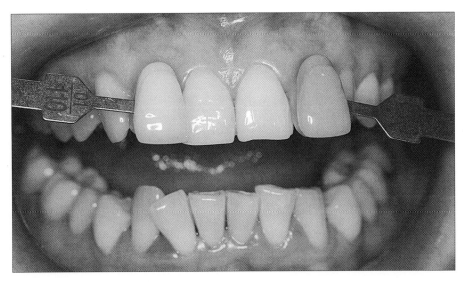

Figure 4.21 Value can be more easily determined from black and white photographs.

becomes able to define chroma scales fairly accurately with practice. To increase accuracy, one can extrapolate by placing a figure after the decimal point, thus expressing gradations of chroma in the following fashion: A3.2; A3.4 or A2.5 A2.8; A2, for example.

Translucency

Translucency is definitely one of the most difficult parameters to explain, and is even harder to quantify. It is almost as important as value, and plays a decisive role in light transmission phenomena.

Unfortunately, shade guides only offer standard translucency, generally at a lower level than that seen in natural teeth; this restricts their suitability for conveying such an essential quality. Quite apart from this consideration, shade guides can never give the right information on the translucency of a tooth, which depends partly on the dental enamel and, to a lesser extent, on the dentin. Opalescence is another associated factor.

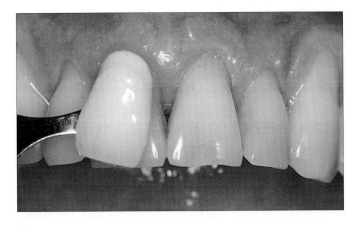

(**a**)

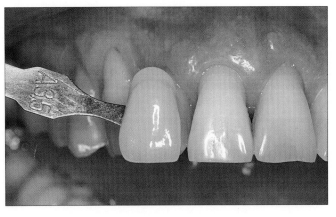

(**b**)

*Figure 4.22 Using the Vita shade guide, it can be seen that value and chroma are associated factors: (**a**) shade tab is too high in value and low in chroma; (**b**) shade tab has higher chroma and lower value.*

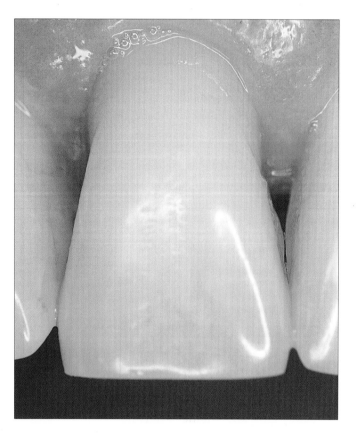

Figure 4.23 Type A tooth: only slightly translucent.

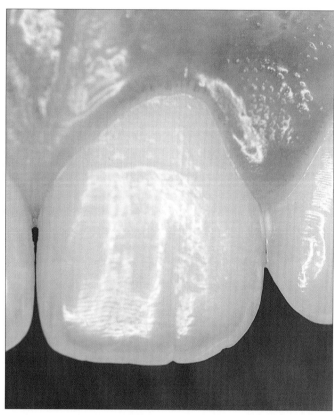

Figure 4.24 Type B tooth: translucent incisal edge.

Translucency of teeth varies from one individual to the next. It can also be highly susceptible to changes with age. Dental enamel and dentin will likewise undergo a great many age-related transformations. The enamel of a new tooth is not very translucent, and the dentin is very opaque. The enamel of an older tooth thins and grows more translucent or even transparent; the dentin becomes less opaque but more saturated.

Translucency has been thoroughly researched by Sékine et al (1975), who conducted an interesting study on 213 human teeth (maxillary incisors; both sexes), describing three types of translucency.

- Type A: little translucency, random distribution in all cases. These are teeth giving no impression of transparency. The laboratory prescription form should state no transparency or barely translucent tooth (Figure 4.23).

- Type B: translucency is found in incisal regions only, in the form of streaks (Figure 4.24).

- Type C: translucency exists at incisal regions and proximal edges (Figure 4.25).

This classification does not, of course, suffice to determine the translucency of all natural teeth precisely: types B and C must be broken down into numerous subdivisions.

It is often useful to record not just the extent of the translucent areas but also their hue, which could range from bluish-white to blue, gray, orange, brown, etc. The assessment of the general translucency of the dental enamel of labial/buccal as well as lingual/palatal surfaces should not be omitted.

In view of the wide range of possible shadings, we use a translucency rating scale ranging from 1 to 5 for the

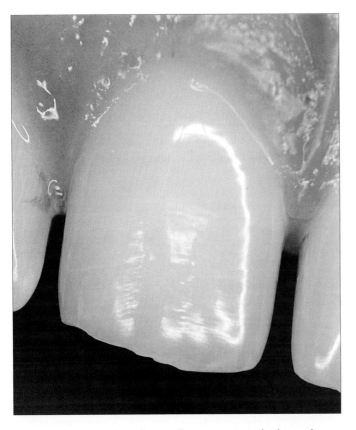

Figure 4.25 Type C tooth: translucency at incisal edge and proximal aspects.

area, the dental practitioner lets the ceramic technician know that the tooth to be reproduced resembles photograph 5 or 6, say. Once in possession of the document, the technician will have an exact visual image of the color and extent of the translucent area to be copied.

Photographic reference systems are an indispensable back-up to shade guides and an important factor in data transmission.

Useful points

- Conventional shade guides can certainly not be described as ideal. They remain too restricted for adequate definition of the four parameters of color – hue, value, chroma and translucency. Some prefer the Chromascop (Ivoclar) guide: at present, this offers 20 shades and a practical arrangement for shade selection. Although a laudable effort, it is still far from completely satisfactory.

- Ceramic color guides are most commonly manufactured from a ceramic material differing from that used in powders. This increases the chances of occurrences of metamerism and hence errors in color matching. Manufacturers must be urged to produce color guides of the same ceramic material as the powders they offer. This has already been achieved in the case of certain existing ceramics. Shofu was the first company to offer a standard Vita color guide made of the same powders as the dental ceramic material, called Crystar (Figure 4.26). Slight differences do occur between the same Vita and Crystar references; however, samples are more saturated overall in the latter. Ivoclar's Chromascop is offered with a full color guide system, which is very comprehensive; unfortunately, however, it is only this full system that corresponds to the IPS dental ceramic from the same manufacturer (Figure 4.27).

sake of simplicity, with 1 representing a low degree of translucency and 5 corresponding to highly transparent enamel. One might, for example, express data on the translucency of a tooth as type B: translucency T3 for a tooth exhibiting incisal translucency only in the bluish-white range and middle intensity.

A photographic reference system undoubtedly remains the best guide for conveying these essential data. One simply assembles high-quality photographic prints in an album showing different patterns of the most commonly found arrangements, shapes, colors, translucency levels, and types of surface texture and luster. These photographic references obtained from natural teeth must be classified and numbered in chronological order. In the case of translucency, we have chosen several steps representing the different stages that we are called upon to repeat most commonly. To convey the appearance and the extent of the translucent

The spectrophotometric study performed by Yamamoto (1992) on natural tooth color and color pads is very informative. It states that most teeth are of hue A on the Vita color guide, and a high proportion are between A2 and A3.5. Only very low proportions of hues B, C and D occur. We have come to precisely the same conclusions: we select 80% of our hues from group A.

The three dimensions of color – hue, value and chroma – cannot be viewed by the human eye with the same impact. Arranged in order of importance, value

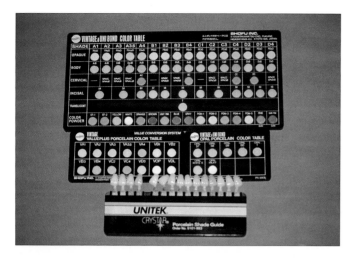

Figure 4.26 The Unitek shade guide, plus shade guide system.

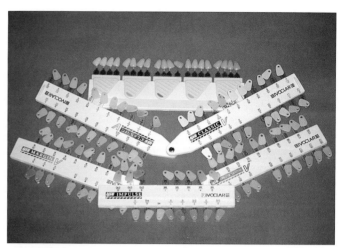

Figure 4.27 Chromascop shade guide, plus shade guide system.

will come first, followed by chroma and then hue. According to Yamamoto, value is three times as important as hue and twice as important as chroma. To complete these conclusions, it is logical to place translucency just after value but well before hue and chroma. It should also be mentioned that the higher the value and the lower the chroma of a tooth, the less importance will hue have; it is only actual appreciation of value and degree of translucency that count. This is often the case for A1 or B1 teeth. Conversely, the lower the value and the higher the chroma (A4 teeth or above), the more important will hue and translucency be.

Shade selection should also take account of other factors that are particularly difficult to quantify, such as

- fluorescence;

- the influence of the color of surrounding tissues, which impart a purplish-red shade within the mouth;

- the color of tooth substrate or metal supports;

- the degree of opacity or translucency of the bonding or luting cement;

- the type of ceramic material used.

To summarize, it should be remembered that the four dimensions defining color generally differ in importance: value remains the most and hue the least important among them.

Opalizers, opalescence and the opalescent effect

All translucent materials and, more particularly, dental ceramics as well as natural teeth contain so-called opalizers. Opalizing materials most commonly take the form of fine or extra fine particles. The translucency created by these fine powders will depend on the amount, grain and composition of the opalizers. Dental enamel and incisal ceramic powders contain very low amounts of opalizing particles, for example; natural dentin and dentin powders contain slightly more, and will appear more opaque; opaque powders or dentins contain even more, and this will obviously have a great influence on light transmission.

Opalizing particles produce a light-scattering effect in the tooth and dental ceramic, which will vary in degree depending on their refractive index and the size and quantity of particles. The greater the scattering, the more opaque will the material look; conversely, the less

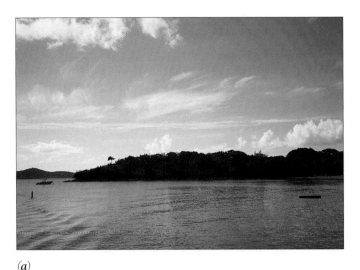

(a)

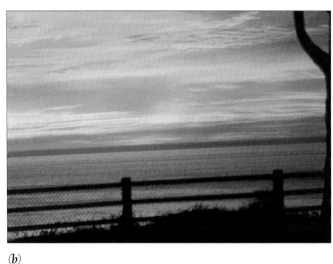

(b)

Figure 4.28 (**a**) *The sky is blue during the daytime, but* (**b**) *red or orange at sunrise and sunset: this difference is associated with a physical phenomenon involving the scattering of light from the sun.*

the scattering, the more translucent will the material appear. Thus no scattering occurs with a sheet of glass; nearly all light rays pass through the glass, which will appear transparent. In our 'transparent' ceramics, there are practically no opalizing particles and hence little diffraction, so that almost all light rays pass through the ceramic material.

The following opalizing substances with a refractive index differing from that of the remainder of the powder are used in ceramic powders to create different pastes, whether transparent, enamel, dentin or opaque: titanium oxide (TiO_2; refractive index 2.52, i.e. a very high index), zirconium oxide (ZrO_2; refractive index 2.2), and tin oxide (Sn_2O_2; refractive index 2.0). It should be noted that the more the degree of chroma of a powder increases with the addition of color pigments, the more will the material decrease in translucency, since the refractive index of pigment particles, differing from the ceramic matrix, will also exert an opaquing effect.

As noted by Yamamoto (1992) – and as discussed in Chapter 5 – teeth increase their chromaticity with age through saturation of the tissues, but, at the same time, the tissues in general and the enamel in particular become increasingly translucent.

Unfortunately, saturated shades are less translucent than non-saturated tints in most ceramic powders.

Modern ceramics such as Vintage (Shofu) appear to take account of this; it should be noted that the translucency of highly saturated complete color sets has been markedly improved.

It can thus be concluded that the part played by opaquing substances in the translucency of dental ceramics is decisive.

It is apparent that the smaller (and more numerous) the particles, the greater is the frequency of diffusion, which imparts a more or less opaque appearance to materials. However, if opaquing particles are particularly small – less than the wavelength of light – and with not too high a density and good distribution, then an opalizing, not an opaquing, effect will be obtained.

Opalescent effect

This effect stands out particularly in natural teeth as well as in the famous opal stone. Opals appear blue with reflected light and reddish-orange with transmitted light. Teeth also show opalescence. This opalescent effect is due to a particular type of light diffraction related to the presence of very fine and perfectly homogenous particles.

In natural teeth, very fine particles occur, particularly in the enamel, in the form of hydroxyapatite crystals,

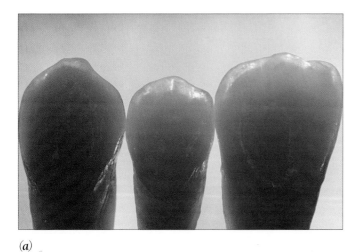

(a)

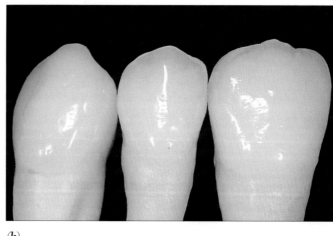

(b)

Figure 4.29 Illustration of opalescence in teeth made of Duceram-LFC (Ducera) ceramics. (**a**) In transmitted light, the transparency at the incisal edge shows up as orange-tinted. (**b**) In reflected light, the transparency at the incisal edge shows up as blue-tinted.

averaging 0.16 µm long and 0.02–0.04 µm thick, which are responsible for the opalescent effect. Teeth will display varying degrees of opalescence, according to the distribution of these crystals. They will therefore show blue glints, especially at the incisal edges; with transmitted light, an orange-yellow shade will be observed, however.

To explain this physical phenomenon (the Tyndall effect), which is also responsible for blue skies during the day and orange-tinged sky at dusk (Figure 4.28), we return to certain basic concepts regarding light reflection and scattering. A (tooth) surface will, via the fine particles, reflect short (400 nm) wavelength (i.e. blue) rays; the other (600–700 nm) wavelengths of the light spectrum will be absorbed. Thus the tooth will show certain bluish areas. Transmitted light, on the other hand, gives the tooth an orange-red appearance, since short wavelengths have been reflected, and the observer will only see light at longer wavelengths (600–700 nm).

If the tissue composition alters, as with heavily discolored (e.g. tetracycline-stained) teeth, this opalescence may greatly diminish or even disappear, imparting some degree of opacity to the teeth.

This opalescent effect can now be re-created using modern ceramics, especially low-fusing varieties such as Duceram-LFC (Ducera) (Figure 4.29). To produce this effect artificially, very fine and, above all, opaque particles with a refractive index differing from that of the ceramic paste should, in theory, be mixed with the basic powder. During subsequent firings, however, the risk of homogenization can arise through dissociation of the fine particles within the ceramic matrix, with loss of the opalescent effect, and having disastrous incidental effects on translucency and hue. The homogenization effects due to these low-fusing powders can be suppressed by adding fine zirconium oxide particles, which, in theory, are only destroyed at temperatures over 700°C, that is 50–100°C above the firing temperature range for these ceramic materials. In all other ceramics the opalescent effect will be considerably affected by firing temperature and the number of firings.

Counter-opalescence

This phenomenon is particularly noticeable on metal ceramic bridges. The incisal edge appears bluish whereas proximal edges look dark and mainly orange-yellow, despite the use of opaline ceramics in these two areas. The explanation of counter-opalescence is that light will be reflected because of opacity, and the transmitted light will give the tooth an orange shade.

How to avoid counter-opalescent effects
• By avoiding too shallow a depth of ceramics.

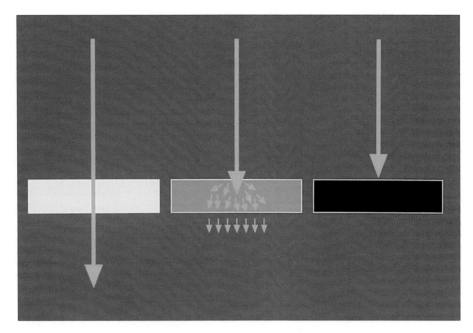

Figure 4.30 Transparent bodies allow light to pass through. Translucent bodies allow light both to pass through and scatter it. Opaque bodies do not let light through.

- By using opaque dentins and a build-up technique proceeding in successive layers (stratification) with dentins of gradually declining saturation to inhibit internal reflection effects.

- By using darker opaque materials to increase absorption with a ridged effect, which is important for 'breaking' the reflection, thus promoting a light scattering effect on contact with the surface.

- By avoiding over-fired opaque materials, which become smooth and shiny. A matt, ridged appearance should be opted for, obtained by lower firing temperatures.

Reflection, refraction and light transmission

The complex phenomena associated with light transmission within a natural tooth or ceramic material can best be understood by returning to the laws of reflection and refraction of light (Figure 4.30).

Reflection

When a light ray originating from an environment with refractive index 1 strikes a surface of refractive index 2, this results in a ray that is reflected in environment 1 and a ray undergoing refraction in environment 2. The angles of incidence and reflection will always be identical. However, the angle of refraction will be proportional to the refractive indices of the materials crossed by the light rays.

Under certain circumstances, where all stray light is reflected by the surface, total reflection will take place—a phenomenon occurring where the angle of incidence exceeds the angle for which all rays will be reflected (the critical angle). This explains why whitish areas seem to appear on teeth; these are in fact nothing more than the results of the full reflection of light rays. The same applies to the incisal edges, where a very fine white edge occasionally appears (the 'halo' effect), breaking up the bluish look of the edge. However, this stems from a much more complex phenomenon, and depends on the angles of the incisal edge (Figure 4.31).

Thus total reflection or none at all, i.e. refraction, may occur, depending on the angle of incidence.

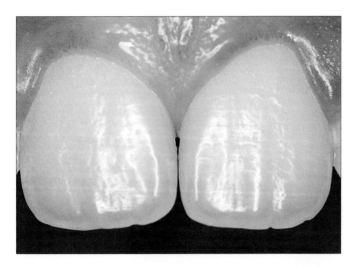

Figure 4.31 The appearance of a whitish border is associated with the angle at the incisal edge.

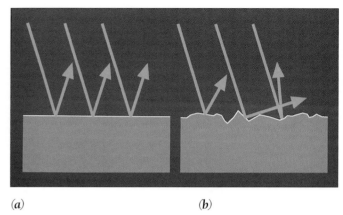

(*a*)   (*b*)

*Figure 4.32 When parallel light rays hit a flat opaque surface, the reflected rays remain parallel to each other (**a**), whereas when the surface is uneven, they are scattered in several directions (**b**).*

The angle of incidence must then exceed the critical angle for the effect of total reflection to be used in ceramics. To create this total reflection at the ceramic edge of a front tooth, for example, the angle of the incisal edge of the adjacent natural tooth should not be faithfully reproduced but actually reduced by 5°, since the critical angle of enamel is 37°, compared with 32° for ceramics.

Useful points

- All substances have different refractive indices, and thus surface reflection properties.

- The lower the refractive index, the less will the surface reflect light. Hence a tooth (refractive index 1.65) always appears more luminous than ceramics (refractive index 1.50), of whatever variety and however assembled, when viewed under the same light. It is important to remember this during shade selection.

- When a tooth or ceramic material is coated with a film of saliva, one should never take the actual refractive index of the surface into account, but rather the relative refractive index, which will always be lower. This explains why a natural or ceramic tooth coated with a film of saliva always appears less luminous. It should be remembered that

$$\frac{\text{refractive index of environment 1}}{\text{refractive index of environment 2}} = \text{relative refractive index}$$

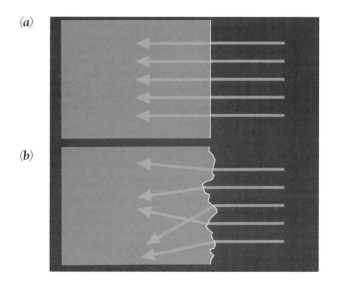

(*a*)

(*b*)

*Figure 4.33 When parallel light rays hit a flat transparent surface, they remain parallel (**a**), whereas when the surface is uneven, they are scattered in a number of directions (**b**).*

Influence of surface appearance on light reflection effects

When light strikes a smooth, flat, opaque body, the reflected rays will all be parallel (Figure 4.32a). If the body is rough, the reflected rays will no longer be parallel (Figure 4.32b) – a true scattering of these reflected

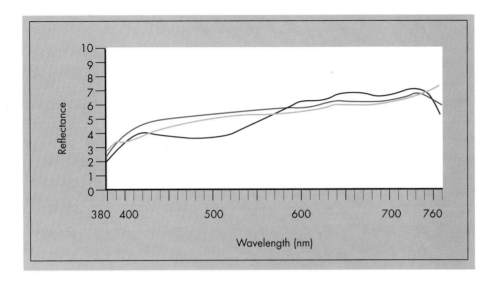

Figure 4.34 Reflectance curves of dental enamel (red), a dental ceramic (blue), and a restorative resin (yellow), all of the same shade, showing evidence of metamerism.

light rays takes place. When light strikes a smooth, flat, transparent body, the transmitted rays will all be parallel (Figure 4.33a). If the body is rough, the transmitted rays are diverted in multiple directions or 'diffused' (Figure 4.33b). Thus the visual aspect of the surface is modified by the surface geometry.

The texture of natural teeth is made up of a set of larger- and smaller-scale surface fluctuations, which have a considerable impact on reflection and hence on tooth color, which will additionally undergo age-related alteration. The more ridged is the tooth surface, the less translucent will it be. Surface defects will have to be increased to reproduce a new, nontranslucent tooth in ceramics; to reproduce an older tooth, the reverse applies.

Metamerism

Two surfaces or colors are said to be metamers when they have non-matching spectral analysis curves, but appear to have identical colors under certain lighting conditions. Two objects, such as an artificial and a natural tooth, can therefore appear correctly color-matched under certain lighting conditions but have different colors under changed lighting conditions. Shade guides, dental ceramics and natural teeth are three different substances, and therefore have a high potential for exhibiting metamerism. The practitioner

should be aware of this potential, and should take steps to minimize it (Figure 4.34).

How to reduce metamerism

- By lobbying manufacturers for ceramics with spectral curves as close as possible to those of natural teeth.

- By working under regulated light sources and always matching shades under the following three different sets of lighting:
  - daylight;
  - the artificial lighting of the surgery;
  - dim light.

- By having the shade selected checked by someone else (the dental assistant or ceramic technician). The shade most closely approximating the choice of the two 'observers' will often be the best match.

- By testing one's vision, and more particularly color vision, periodically.

- By shade selection using shade guides of the same material as the dental ceramics.

- By limiting surface staining.

A match that looks right under all three different types of light will always prove better than one appearing correct under any one of these – even daylight.

References

Billmeyer FW Jr, Saltzmann M, *Principles of Color Technology.* New York: Interscience, 1967: 1–23.

Clark EB, An analysis of tooth color. *J Am Dent Assoc* 1931; **18**: 2093–103.

Clark EB, Tooth color selection. *J Am Dent Assoc* 1933; **20**: 1065–73.

Hayashi T, *Medical Color Standard V: Tooth Crown.* Tokyo: Japan Color Research Institute, 1967.

Munsel AH, *A Color Notation, 2nd ed.* Baltimore, Munsel Color Company, Inc, 1961: 15–20.

Nakagawa Y et al, Analysis of natural tooth color. *Shikai Tentr* 1975; **46**: 527.

Preston JD, Bergen SF, *Color Science and Dental Art: A Self-Teaching Program.* St Louis: Mosby, 1980.

Ronchi V, *The Nature of Light.* Cambridge: Harvard University Press, 1970: 265.

Sékine M et al, Translucent effects of porcelain jacket crowns. 1: Study of translucent layer pattern in natural teeth. *Shika Giko* 1975; **3**: 49.

Sproull RC, Color matching in dentistry. Part I: The three dimensional nature of color. *J Prosthet Dent* 1973a; **29**: 416–24.

Sproull RC, Color matching in dentistry. Part II: Practical applications of the organization of color. *J Prosthet Dent* 1973b; **29**: 226–66.

Ubassy G, *Shape and Color: The Key to Successful Ceramic Restorations.* Berlin: Quintessence, 1993.

Winter R, Visualizing the natural · dentition. *J Esthet Dent* 1993; **5**: 103–17.

Yamamoto M, The value conversion system and a new concept for expressing the shades of natural teeth. *QDT Yearbook* 1992; **19**: 9.

CHAPTER 5

Color of Natural Teeth

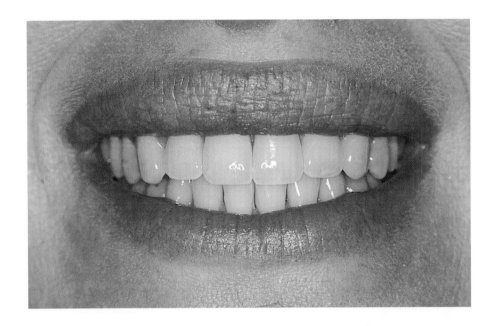

It is advisable to make time, whenever possible, to examine not just the shape and color of the teeth, but also their spatial arrangement and integration in relation to the smile and facial features.

The anatomical features common to teeth belonging to the same arch must be identified, as well as their arrangement, shape and color and their relationship to the patient's facial characteristics (Figure 5.1). All these aspects must be studied meticulously to build up the observation techniques, which will be refined with experience. Methodical observation requires awareness of general facial characteristics, and the relationship between the lips and the teeth, especially the smile line, formed by natural lip movement. Attention should then be focused on an individual tooth, outlining its overall shape, the height of contour, emergence profile, transition angles, appearance of the incisal edge, shape of the collar and surface appearance (texture, defects and color). Lingual surfaces should be examined just as meticulously. Tooth color must then be assessed by attempting to determine the four parameters mentioned in Chapter 4, using the standard shade guides. All these data will be required to fill in the patient's record and laboratory form correctly (Figure 5.2).

Observations should always be made from two angles: direct and sideways. The sideways view allows for better appreciation of transition angles,

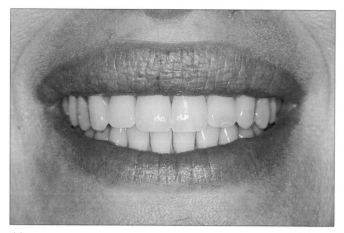

(a)

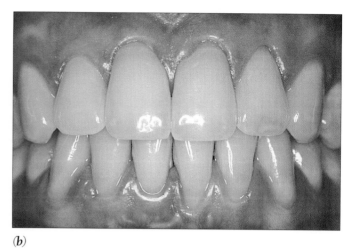

(b)

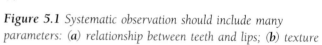

Figure 5.1 *Systematic observation should include many parameters: (**a**) relationship between teeth and lips; (**b**) texture and transition angles, and (**c**) color.*

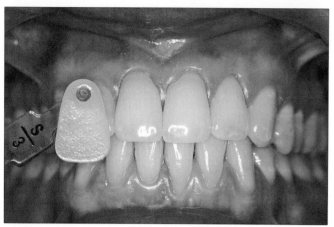

(c)

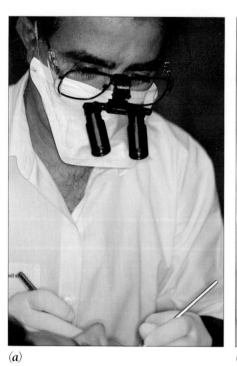

(a)

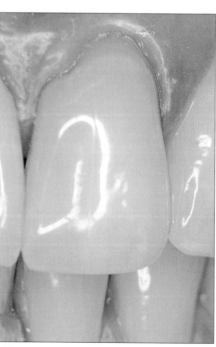

(b)

Figure 5.2 (**a**, **b**) *An accurate and detailed examination of a tooth can only be made with the aid of powerful magnifying glasses (5X).*

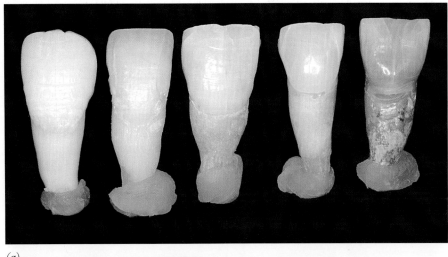

(a)

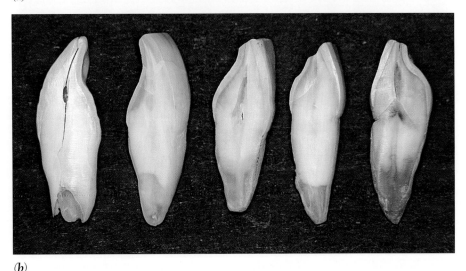

(b)

Figure 5.3 *Teeth illustrated at different ages, showing how surface conditions and different tissues evolve: (a) facial view; (b) cross-section.*

contours, emergence profiles and, occasionally, the appearance of certain defects, such as cracks or fissures. This basic training should be conducted regularly, and the eye should gradually become used to analyzing the different parameters when viewing a tooth.

Natural tooth color

The color of natural teeth is affected by several parameters. It depends on the thickness, composition and structure of the tissues forming the tooth. These three parameters will evolve considerably through life, thereby influencing tooth color (Figure 5.3).

The tooth consists of the following main tissues – tooth pulp, dentin and enamel. Each of these tissues possesses different optical properties (Figures 5.4–5.8).

The pulp

The pulp, usually a dark-reddish color, may be observed in the center of the tooth. The volume occupied by the pulp varies considerably with age, being larger in young

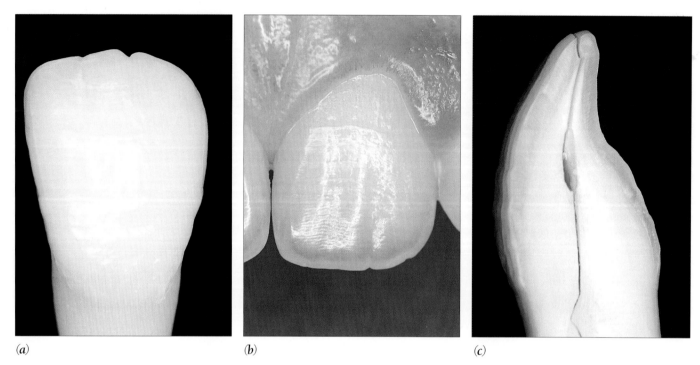

(a)   *(b)*   *(c)*

Figure 5.4 *Young teeth:* (**a**) *these are very light, and the enamel displays rich texture and a high degree of translucency.* (**b**) *This is undoubtedly the type of tooth that is hardest to recreate in ceramics.* (**c**) *The cross-section reveals highly colored opaque dentin, and hardly any transparent dentin.*

teeth, and this has an influence on the overall color, imparting a pinkish appearance, often prominent on the lingual surfaces. The pulp cavity narrows significantly in the course of time, and its influence over the shade of the tooth is diminished.

The pulp is considered the most vital part of the tooth. It is through activity within the marginal zone that dentin develops during tooth formation, as well as throughout the life of the tooth (secondary physiological dentin).

Dentin

Dentin, the most important dental tissue in terms of color, surrounds the pulp cavity. Under normal circumstances, it is covered either with enamel or cement. Dentin consists of minerals (approximately 70%, primarily hydroxyapatite), organic material (20%) and water (10%). The low mineral content of dentin compared with enamel and the high proportion of organic substances explains the relative opacity of primary dentin. A considerable number of narrow and elongated cavities, or dentin tubules, run through it. These tubules, peculiar to primary dentin, lead to selective diffraction of light, whereby certain rays will be reflected and others absorbed. Such diffraction results in the opacity of primary dentin. This dentin may evolve with age, forming secondary physiological dentin, or dentin of other types, displaying different structures and compositions, which will affect the optical properties of these tissues.

Secondary physiological dentin: This continues to form throughout life, but is only deposited sporadically. It has a higher mineral content than primary dentin and is less opaque. It also has a higher degree of chromaticity.

Sclerotic dentin: This is manifested as the response of the dental pulp to caries or trauma. It is often more saturated than primary and secondary dentin, and is limited to the site of trauma.

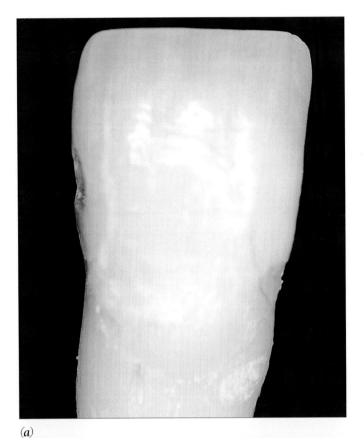

(a)

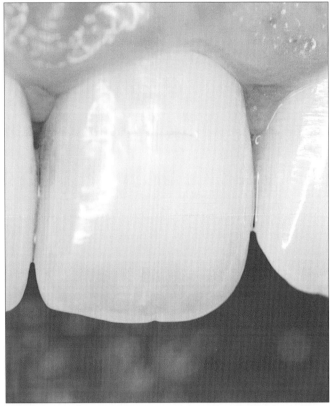

(b)

Figure 5.5 *Adolescent teeth: (**a,b**) the enamel still displays some horizontal striae as well as a high degree of translucency and opalescence. (**c**) The cross-section shows secondary dentin and a border of transparent dentin at the dentinoenamel junction.*

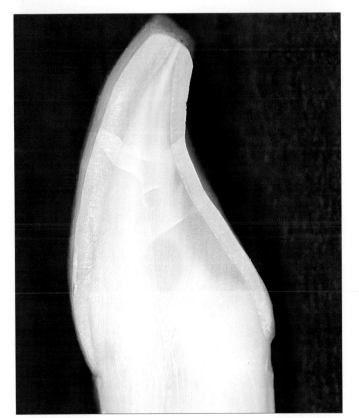

(c)

Transparent dentin (Majito's 'brilliance zone'): A hyper-mineralized zone may appear as the tooth ages, which infiltrates dentin tubules and eliminates Tomes' fibers. It particularly affects the roots, which become highly transparent, so that the inner coloring sometimes shows through the cement and the gingiva (appearing most commonly as a gray or bluish shade in the case of highly pigmented pulpless teeth). A highly characteristic zone may also form at the dentinoenamel junction. This dentin shows different levels of translucency, and sometimes can even be fully transparent.

This zone has a high mineral content and plays an important role in light transmission phenomena. It performs, in fact, like an optical fiber, and helps to increase the transparency of the teeth. This transparent

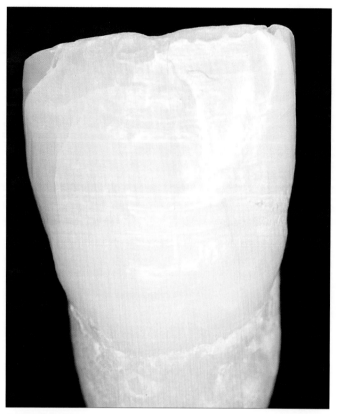

(a)

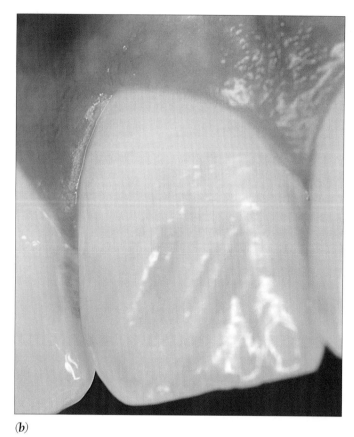

(b)

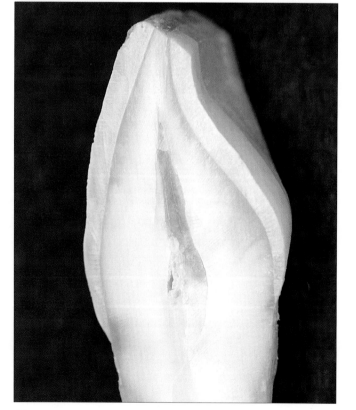

(c)

Figure 5.6 *Adult teeth: (**a,b**) The incisal edge is heavily worn and the shade more impregnated with orange-yellow. (**c**) The cross-section shows major tissue changes, with secondary dentin present and major sclerotic dentin formation.*

dentin at the dentinoenamel junction is more prevalent in aging than in young teeth.

Enamel

This is the hardest and most mineral-rich tissue in the body. It is made up of 95% minerals and 5% water and organic matter. The high mineral content and the nature and arrangement of the hydroxyapatite crystals make this tissue hard, brittle, translucent and radio-dense.

The optical appearance of tooth enamel depends on its composition, structure, thickness, degree of translucency, opalescence and surface texture.

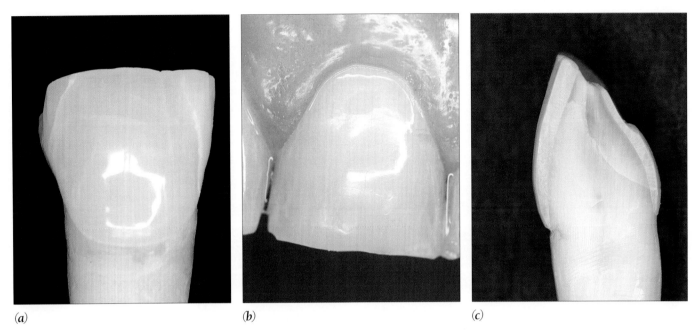

(a) (b) (c)

Figure 5.7 *Aging teeth: the enamel is thinner, very smooth and very transparent. Pulp volume is greatly reduced and much secondary dentin is present. (a) Extracted tooth; (b) in vivo; (c) cross-section.*

As with dentin, all of these parameters will evolve during the life of a tooth (thus affecting the optical properties of the enamel). The enamel varies in thickness between the three different portions of the tooth:

- In the **incisal third** the thickness of the enamel may reach 1.5 mm. In young teeth the edge is often made up of enamel only, which lends this region a special translucency, often making the incisal edge appear bluish by creating an opalescent effect. This translucency extends to the proximal surfaces in some cases.

- In the **middle third** the enamel thins out and the tooth becomes less translucent.

- In the **cervical third** the enamel can become very thin (0.2–0.3 mm), and, with only a fine layer present, this tissue becomes highly transparent and the color of the underlying dentin shows through, thus creating a considerably more opaque effect.

Thus the optical properties of tooth enamel depend on its thickness as well as its composition. In a young tooth the enamel has a lower mineral content and is very thick, creating the optical effect of slight translucency; the tooth thus appears very high in value. In an older tooth the enamel becomes mineral-rich and thinner due to natural wear. This is conveyed by the optical effect of very pronounced translucency or even transparency, which will then allow the color of the underlying dentin to show through.

Reasons for variation in natural tooth color

Natural tooth color, as already explained, depends on the composition, structure and thickness of the dental tissues. Any change, transformation, or alteration in any of these tissues, whether mechanical, chemical or biological, will bring about a change in tooth color.

Natural tooth is generally a true color mosaic, in the 'yellowish-white' range. This harmony of color varies from one individual to the next and even from one tooth to another. The reasons for these chromatic variations, as already explained, are dependent on a number of considerations, and the hereditary factor also plays an important role.

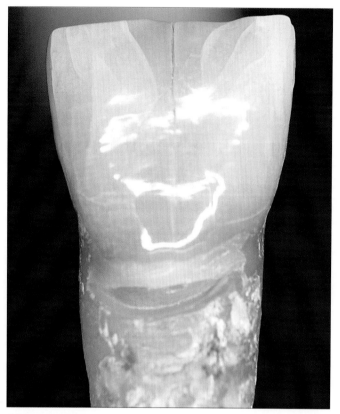

(a)

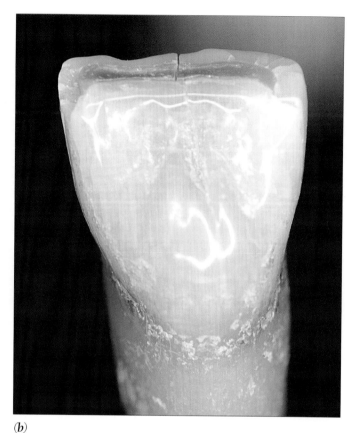

(b)

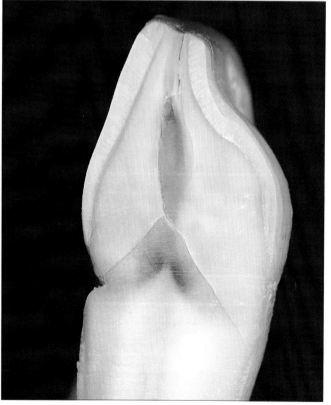

(c)

Figure 5.8 *Aged teeth: (**a**, **b**) the enamel is even thinner and transparent; one heavily colored fissure and numerous crevices are evident. (**c**) In cross-section it can be seen that the dentin has undergone many changes; it has become vitrified, very translucent and pigmented by filtration. Note the extent and the transparent shade of the dentinoenamel junction.*

Difference in topographical locations also lead to variations in the crystalline arrangement of each tissue during the mineralization phase, and this has repercussions on light transmission. The quality of mineralization remains under the control of vitamins, such as A and D, hormones such as pituitary, thyroid and parathyroid hormones, and nutrition, which must, for example, ensure a regular and adequate supply of calcium and trace elements such as fluoride.

The eruption of a tooth in the dental arch does not signal the end of the evolution process. Mineralized tissues are subject to numerous exchange processes. They connect to the blood supply via the dental pulp, and to the oral environment via the saliva. Tetracycline-induced staining is a good example of substance transfer to the dentin tissue

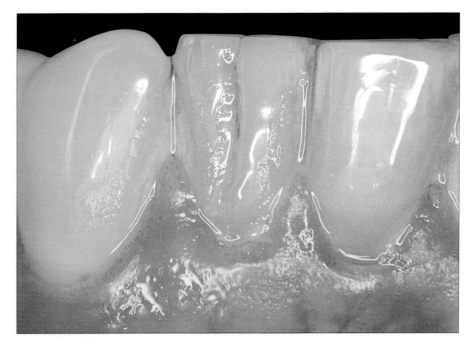

Figure 5.9 *Typical appearance of a fissure in the enamel.*

via the blood circulation. Enamel, too, can let stains through because of its porosity and surface defects (cracks and fissures). Some authors believe that these defects could also be a point of entry for microbial infiltration.

At this point, a clear distinction should be made between cracks and fissures, since these are often confused.

Fissures: also known as 'enamel lamellae', are sites of rupturing or fracturing, often produced when the brittle enamel matures (Figure 5.9). These defects, which extend to varying depths, may propagate to the dentinoenamel junction or even beyond it in some cases. A keratin-like organic tissue exists within the fissure, and can easily be stained by exogenous stains. The passage of these stains may extend to the dentin.

Cracks: these also occur in enamel, and most commonly arise as a result of occlusal trauma and mastication.

Enamel tissue, with its lack of resilience, may fracture under certain types of mechanical or thermal stress. These cracks appear as streaks or opaceous white surfaces. The crack, a space often filled by air or water, divides the two enamel surfaces, and this produces a diffraction site for light rays passing through the enamel. This type of defect

increases enamel permeability. In some cases these cracks are infiltrated by external coloring substances and appear as white, orange or brown streaks.

Thus, as teeth come under influences from the internal and external environment from the point of formation and throughout their existence, they will be subject to numerous color changes.

Mechanisms of tooth staining

The relative permeability of dental enamel via cracks and fissures is not the only factor enabling exchange with oral fluids. The organic constituents at interprismatic sites also contribute to such exchanges.

Color pigments contained in drink and foodstuffs (known as 'chromophores') will become attached to the organic tissues contained in interprismatic sites and fissures by chemical binding of their hydroxyl and amino groups. In addition, binding between these pigmented substances and calcium ions forms new molecules varying in size and optical effect.

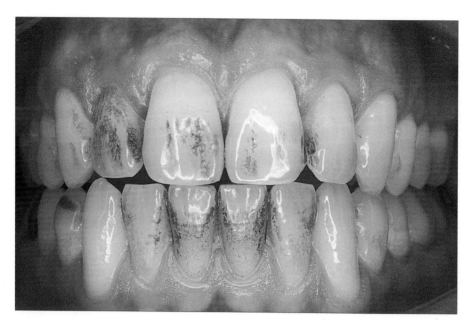

Figure 5.10 Tobacco-induced staining.

Tea and coffee are two good examples of drinks that stain. Tea contains quercetin, a pigment containing five hydroxyl groups that form stable attachments to the interprismatic organic substance.

In the same way, but by an endogenous route, certain pigmented groups contained in tetracyclines, in particular hydroquinones, become attached to dentin tissues, forming a complex with calcium ions of the mineral framework. They may also become attached to collagen. Hydroquinones occasionally change into quinones, producing a stronger chestnut-brown staining. This change in the shade of the chromaphore pigment reflects oxidation of the hydroquinone,· which can be produced by light, for instance. It has also been noted (Walton et al, 1982; McEvoy, 1989a,b) that the photo-oxidation resulting from extended dental exposure to sunlight could darken some incidences of tetracycline staining.

Many pigments, such as metal oxides, can, by the same process, via either endogenous or exogenous routes, become attached to dental tissues, with which they react to produce complexes of varying stability. Depending on the degree of binding, they may be partially or completely oxidized by certain physicochemical treatments. Hydrogen peroxide remains the preferred chemical treatment. It has an oxidizing effect on chromophore groupings, and on double bonds in particular. It will make these complexes either partially or wholly soluble, resulting in attenuation or disappearance of the staining.

Reasons for staining

Natural tooth staining can be classified in several ways:

- according to stain origin (external or internal);

- according to color;

- according to pathological (or non-pathological) nature.

It is often difficult to fit the great diversity of stains into such fixed classifications, and this text will outline the most characteristic and frequently encountered stains, rather than giving an exhaustive list.

External staining

External staining is due to:

- stains contained in food or drink, such as tea or coffee;
- all forms of tobacco (whether cigarettes, pipes, chewing tobacco or other: Figure 5.10);

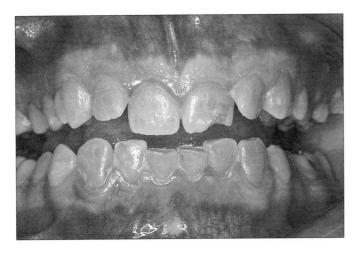

Figure 5.11 Dentinogenesis imperfecta.

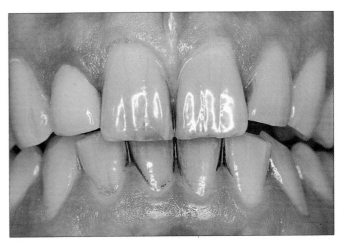

Figure 5.12 *Staining due to natural aging: 20 years later the ceramic material on the maxillary right lateral has not changed color, but the natural teeth have become stained.*

- chromogenic bacteria, which cause green, brown or black staining, most commonly seen in the cervical area in small children, for example;

- chemicals such as the chlorhexidine contained in certain mouthwashes, which produce unsightly blackish-brown deposits.

Theoretically, external staining affects the enamel surface only. However, in some instances external agents can penetrate deep into the enamel and stain it, sometimes actually reaching the dentin. When cementum is exposed, it too can be subjected to staining.

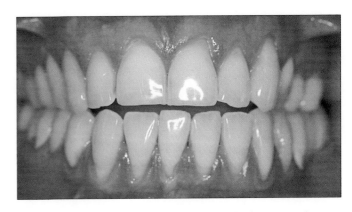

Figure 5.13 *A 40-year-old female patient displaying regular dental chroma – a case that is likely to respond extremely well to chemical bleaching.*

Internal staining

Internal staining may be:

- genetic, as in the case of amelogenesis imperfecta or dentinogenesis imperfecta, with disastrous staining, sometimes involving all the teeth (Figure 5.11);
- prenatal, resulting from an illness contracted by the mother, such as German measles, congenital syphilis, a severe onset of anemia, etc;
- postnatal, due to excessive intake of fluoride or medication such as tetracycline.

Prenatal and postnatal staining are now declining in the Western world as pediatricians and gynecologists become aware of the problem.

It is staining of internal origin that most commonly affects enamel and dentin. This is much more serious than external staining, and requires very different treatment.

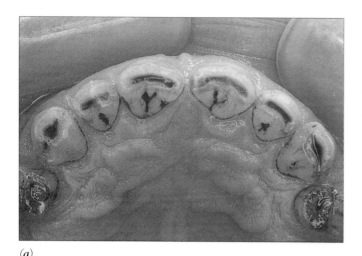

(a)

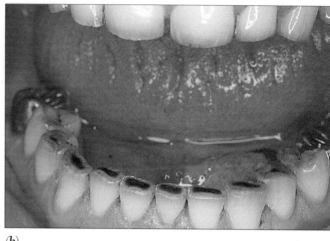

(b)

Figure 5.14 *Worn teeth can easily let in staining agents: with this pipe smoker, the tobacco stain has filtered deep into the dentin of both* (**a**) *maxillary and* (**b**) *mandibular teeth.*

Age-related staining

Aging constitutes a good example of staining resulting from a combination of many different causes (Figures 5.12 and 5.13). It inevitably involves physiological transformation of the tissues in addition to mechanical and chemical insult. The enamel becomes more translucent, the dentin undergoes transformation, and the pulp narrows. Different parameters will act in widely varying degrees to accelerate fading, yellowing and darkening of the teeth, including some types of dental treatment, external staining induced by foodstuffs and tobacco, receding gingiva, trauma and medication. Visually, all these factors will have an adverse effect on light transmission, affecting hue, chroma, value and translucency.

Staining due to natural aging of the teeth is highly responsive to chemical whitening treatment.

Iatrogenic staining

Many surface abrasion sites can be seen on the cusps and occlusal edges, particularly in the presence of bruxism or parafunctional activity. Teeth that have been ground in this way allow areas of dentin to show through, and these can be infiltrated by external stains very rapidly.

This type of staining often occurs in incisors, and, most frequently on the lower incisors, creates the appearance of aged teeth (Figure 5.14). Cracks and fissures may also take up color and affect the shade of the teeth. The dental contour, texture and luster can also be altered by

- excessive brushing;

- abrasive toothpaste;

- acids contained in food and drinks;

- gastric reflux, e.g. in anorexia and bulimia, where the pH of the saliva becomes very acid and literally etches the enamel, lending it a particularly dull and flat appearance.

Thus some problems can be prevented by elementary hygiene advice and dietary recommendations.

Trauma

Dental insult can bring on varying degrees of pulp hemorrhage. If this is local, the blood flows into the tubules, releasing hemoglobin, the breakdown of which

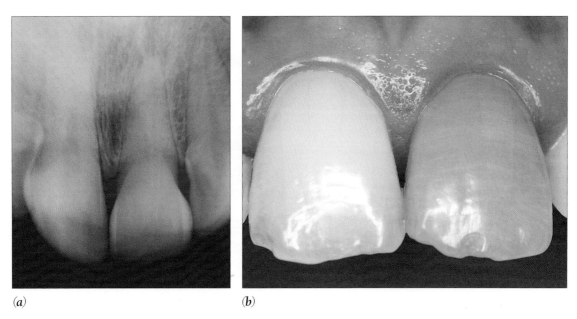

(a)   (b)

Figure 5.15 (**a**) *Radiograph of maxillary central incisor that has undergone major trauma. The root canal cannot be identified and is probably totally calcified.* (**b**) *The minor hemorrhage upon impact evidently was enough to discolor the tooth permanently.*

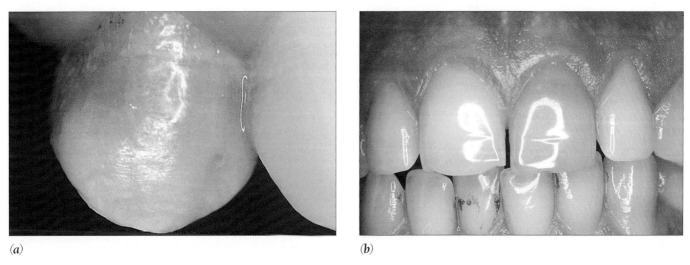

(a)   (b)

Figure 5.16 (**a, b**) *Major discoloration often observed in non-vital teeth.*

releases Fe²⁺ ions that may bind with oxygen to produce iron oxides. In some cases, these oxides combine with sulfur to give a dark-gray ferrous sulfide.

A major pulp response is often associated with this minor hemorrhage, resulting in production of secondary dentin, at the expense of pulp size, and is occasionally sufficient to obliterate the pulp space (Figure 5.15).

The appearance of the tooth will change according to the degree of trauma (Figure 5.16). Generally, it will appear more saturated and more opaque. Gray staining is associated with hemorrhage and hemoglobin breakdown products, and orange shades with the formation of dentin.

Treatments for discolored vital teeth include prosthetic reconstruction using laminate veneers, jacket crowns, or even metal–ceramic crowns for excessively stained teeth. Chemical treatments are often ineffective.

Major hemorrhage

A reddish color will appear on the tooth immediately after insult, signaling flooding of the tubules with blood. Depending on how the Fe^{2+} ions contained in the hemoglobin react, the teeth turn progressively from pink to orange and then to brown, blue and finally gray. The type and intensity of the discoloration will depend on the length of time between the teeth becoming non-vital and endodontic treatment. Unfortunately, in some cases, signs of pulp hemorrhage following insult may not be observed. Nevertheless, the tooth may be non-vital, and if root canal treatment does not take place quickly, necrotic breakdown products of the neurovascular complex will take on varying degrees of a brownish-gray color, which they will then pass on to the dental tissue.

Chemical treatments work extremely well on staining caused by the continuing presence of necrotic tissue, but are much less effective for iron (oxide and sulfide) staining.

Iatrogenic dental treatment In over 50% of cases, major staining results from the caries itself and the treatment of caries. All dental practitioners should take this to heart, since observation of a few basic laws of hygiene, good prophylaxis, regular checks and appropriate treatment could reduce this percentage considerably.

Caries

Dental caries is the primary cause of unesthetic pigmentation (Feinman et al, 1987), followed by dental tissue breakdown products, entry of bacteria, stains and dyes, and finally foodstuffs. Cavities must be thoroughly cleaned out before filling. Unfortunately, infiltration by certain pigments stains the enamel and dentin irreversibly.

Endodontic treatment

Some pulp hemorrhage may occur during the course of endodontic treatment. Such hemorrhage is now known to lead to production of Fe^{2+}, and care must be taken to eliminate this by careful conditioning and cleansing of the root canal and pulp cavity before any canal obturation takes place. Any hemorrhage that occurs during the process of filling may lead to staining of the

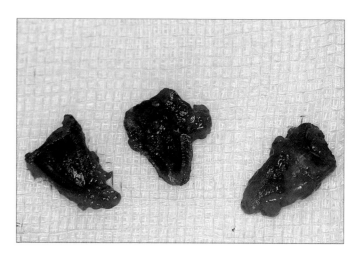

Figure 5.17 Extracted tooth fragments: damage from corrosion can be noticed.

root and coronal dentin in the months or years to come. Root staining can cause major esthetic defects (especially when the gingival tissue is thin). It is technically possible to treat discolored roots chemically, but more clinical evidence is required on safety aspects.

Incomplete removal of necrotic tissue can be an additional cause of staining in the course of endodontic treatment. It sometimes happens, particularly in young teeth in which access cavities have been ill-prepared, that tissue residues can be left in the pulp horns, and their breakdown products inevitably stain the teeth. Fortunately, such staining is highly sensitive to chemical bleaching.

Root canal filling materials

These may diffuse into dental tissue and produce staining. Each substance may be identified by the color it imparts to the tooth: silver cones, for example, cause black staining through oxidation, most commonly affecting the roots. Arsenic anhydride can also induce staining, and this alone should preclude its use. It causes necrosis, and this will inevitably promote occurrence of pigmentation, which will filter into the dentin tissue under temporary fillings.

Restorative materials

Restorative materials may be responsible for a wide variety of stains. Silver amalgam restorations cause bluish-gray staining of teeth, reaching to varying depths, and sometimes even the surrounding mucosa can be

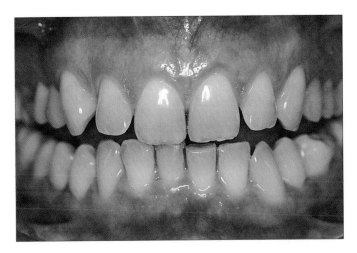

Figure 5.18 An even, yellow staining induced by tetracycline – 1st degree.

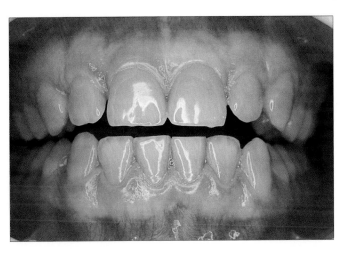

Figure 5.19 An even staining by tetracycline, with a brownish-gray shade – 2nd degree.

affected through ionic migration or by corrosion. Regardless of the issue of any biological risk of this migration, it may prove esthetically disastrous, especially in the anterior teeth. The severity of this staining depends upon the composition of the alloy used, how it is applied, and, above all, on the seal it provides. Even under entirely optimal conditions, bluish-gray staining will always show through the tissue generally, and through the enamel in particular. In view of this, it is best to avoid the use of silver amalgam in anterior teeth, and confine its use to posterior teeth.

Glass-ionomers, silicates and non-sealing composites may also lead to staining by percolation of fluids. Well-made metal (gold or nickel–chrome) inlays do limit dental staining, but are unsightly in visible areas.

At present, ceramics appear to be the most esthetically suitable filling material in view of their high degree of biocompatibility and visual properties. Unfortunately, questions of cost and the relative complexity of ceramic application have hitherto prevented their use from becoming widespread.

Corrosion of alloys in the oral environment is a major factor that leads to staining and discoloration, and the introduction of different metal compounds into the mouth will increase the risk. The combination of a steel post with an amalgam build-up, covered by a gold crown, has a high corrosive potential. Often, when extracting such teeth, it is noticed that the root is completely blackened and the dentin might show degradation (Figure 5.17). Great care should therefore be taken over coronal reconstruction, using either cast dowel cones (made of the same metal) or titanium posts.

Tetracycline-induced staining

In 1958, Schwachman et al postulated that tetracycline – or at least certain of its constituents – could cross the placental barrier and become attached to fetal tissues that are in the process of mineralization: this will include the teeth in their various developmental stages. It was only in 1963, over 20 years after the launch of this antibiotic, that the Food and Drugs Administration (FDA) issued a warning against it, because of its potential to stain teeth.

Tetracyclines produce very variable effects on the teeth: a mere yellow even staining, minor or major brownish-gray staining, or the formation of streaks. The degree of tooth staining depends on the duration and dosage of substance uptake, the patient's stage of development (age) and the variety of tetracycline involved. Most writers advise against using the antibiotics at the onset of primary incisor formation, that is, from the fourth month of gestation until completion of the formation of the incisor canine array at the age of 7 or 8 years. Antibiotics taken during this period produce discoloration of the primary and permanent teeth. According to Bevelander (1964), the location of staining, particularly when it takes the form of streaks, provides a precise guide as to the onset of this medication. Goldberg et al (1987) suggest that the risk of staining is greater during odontogenesis, but occurrences of discoloration in

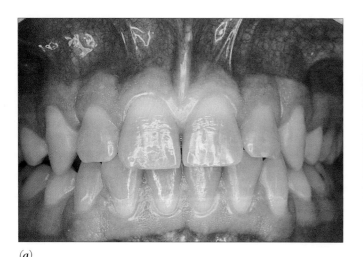

(a)

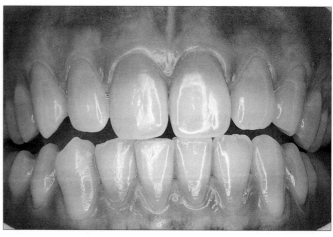

(b)

Figure 5.20 (a, b) Major, irregular tetracycline staining with gray streaks present – 3rd degree.

adults cannot be entirely excluded, given the constant state of demineralization and remineralization at the enamel surface. Lambrou et al (1977) confirmed that, even in fully mineralized enamel with no initial tetracycline content, the substance may still become incorporated during phases of remineralization. Poliak et al (1985) described four cases of staining in adults after taking minocycline. The possibility of tetracycline staining in adults, although rare, should be kept in mind. The mechanisms underlying the onset of such discoloration remain uncertain, but it would appear that other products could also play a part in altered tooth color. This process could be associated with high dental iron content, level of porosity, surface defects, and so on.

Tetracyline-induced discoloration is caused by chelation between the antibiotic and, especially, calcium ions, to form a calcium orthophosphate–tetracycline complex. This antibiotic inhibits protein synthesis. Its capacity for binding with nickel, manganese, zinc, nitrate and aluminum, and with iron and calcium in particular, leads to the formation of numerous complexes. The staining produced by formation of these complexes is characterized by fluorescent properties and ultraviolet light absorption spectra that differ strongly from the corresponding properties in normal teeth.

Staining can vary a great deal, depending on the type of antibiotic used: brownish-gray in the case of chlortetracyclines such as aureomycin, yellow in the case of dimethylchlortetracyclines. Exposure to light leads to the darkening of some tetracycline staining through light-induced oxidation. This depends on the type of tetra-

cycline involved and the photochemically oxidized substances obtained (Walton et al, 1982). Moreover, Stewart demonstrated in 1973 that tetracycline molecules embedded in the skeleton were capable of migrating into the dentin through the blood. This delayed accumulation of tetracycline in the dentin, as well as the intradentin photochemical oxidation of these new calcium–tetracycline complexes, probably explains incidences of post-treatment relapse.

It may prove useful to classify the wide variety of discoloration observed with tetracycline for the purposes of diagnosis and treatment. Boksman and Jordan's classification (1983) gives four levels of discoloration.

1st degree: with slight yellow or light-brown staining, even, and free of streaks, bleaching treatment proves very effective (Figure 5.18).

2nd degree: in the case of average staining ranging between yellow, light-brown and slightly gray shades, where there is greater saturation but the color remains even and free of streaks, here, too, chemical treatment proves effective (Figure 5.19).

3rd degree: once the staining becomes uneven and gets to the point of even greater saturation (whether gray, dark-brown, blue or indigo) and with streaks or surfaces with particularly high saturation, bleaching treatment can no longer be advocated as the best therapy. Regardless of the number of sessions that are devoted to removal of staining, only attenuation of this stain rather than total elimination can gener-

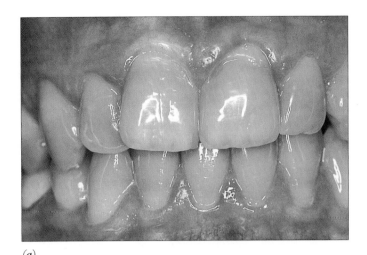

(a)

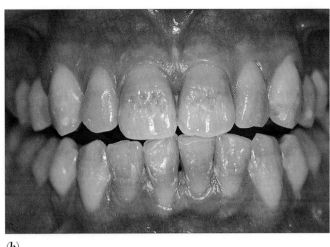

(b)

Figure 5.21 (a, b) Major tetracycline staining with very persistent gray streaks – 4th degree.

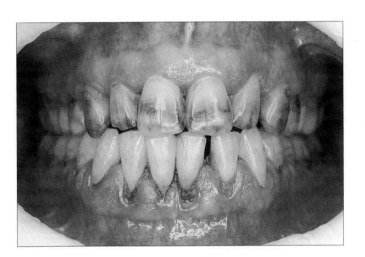

Figure 5.22 Brown staining due to excess fluoride (simple fluorosis).

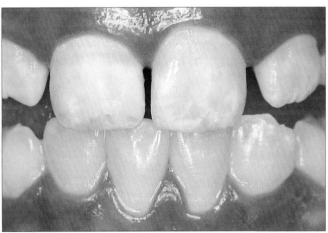

Figure 5.23 Opaque fluorosis.

ally be achieved. The visual qualities of this heavily discolored tissue are often poor, moreover, so that even white teeth will always have a colorless, opaque appearance (Figure 5.20).

4th degree: this classification covers all exceptional types of staining, including highly saturated teeth, with a patchy or streaky arrangement. These teeth most frequently require prosthetic treatment, and can never be treated successfully by chemical means (Figure 5.21).

Fluorosis

Fluoride action is basically dose-dependent. A low dosage of fluoride provides some protection against caries. At too high a dose it can cause brown staining, white patches and surface hypomineralization, up to the point where the enamel surface becomes very porous and a highly characteristic mottling appears. Fluoride produces its staining effect mainly during formation and calcification of the enamel, that is,

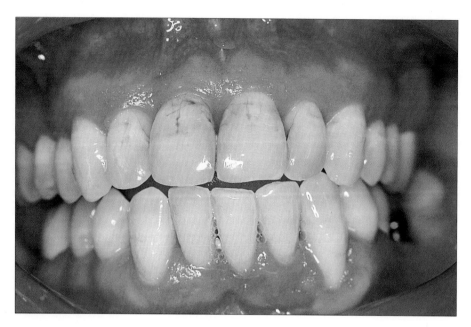

Figure 5.24 Fluorosis with surface porosity.

between the fourth month of gestation and the age of 8 years. Most lesions affect permanent teeth, showing a preference for molars and premolars. These lesions can extend to all the teeth, including deciduous teeth, depending on fluoride concentration, genetic predisposition, developmental stage and duration of exposure.

Fluoride exerts its action on the ameloblasts, in which it produces an adverse metabolic effect. Takuma et al (1983) note that in fluorosis, secretory and post-secretory ameloblasts are affected. According to Shinoda (1983), disruptions of amelogenesis apply mainly to the maturation rather than the secretion phase, thus bringing about modifications to the matrix of fluorotic teeth. Accordingly, tooth enamel affected by fluorosis has been found to contain a consistently high proportion of immature matrix proteins (Fejerskov et al, 1984) responsible for the individual type of staining.

Fluorosis can appear under a number of different guises, and has been classified as follows (Feinman et al, 1987):

- *Simple fluorosis.* These teeth show brown staining, smooth enamel and no surface defects (Figure 5.22).

- *Opaque fluorosis.* These teeth show gray staining or whitish stains of varying opacity. These patches are most commonly surface-deep, and can be effectively treated using microabrasion techniques (Figure 5.23).

- *Fluorosis combined with porosity.* Highly characteristic mottling of the surface, which may take different forms, can be observed (Figure 5.24).

References

Bevelander G, The effect of tetracycline on mineralization and growth. In: Staphe PH (ed) *Advances in Oral Biology, Vol 1.* London: Academic Press, 1964.

Boksman L, Jordan RE, Conservative treatment of the stained dentition: Vital bleaching. *Aust Dent J* 1983; **28**: 67–72.

Feinman RA, Goldstein RE, Garber DA, *Bleaching Teeth.* Chicago: Quintessence, 1987.

Fejerskov O, Josephsen K, Nyvad B, Transmission and scanning electron microscopical studies of human enamel surfaces at time of eruption. In: R W Fearnhead, S Suga (ed) *Tooth Enamel IV.* Amsterdam:Elsevier, 1984.

Goldberg M, Fortier JP, Guillot J et al, Colorations de l'émail dentaire. *Actual Odontostomatol (Paris)* 1987; **157**:99–118.

Lambrou D, Tahos BS, Lambrou KD, In vitro studies of the phenomenon of tetracycline incorporation into enamel. *J Dent Res* 1977; **56**:1527–32.

McEvoy SA, Chemical agents for removing intrinsic stains from vital teeth. I Technique development. *Quintessence Int* 1989a; **20**:323–28.

McEvoy SA, Chemical agents for removing intrinsic stains from vital teeth. II Current techniques and their chemical applications. *Quintessence Int* 1989b; **20**: 379–83.

Poliak SC, Digiovanna JJ, Gross EG et al, Minocycline associated tooth discoloration in young adults. *JAMA* 1985; **254**:2930–32.

Schwachman H et al, The effect of long-term antibiotic therapy in patients with cystic fibrosis of the pancreas. *Antibiot Annu* 1958–1959:692–99.

Shinoda H, Effects of long-term administration of fluoride on the enamel formation in rats. In: S Suga (ed) *Mechanisms of Tooth Enamel Formation.* Tokyo: Quintessence, 1983.

Stewart DJ, The reincorporation in calcified tissues of tetracycline released following its deposition in the borre of rats. *Arch Oral Biol* 1973; **18**: 759–64.

Takuma S, Furi A, Tomoda F et al, Ultrastructural studies of disturbance in amelogenesis induced in rat incisors by fluoride and strontium administration. In: S Suga (ed) *Mechanisms of Tooth Enamel Formation.* Tokyo: Quintessence, 1983.

Walton RE, O'Dell NL, Myers DL et al, External bleaching of tetracycline stained teeth in dogs. *J Endodont* 1982; **8**: 536–42.

CHAPTER 6

Treatment of Tooth Discoloration

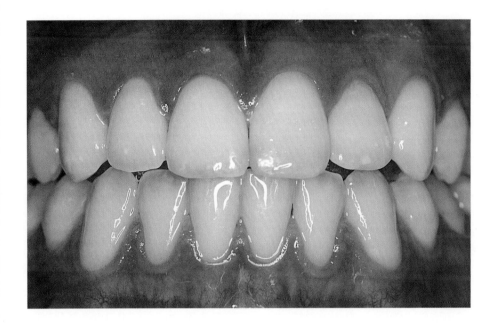

Five methods of treating discoloration and staining in natural teeth exist at present: microabrasion, chemical bleaching, direct application of composites, laminate veneers, ceramic and metal–ceramic crowns. Considerations of intensity, spread and depth as well as cost of treatment will determine which of these five techniques should be applied. Combinations of two or three different treatments can often be used for certain types of staining (microabrasion, bleaching and ceramic laminates, for example).

This chapter is devoted exclusively to various chemical treatments of discoloration. Two further chapters will be devoted to ceramic laminate veneers and jacket crowns (Chapters 9 and 10 respectively), although these can be combined with chemical techniques.

Historical perspective

Hydrochloric acid and hydrogen peroxide are the two main chemical agents used to treat many types of internal and external staining in both vital and pulpless teeth. These two substances have been used either jointly or individ-

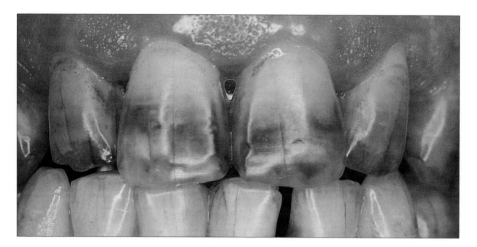

Figure 6.1 *Enamel discoloration caused by excess fluoride.*

ually for over 100 years, sometimes in conjunction with other chemicals, thus providing a variety of treatment options that can benefit from a synergistic effect. Rather than mentioning all available chemicals for altering tooth color, this chapter will concentrate on those making it possible to develop simple, practical and effective treatment methods.

The first relevant publication appeared in 1877, when Chapple described the use of oxalic acid in the treatment of certain types of tooth discoloration. Two years later, Taft suggested a chlorinated solution (Labarraque solution) for similar purposes. Weskale (1895) favored mixing hydrogen peroxide and ether for the treatment of discolored teeth. To make the treatment more effective, the solution was activated by an electric current. It was not until 1918 that Abbot introduced an effective method using heat- and light-activated 37% hydrogen peroxide, which was to provide the foundation for present-day techniques. Two years before that, in 1916, Kane had discovered that the excess fluoride contained in water from differing sources could produce discoloration of the enamel (Figure 6.1), with differing degrees of (normally superficial) staining. Following this discovery, Kane tried to remove the staining from teeth by applying a cotton wool pad soaked in hydrochloric acid, heated over a flame. Since that time there have been two different courses of treatment for mainly fluoride-induced staining:

- the Kane school of thought, which favors the use of microabrasion techniques;

- the Abbot school of thought, which favors purely chemical (hydrogen peroxide) treatment.

Many improvements to the Kane technique followed, including the modification of McInnes (1966). He introduced a new solution, named after him and made up of a fresh mixture of 5 ml 36% hydrochloric acid, 5 ml 30% hydrogen peroxide and 30% ether. He applied this solution to the discolored tooth surface using a simple cotton wool pad. After 16–20 minutes of application, the teeth were rinsed with water and then neutralized using a sodium bicarbonate paste. He emphasized, even then, the need to polish the teeth after treatment. McCloskey (1984) recommended the use of a dilute (18%) solution of hydrochloric acid only, which he rubbed onto the enamel using a cotton wool ball, as MacInnes had done. Croll and Cavanaugh (1986) suggested combining 18% hydrochloric acid with pumice and rubbing in this paste using wooden rods for 5 seconds at a time, followed each time by rinsing with water. In 1990, the work of Croll and Cavanaugh led to the introduction of a new product named 'Prema' (Premier), consisting of a ready-to-use mixture of 10% hydrochloric acid and pumice. Miara et al (1991), having tested citric, hydrochloric, phosphoric, nitric and other acids, as well as numerous hydrochloric-acid- and hydrogen-peroxide-based mixtures at different concentrations, introduced the Micro Clean (Cédia) microabrasion system. This consisted of a mixture of hydrochloric acid, pumice and a low concentration of hydrogen peroxide applied over 5–10 second periods to the teeth

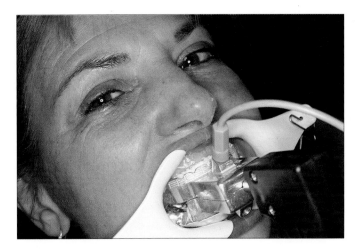

Figure 6.2 Thermochemical bleaching technique: BV bleaching.

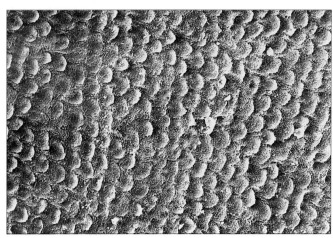

Figure 6.3 Hydrochloric acid produces surface demineralization of the enamel, as seen in this SEM photograph (×1500).

undergoing treatment, using small rubber caps attached to an alternating contra-angle handpiece.

Tooth bleaching techniques using heat-activated hydrogen peroxide fell into disuse for a considerable time. However, once tetracycline staining became prevalent during the 1970s, these techniques were reactivated. Arens (1972), in particular, was instrumental for this trend, followed by Feinman et al (1989), who can claim to have been the first to give a thorough definition of the technique and, more particularly, its field of application.

In the 1980s, Zaragoza, backed by a team of dentists, pharmacists and chemists, introduced a new thermochemical technique, named 'BV bleaching' (Figure 6.2). He used a special enamel preparation before applying 70% hydrogen peroxide, activated by heating in a 'thermo-tray'. Despite its interesting results, this treatment has now fallen into disuse because of practical considerations. It is somewhat cumbersome and requires special equipment. Moreover, highly concentrated hydrogen peroxide solutions require very careful handling, as well as major safety precautions, and carry a higher risk factor for the teeth and the surrounding tissue than solutions of lower concentration. It is important to note that the latest European guidelines forbid the use, in the mouth, of cosmetic products containing more than 0.1% hydrogen peroxide. As a result of this, bleaching of teeth is banned in certain countries where it is considered to be a cosmetic treatment – this is the case, for example, in the UK. In most other EU countries the question is unresolved, but the treatment is not banned.

In the last decade, most workers have resorted to the use of gels, which are easier to handle, and hydrogen peroxide concentrations of 20–37%. These preparations are activated either chemically or by light.

Alongside these traditional bleaching techniques, Haywood and Heymann (1989) recommended the use of a 10% carbamide peroxide gel (equivalent to 3.6% hydrogen peroxide), applied via fine plastic trays for the patient to wear several hours per day over a 1–2 week period. This marked the birth of a new technique, which could claim to be simple and, above all, to rely on bleaching substances at very low concentrations. This technique is now meeting with considerable success, as confirmed by the numerous products in this category that are currently appearing on the market.

Other improvements to chemical treatments for stain removal will doubtless be made in the future, primarily at the product and application level.

Practitioners thus have three chemical techniques presently available for the treatment of dental discoloration:

- microabrasion;

- office bleaching using self-, light- or heat-activated 20–37% hydrogen peroxide-containing gels;

- patient-administered home bleaching using carbamide peroxide gels.

The choice of which chemical treatment to apply will depend on the source, form, extent, type, color and site

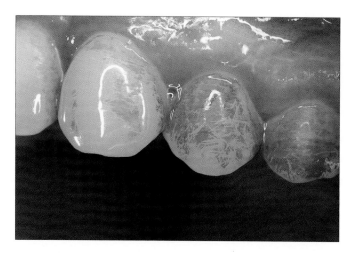

Figure 6.4 Staining due to the tannin contained in tea.

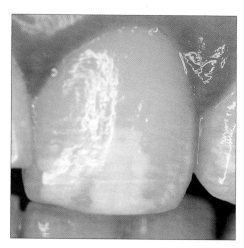

Figure 6.5 White stains.

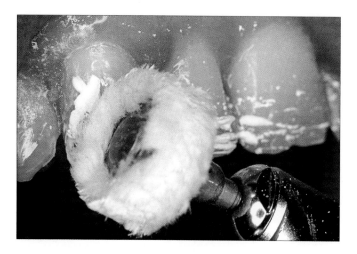

Figure 6.6 All rotating instruments carry the risk of splashing and spillage, and are not recommended for this procedure.

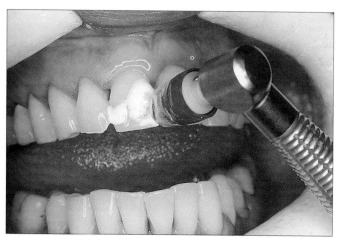

Figure 6.7 Use of an alternating contra-angle handpiece reduces the risk of spillage.

(whether superficial or deep) of staining. Some chemicals have a surface action, while others penetrate more deeply. They can act either selectively or non-selectively on different types of staining.

Microabrasion

Action of hydrochloric acid

The action of hydrochloric acid should be properly understood in order to identify the exact indications for

and constraints on this method. At concentrations of 18–36%, hydrochloric acid causes surface demineralization of the enamel (Figure 6.3). The degree of enamel loss can be controlled accurately and safely by utilizing the correct concentration, procedure and application time. The effects of hydrochloric acid are always non-selective and superficial. They may be augmented by:

- the addition of an abrasive, such as pumice;

- temperature;

- chemicals such as hydrogen peroxide and ether.

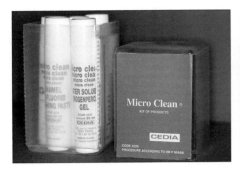

Figure 6.8 *Micro Clean kit (Cédia).*

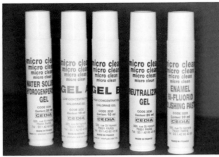

(**a**)

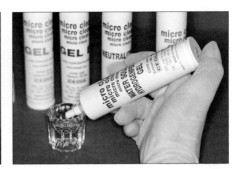

(**b**)

Figure 6.9 (**a**) *The Micro Clean kit consists of five substances: blue: 10% hydrogen peroxide gel; green: dilute hydrochloric acid gel; red: concentrated hydrochloric acid gel; mauve: neutralizing gel; orange: polishing paste containing fluoride.* (**b**) *The conditioning system is particularly practical.*

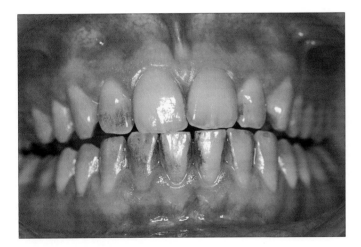

Figure 6.10 *Patient exhibiting tooth staining due to external deposit of nicotine.*

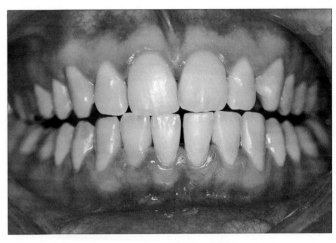

Figure 6.11 *Teeth following a microabrasion session and dilute hydrochloric acid gel.*

Figure 6.12 *Result following careful polishing.*

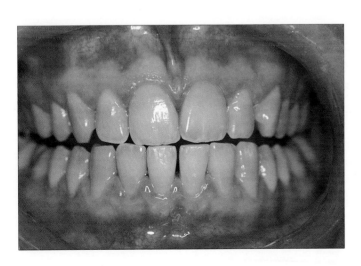

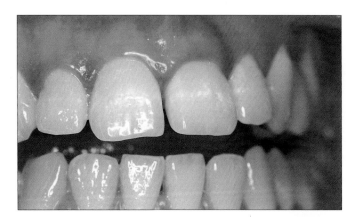

Figure 6.13 Young patient exhibiting white spots of mild decalcification resulting from the application of orthodontic brackets.

Indications

This surface-acting, mechanochemical and somewhat destructive process can bring about non-selective removal of:

- all staining from external sources (tea, coffee, tobacco) (Figure 6.4);

- surface staining (film, whitish patches) (Figure 6.5);

- multicolored (brown, gray or yellow) defects.

This technique remains completely ineffective for deep-lying stains, especially age-related discoloration or tetracyline-induced staining. The method can be used successfully in conjunction with chemical bleaching techniques.

Application

Present-day microabrasion systems must comply with certain requirements.

- They must use substances in the form of water-soluble gels, for ease of application.

- They must offer simple, effective application procedures, limiting the risk of spillage or splashing as much as possible (Figures 6.6 and 6.7).

- They must offer the option of adapting the concentration to suit the lesion being treated.

The controlled microabrasion technique using the Micro Clean system (Figure 6.8) fulfils these requirements at present. Without actually changing tooth color, it enables permanent elimination of patches, coatings, stains and deposits at the surface or in superficial areas of the dental enamel. It also produces a slight brightening effect due to the presence of hydrogen peroxide.

Micro Clean may be applied in two different ways, according to the hydrochloric acid concentration used (Figure 6.9).

Elimination of extrinsic stains: tobacco, coffee, etc.

A low-concentration mixture consisting of a mild hydrochloric acid gel, a special abrasive and a 10% hydrogen peroxide gel is used (Figures 6.10–6.12). This mixture

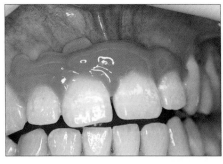

Figure 6.14 Isolation of the soft tissues by using a lip retractor and the application of a light-cured Paint-On Dental Dam (Den-Mat).

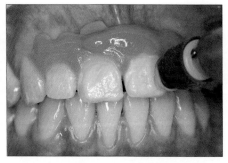

Figure 6.15 Microabrasion with high-concentration gel using an alternating handpiece.

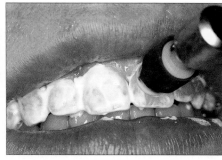

Figure 6.16 After neutralizing, the teeth are very carefully polished.

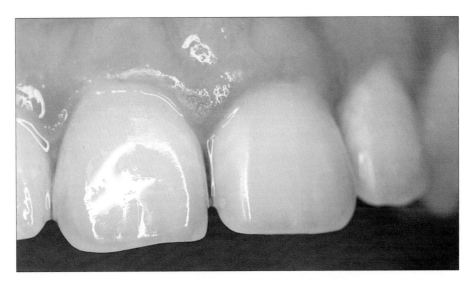

Figure 6.17 The white spots have been completely removed.

should be applied for 5 seconds at a time, followed by rinsing with water. It is applied by means of a rubber cup attached to an alternating contra-angle handpiece. In view of the low concentrations used and the brief application time, use of some gingival protection may not be necessary, but could be considered. The depth of enamel layer lost is very minor, measuring only a few micrometers for each 5-second sequence. To complete the treatment, a sodium bicarbonate-based neutralizing gel is left on the gingivae and the teeth being treated for a few minutes, in order to neutralize the acidic action of the mixture.

Microabrasion is always followed by thorough polishing with a paste used for polishing natural teeth.

Elimination of intrinsic stains: white spots, film or superficial staining

In the case of intrinsic stains (Figures 6.13–6.17), a certain amount of enamel will inevitably have to be removed by chemical or mechanical abrasion. A high-concentration mixture is therefore used, made up of a relatively strong (18%) hydrochloric acid gel, pumice and 10% hydrogen peroxide. Because of the acidity of the compound, the dentist and auxillaries involved in the treatment must take protective measures by wearing gloves, masks and spectacles. The patient, too, must be protected, in order to avoid any contact between the mixture and the soft tissue:

- protective spectacles and possibly lip retractors should be used;
- there should be gingival protection by means of a rubber dam or other simpler systems such as the light-cured Paint-On Dental Dam (Den-Mat) or cyanoacrylate (Futura Medical).

Having taken these protective measures, the mixture should be applied for 5 seconds at a time, followed by rinsing. After application of the high-concentration solution, a neutralizing gel should be placed on the site and left there for several minutes, again followed by thorough rinsing.

To avoid any sort of spillage, one should use an alternating contra-angle handpiece, rather than standard rotating instruments. Another option is to use a 10:1 gear reduction slow-speed contra-angle handpiece. Manual application using cotton wool or even a dispenser, as suggested by Croll and Cavanaugh (1986), remains much less effective, although it is still preferable to the use of a normal rotatory contra-angle handpiece.

Effects of chemical treatment

The authors conducted a scanning electron microscope study assessing damage to the enamel and capacity for penetration by the hydrochloric acid mixture. The effect on enamel depends on the acid concentration and the length of the application time, with the rate of the alternating movement remaining constant (Figures 6.18

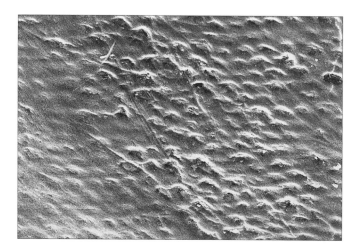

Figure 6.18 SEM appearance of untreated enamel (young tooth) displaying the perikymata and characteristic appearance of prisms at the enamel surface (× 460). (Courtesy of Dr Y Haikel.)

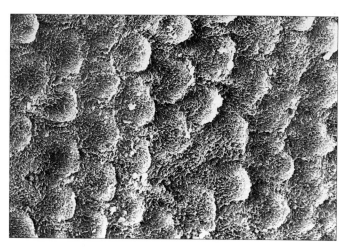

Figure 6.19 Enamel treated with hydrochloric acid, showing demineralization of the surface layer, enlargement of bands, and prisms with typical appearance of acid etching (Sylverstone's type II) (SEM, × 1500). (Courtesy of Dr Y Haikel.)

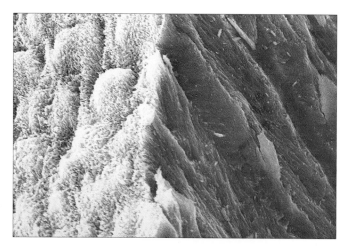

Figure 6.20 Enamel treated with hydrochloric acid and then fractured; no deep demineralization noted (SEM, × 1900). (Courtesy of Dr Y Haikel.)

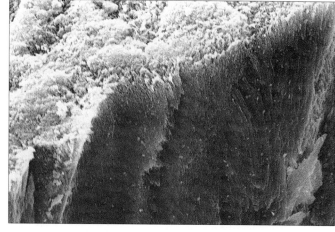

Figure 6.21 Enamel treated with hydrochloric acid and then fractured; higher magnification shows that acid penetration remains very superficial (SEM, × 2900). (Courtesy of Dr Y Haikel.)

and 6.19). For every four or five sequences lasting 5 seconds, enamel loss is several micrometers up to some tens of micrometers for high concentrations. This abrasion remains centered around the treated area; the solution does not penetrate far enough into the enamel to reach the dentin zone. Other research demonstrates that these solutions do, in fact, remain local, only penetrating very slightly into the enamel (Figures 6.20 and 6.21). According to Baumgartner et al (1983), applying a mixture of 36% hydrochloric acid and 30% hydrogen peroxide did not seem to have an adverse effect on the pulp. Griffin et al (1977), using a mixture of

Figure 6.22 *Enamel treated with hydrochloric acid and polished: the demineralized surface layer has completely disappeared and there is a flatter look than with non-treated enamel (SEM, ✕ 600). (Courtesy of Dr Y Haikel.)*

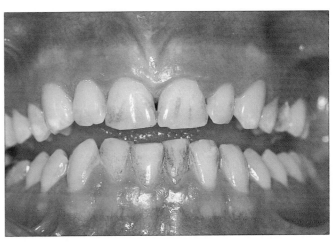

Figure 6.23 *This patient had been drinking 1–2 litres of carbonated beverages per day for several years, which rendered his enamel more porous and promoted disastrous build-up of extrinsic coloring agents.*

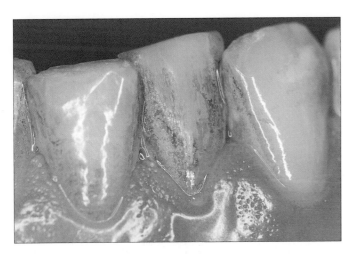

Figure 6.24 *Close-up view of mandibular incisors: ridging of the enamel surface and impregnation by extrinsic coloring agents.*

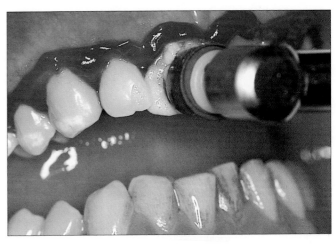

Figure 6.25 *Microabrasion of maxillary teeth.*

hydrochloric acid and hydrogen peroxide labeled with phosphorus-32, noted that neither of these substances penetrated through the enamel to reach the dentin area. They proceeded to show that neither hydrochloric acid nor the combination of hydrochloric acid, hydrogen peroxide and ether increase the natural permeability of enamel and dentin. They attribute the occurrence of surface demineralization solely to the action of hydrochloric acid, which has a true eroding effect. The enamel, if adversely affected by the treatment, can thus regain its usual surface quality after careful polishing (Figure 6.22). In fact, surface quality has often been

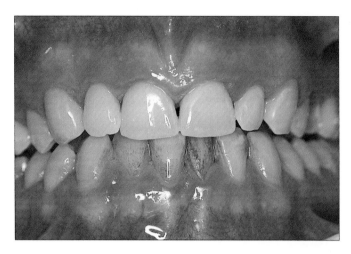

Figure 6.26 The effectiveness of microabrasion can be appraised after polishing.

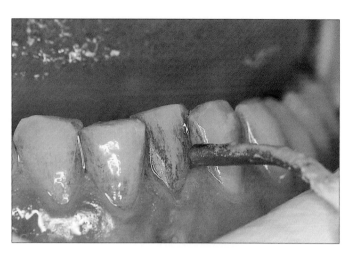

Figure 6.27 The mandibular teeth are cleaned by ultrasonic scaler and then polished.

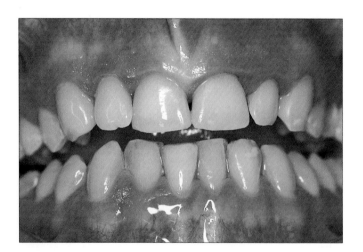

Figure 6.28 Better luminosity value is noted in microabraded teeth.

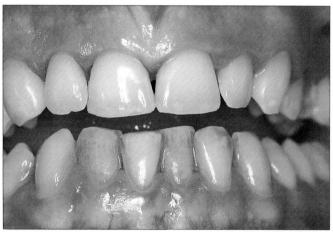

Figure 6.29 Three weeks later, the microabraded maxillary teeth are perfectly clean. The lower teeth are stained once again, however, illustrating the improved surface quality of the maxillary teeth following microabrasion.

found to improve following microabrasion and careful polishing (Figures 6.23–6.31) – an observation confirmed by the authors' electron microscope study.

A smoother enamel surface reduces accumulation of dental plaque and alters the visual quality of the surface; this has direct repercussions on tooth color. The operator should be aware of this, because reducing the enamel in depth and, especially, making it smoother and shinier does not result in whitening (or increasing the 'value') of the tooth. Quite the reverse is the case: a smooth and shiny enamel surface will tend to reduce value in the incisal region and allow an increase in the effects that show

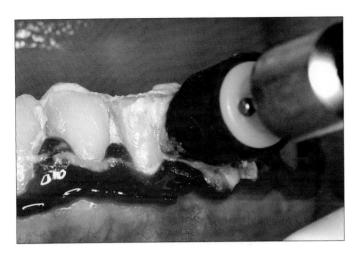

Figure 6.30 *Microabrasion of the lower teeth.*

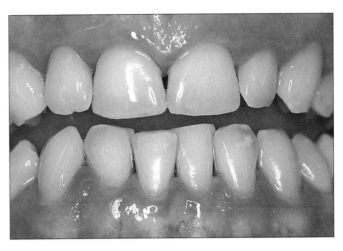

Figure 6.31 *Three weeks postoperatively; no extrinsic staining is evident.*

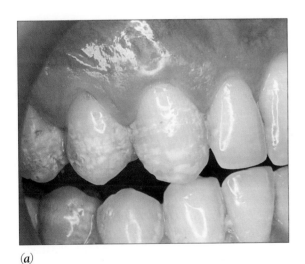

(a)

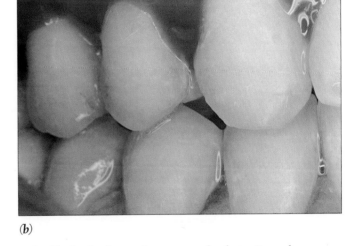

(b)

Figure 6.32 *(a) Mottled enamel due to fluorosis; (b) removal of a considerable depth of enamel to remove dysplasia. It can be seen that heavily microabraded teeth often increase in chroma and, particularly, in opacity.*

through from the underlying dental tissue, resulting in greater chromaticity and opacity. Highly polished enamel will always be more translucent than rough enamel.

Heat sensitivity following chemical treatment is comparatively rare, and disappears after a few days. However, large fissures or cracks could allow infiltration of hydrochloric acid and hydrogen peroxide, making the tooth highly sensitive.

Controlled microabrasion now provides the means of treating certain cases of fluorosis successfully (Figure 6.32). But, most of all, it reverses superficial enamel stains (Figure 6.33) and serves to complement different dental whitening techniques (Figures 6.34–6.37).

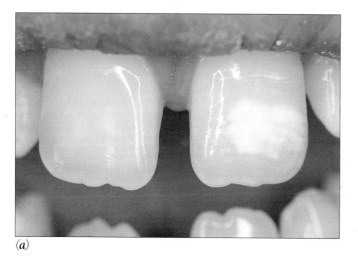
(a)

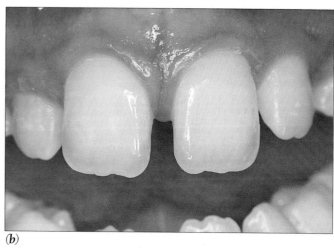
(b)

Figure 6.33 (a) *Left central incisor exhibiting white spot (enamel hypoplasia).* (b) *After microabrasion treatment, the white spot was removed and the tooth resumes its normal appearance.*

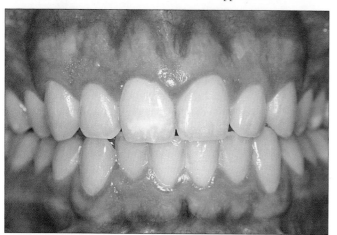

Figure 6.34 *These generally discolored teeth also exhibit 'white spot hypoplasia.*

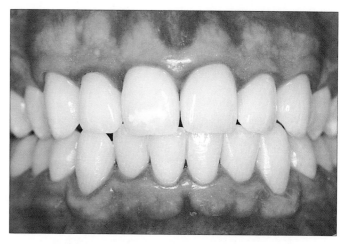

Figure 6.35 *Following one week of home bleaching; the teeth are brighter, but the white staining has not disappeared.*

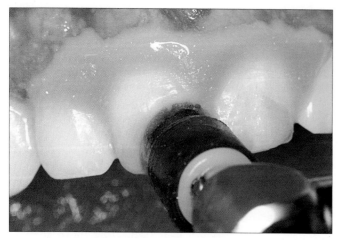

Figure 6.36 *Microabrasion of right central incisor.*

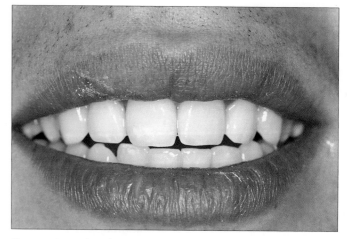

Figure 6.37 *The white spot has been almost completely corrected and color has improved.*

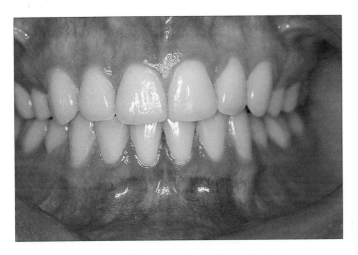

Figure 6.38 25-year-old patient who, after orthodontic treatment, wishes to improve her tooth color.

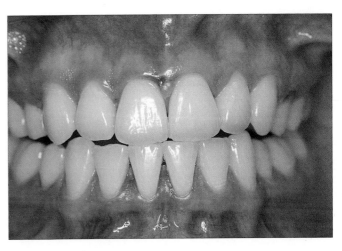

Figure 6.39 Result after two weeks of home bleaching.

Chemical bleaching of natural teeth

Whatever the chosen substance or technique, all current bleaching systems involve the action of differing concentrations of hydrogen peroxide, whether or not associated with prior treatment of the enamel surface.

Although the mechanisms of hydrogen peroxide action can vary slightly from one stain to the next, it generally acts through its oxidizing properties once it begins to decompose under the effects of heat, light or certain chemical activators. Different hydrogen peroxide breakdown reactions have been widely studied by chemists, especially those working in the paper and textile industries. Two reactions have become generally accepted:

- Reaction 1: photodissociation

$$2H_2O_2 \xrightarrow{\text{light, 50–70°C}} 2H_2O + O_2 \qquad (1)$$

- Reaction 2: anionic dissociation $\qquad (2)$

$$H_2O_2 \xrightarrow{\text{basic pH + activator (perborate or persulfate), 30–40°C}} HO_2^- + H^+$$

The first reaction – photodissociation – is induced by light and a rise in temperature. It leads to the appearance of oxygen molecules, which have only minor oxidizing properties. This reaction is the easiest to produce, and is often the primary reaction. The second reaction – anionic dissociation – is produced by a basic pH in the presence of certain activators. It results in the formation of hydroperoxide ions (HO_2^-), which, according to Zaragoza (1983), have markedly superior oxidizing properties. This anionic dissociation is harder to obtain. According to Feinman et al (1991), a third reaction can exist, namely a combination of (1) and (2) that would end in the formation of oxygen and HO_2^- ions. Whatever reaction takes place, hydrogen peroxide breakdown products oxidize the staining agent, thereby attenuating staining. In contrast to hydrochloric acid, the low molecular weight of the hydrogen peroxide breakdown products helps them to pass through the naturally porous enamel.

Hydrogen peroxide will thus have both a surface and a deeper action. Under certain circumstances, it can even reach the dentinoenamel junction and filter into the dentin. Hydrogen peroxide has no abrasive effect, whatever the concentration used, involving as it does oxochrome and chromophore pigments alone, which produce either natural coloring or pathological staining of teeth (Figures 6.38 and 6.39).

The home bleaching introduced by Haywood and Heymann (1989) also acts according to the above mechanisms, since carbamide peroxide, also known as urea peroxide, contains hydrogen peroxide. The hydrogen

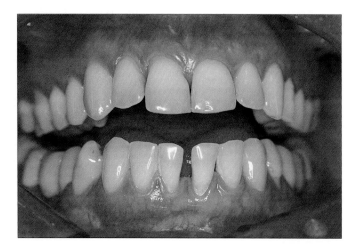

Figure 6.40 Slight staining in a 40-year-old woman.

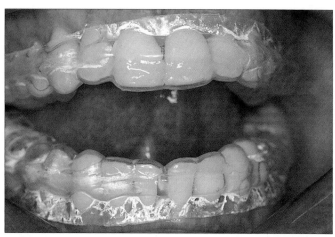

Figure 6.41 Patient using maxillary and mandibular home bleaching trays filled with bleaching gel.

peroxide, stabilized in a glycerol solution, and coupled with urea (carbamide) to form urea peroxide ($CO(NH_2)_2$–H_2O_2), is found in concentrations ranging from 1.5 to 37%. The traditional home bleaching method uses carbamide peroxide at a concentration of approximately 10%, roughly equivalent to 3.6% hydrogen peroxide. Carbamide peroxide solutions currently used in the home bleaching technique take the form of gels of varying thickness, with carbamide peroxide concentrations ranging between 1.5 and 15%. These gels generally contain acid solutions (a phosphoric or a citric acid base), lending them greater durability and stability. They therefore have an acid pH, of between 5 and 6.5; the pH should not exceed 7, since this would have a major effect on their durability. These gels also contain carbopols, which have a double action, enhancing the viscosity of the gel and delaying breakdown of hydrogen peroxide as it meets the saliva. Chemically, carbopol is a polyacrylic acid polymer and therefore very acidic. Trolamine, a neutralizing agent, is commonly added to carbopol to bring down the pH of gels to 5–7.

In general, a good home bleaching material should have

- an average carbamide peroxide concentration of 10%;

- the consistency of a highly viscous gel;

- as neutral a pH as possible, without exceeding the upper and lower limits of 5 and 7 respectively.

A pH of between 5 and 7 does not alter the enamel surface appreciably: major erosive activity requires a pH of less than 4. Acidity can increase dental sensitivity, producing slight areas of surface decalcification. Upon coming into contact with the oral soft tissues, it can also cause irritation or even inflammation. Although saliva acts as a buffer, partially neutralizing acidic solutions, it is advisable to use carbamide peroxide at a pH as close to neutral as possible.

Carbamide peroxide has a simple action: on coming into contact with the saliva, carbamide peroxide breaks down slowly (the breakdown rate depends on the proportion of carbopol present), into urea and hydrogen peroxide; the latter, in turn, breaks down to produce oxygen. The breakdown reaction takes the following form:

10% carbamide peroxide
→ 6.4% urea + 3.6% hydrogen peroxide
→ water + oxygen

Indications

The indications for use of different products will vary widely according to the concentrations used:

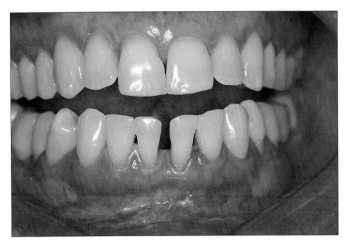

Figure 6.42 After home bleaching the teeth are much brighter .

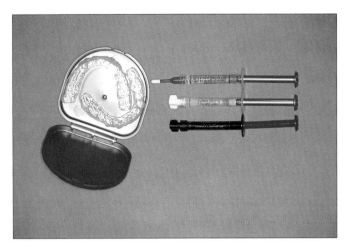

Figure 6.43 Home bleaching equipment (Opalescence): bleaching trays and tubes containing gels.

- for slight staining, especially when age-induced, requiring moderate improvement in color, home bleaching using low concentrations is satisfactory (Figures 6.40–6.42);

- for heavier staining, such as pathological tetracycline-induced stains, or when seeking major color improvement, higher concentrations should be used in the dental office.

A cautious attitude should be adopted as to the outcome of chemical bleaching, rather than raising hopes too high. The precise action of a given chemical on a particular stain can never be predicted accurately. Results can be good or disappointing. It is advisable to start with home bleaching, the outcome of which will be monitored at the end of the first or second week; by then it will be possible to make an accurate assessment of the carbamide peroxide action. If the result proves unsatisfactory, the treatment should be continued with sessions in the dentist's chair using bleaching solutions of high concentrations, often preceded by microabrasion.

Application of home bleaching gels (Figure 6.43)

Once the type, form and degree of staining have been assessed, the patient should be advised (not over-optimistically) of the potential for improvement. Shade guides are a valuable asset for visualizing both the initial and target colors (Figures 6.44–6.46). The patient should also be warned of the various drawbacks of the technique; the need to wear a tray, heat and cold sensitivity, etc.

This treatment consists of various stages. The first session is devoted to conventional clinical examination, with emphasis on the type, shape and extent of staining. After appraisal, careful scaling is performed, followed by photography with and without lip retractors. The set of photographs is completed by including one or two frames with a shade guide inset in order to visualize and quantify the initial color. A shade determination of the initial color should also be made and noted in the patient's record.

Finally, two alginate impressions are taken for making hard plaster casts (Figure 6.47).

In the laboratory, trays are made using calibrated sheets of plastic, heat-molded under vacuum (Figure 6.48).

On the plaster model, the buccal surfaces of the teeth to be treated should be covered with 1–2 mm thick photopolymerizable resin. These coatings will enable the formation of small reservoirs in the tray arrangement (Figure 6.49). The reservoirs will allow increased amounts of the substance to come into contact with the teeth. This space/allowance should stop at about 1–2 mm from the cervical and occlusal edges. It is also advisable to

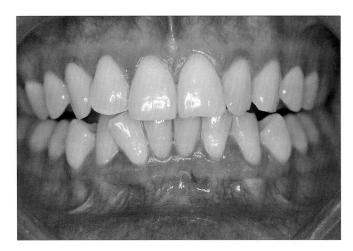

Figure 6.44 *This patient exhibits discolored teeth, and home bleaching treatment is planned.*

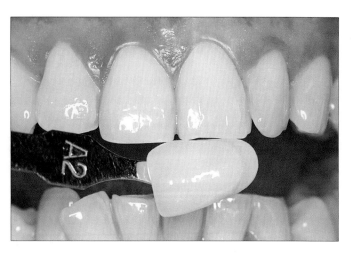

Figure 6.45 *The original tooth color should be identified using the customary shade guide, and recorded.*

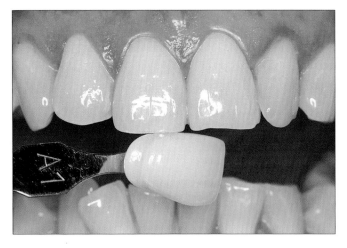

Figure 6.46 *The desired color should be approved by the patient and recorded in photographic or video form.*

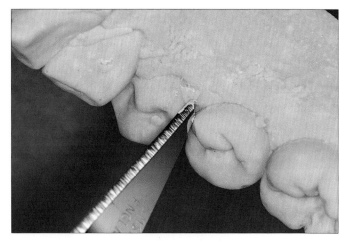

Figure 6.47 *Defects on the plaster model should be removed using a scalpel blade.*

block spaces between teeth using the same resin, thus preventing unnecessary protrusions in the tray that can cause gingival irritation (Figures 6.50–6.52).

The tray is cut off 1–2 mm apical to the gingival line of the teeth. The tray margins must be polished, so the edges are perfectly smooth (Figure 6.53). Some authors recommend an anatomical cut-out matching the edge of the gum (Figure 6.54), but this makes it harder to produce the cut-outs and especially difficult to polish all the edges. Moreover, their sealing properties are not as good, since the tray will often open during application of the product.

The second session is devoted to fitting and adjusting the tray (Figure 6.55), as well as providing accurate explanation to the patient of the procedures to be

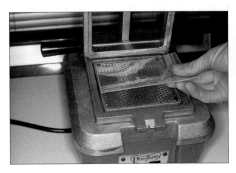

Figure 6.48 *A flexible polyethylene sheet is placed on the thermomoulding apparatus.*

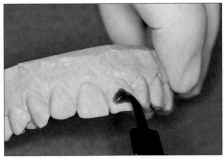

Figure 6.49 *Application of a photo-polymerizable resin to labial surfaces of treated teeth to create 'reservoirs' in the treatment tray that will contain the bleaching gel.*

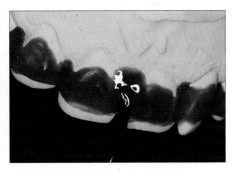

Figure 6.50 *It is important to fill in embrasures on the model using a liquid resin so as to avoid any tight contact with papillae and irritation from the tray.*

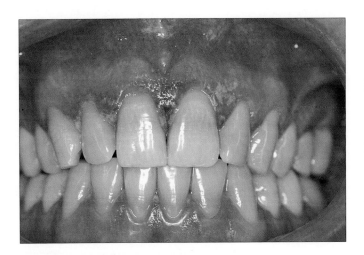

Figure 6.51 *Traumatic ulceration due to friction from a tray fitted too closely at gingival embrasures.*

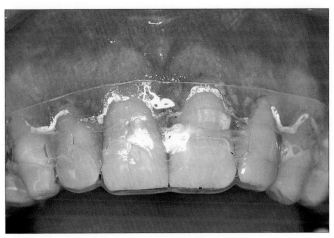

Figure 6.52 *The tray has been remade, the embrasures have been cleared, and the margins of the tray easily clear the cervical area.*

followed. Each product has its own optimum method of use. Product action depends on the proportion of carbopol present. Hence some products have a protracted action and have to be worn overnight, and others, having a shorter action, can be kept on for just 3 hours, preferably renewing the gel every hour. Results will be largely (80%) achieved after 3–4 days; the length

of treatment averages one week or occasionally two, but never longer than three weeks.

The final session is devoted to color monitoring (Figure 6.56) and polishing using a paste for natural teeth (PC4, Cédia). Once the treatment has ended, the patient should wear trays with a fluoride gel for three days (for an average of two hours per day) to increase

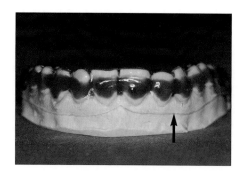

Figure 6.53 *This straight-line cut-out in the tray, apical to the gingival margin (arrow), is simpler to carry out as well as less traumatic and provides a better seal than the anatomical cut-out (Figure 6.54).*

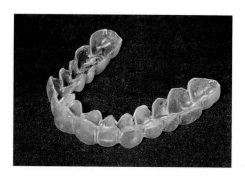

Figure 6.54 *Home bleaching tray with anatomical cut-out. This design is very difficult to perform correctly, and if not done perfectly, the tray quickly becomes irritating and more permeable. This design is not recommended.*

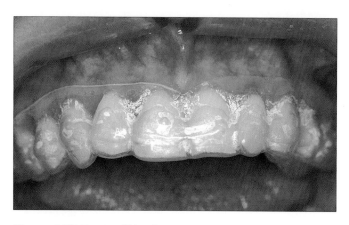

Figure 6.55 *Try-in of bleaching tray.*

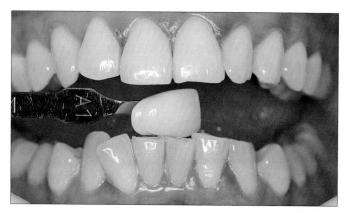

Figure 6.56 *Examination of maxillary anterior teeth after one week of home bleaching treatment. Note the comparison with the A-1 shade tab.*

the rate of remineralization and reduce the risk of sensitivity. In cases of high sensitivity, the addition of fluoride mouthwashes and strontium chloride-based toothpastes might be indicated.

If the patient experiences sensitivity during treatment, a tray with fluoride gel should be worn for one night, and then the normal course of treatment should be resumed.

Follow-up should consist of two or three sessions every six months after scaling.

Generally speaking, it seems advisable to offer this chemical treatment as a combination comprising prelim-

inary scaling, bleaching treatment, polishing sessions and two follow-up sessions after six months, so that the 'contract' adopted lasts for a year (Figure 6.57).

Application of substances at high concentrations

Initially, the authors used Superoxol (35% or 110 vol peroxide), according to the technique described by

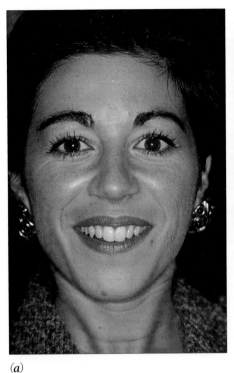

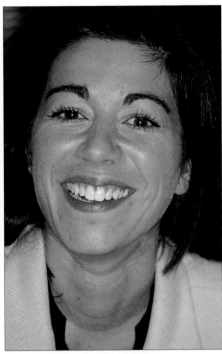

(a)   (b)

Figure 6.57 (a, b) Improvement in tooth color after two weeks of home bleaching treatment.

Feinman et al (1989) (Figure 6.58), and subsequently Zaragoza's (1983) technique (BV bleaching) using chemical preparation of enamel and 70% hydrogen peroxide (i.e. 300 vol) (Figure 6.59). Despite the favorable results obtained with these methods, it no longer seems necessary to use them. These are difficult to handle and invariably cause significant postoperative discomfort for the patient. Limited data are available on their long-term effects and safety. Newer high-concentration bleaching agents are now available that make the procedure easier, effective and less uncomfortable for the patient.

High-concentration bleaching agents should:

* have a concentration range of 20–50%;

* take the form of a gel, preferably prepared just before use.

Methods of activating peroxides
Peroxides can be activated:

* by light (from various sources);

* by heat;

* chemically.

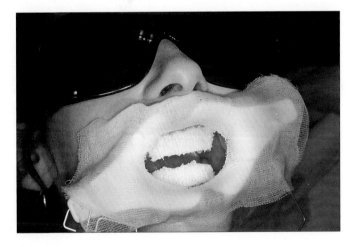

Figure 6.58 Concentrated Superoxol treatment.

An attempt should be made to obtain a mixture with a pH of more than 7 to promote the production of HO_2^- ions.

At present, the two products that closely approach this ideal are Starbrite (Stardent) and Hi Lite (Shofu). Both these products use 35% hydrogen peroxide, mixed with a

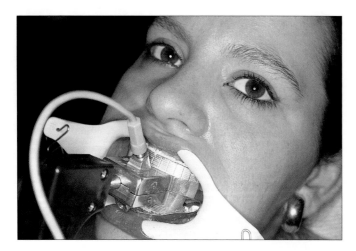

Figure 6.59 BV bleaching treatment.

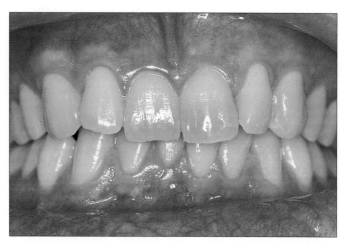

Figure 6.60 This 21-year-old patient exhibits major, evenly spread pathological staining (second-degree tetracycline stain), with heavier staining on the two central incisors.

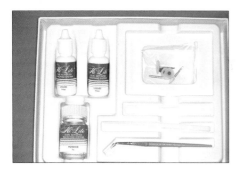

Figure 6.61 Hi Lite (Shofu) tooth bleaching kit.

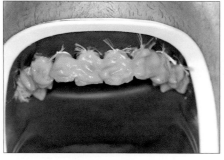

Figure 6.62 The hydrogen peroxide-based gel is applied to the teeth that are isolated by rubber dam.

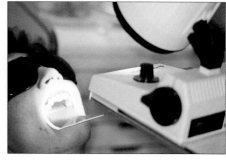

Figure 6.63 Activation using a bleaching lamp.

powder to form a gel. Hi Lite has the original feature of containing a chemical activator promoting faster hydrogen peroxide breakdown (further accelerated by light as well as heat put out by a halogen lamp). Application periods will be of fairly short duration (a few minutes with the halogen lamp and 10–20 minutes without the halogen lamp).

With Starbrite, which contains no chemical activator, the mixture is more effective if light-activated; application periods will be longer, lasting about 20 minutes.

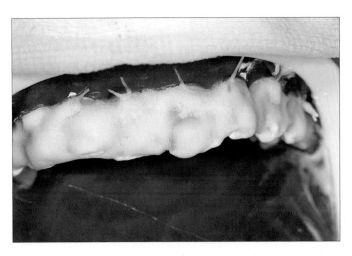

Figure 6.64 After a few (5–6) minutes, the blue mixture changes to a white color. It must then be removed and the procedure repeated.

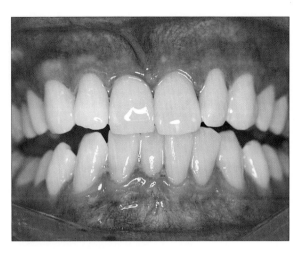

Figure 6.65 The teeth always appear very white and rather opaque immediately after chemical treatment.

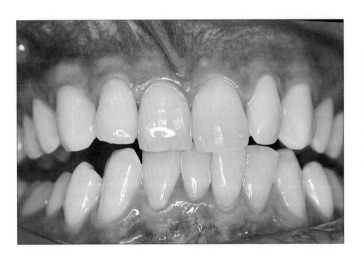

Figure 6.66 The teeth are completely remoisturized and slightly less white one week after chemical treatment, and have acquired a more natural color.

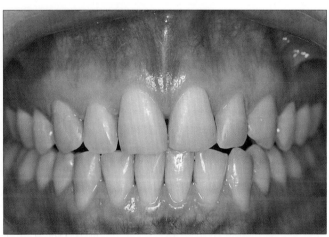

Figure 6.67 Slight, even, tetracycline-induced pathological staining (first-degree tetracycline stain); the surface enamel has a lack-luster look.

Although gingival protection measures are mandatory, the use of gels rather than liquid solutions of hydrogen peroxide minimizes the chances of soft-tissue contact. The viscous nature of gels would also appear to be a factor promoting better penetration of oxidizing ions through the enamel. Gels form a 'blanket' that does not allow easy escape of the oxygen ions. Despite the limited clinical trial data available for gels, they would appear to be better in the case of simpler and less prolonged bleaching sessions.

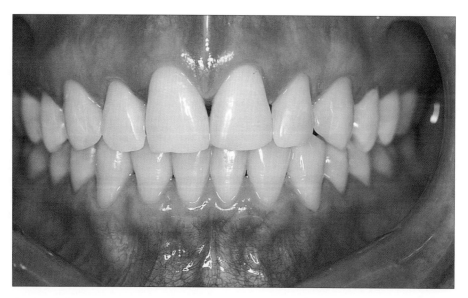

Figure 6.68 Improvement in value and in surface quality thanks to careful polishing.

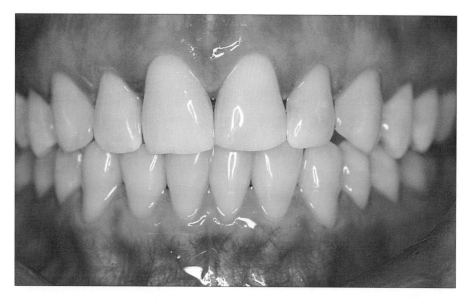

Figure 6.69 Result following two weeks of home bleaching, plus four treatment sessions in the dental office with a concentrated bleaching product.

Hydrogen peroxide acts extremely well on organic staining but much less effectively on stains of inorganic origin, often imparting a gray or blue color to the tooth. It appears that this blue or gray staining tends to reappear sooner than yellow or brown stains, probably because of their origins.

High-concentration chemical bleaching treatment involves the following steps (Figures 6.60–6.69).

First session
During the first session, the following procedures are carried out:

- normal oral examination;

- assessment of staining;

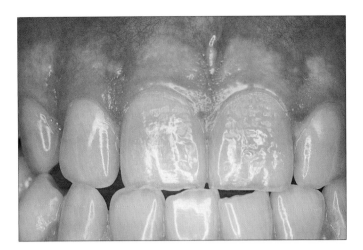

Figure 6.70 A 20-year-old patient with pathological staining associated with dysplasia.

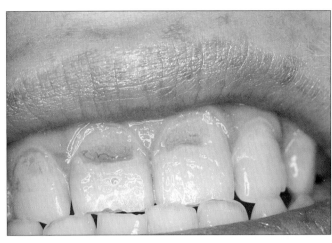

Figure 6.71 Appearance of very extensive areas of demineralization after two sessions of concentrated bleaching. This example illustrates the danger of using concentrated chemicals in the presence of dysplasia.

- careful scaling;

- taking of photographs with and without shade guide for reference purposes.

Second session

The patient is protected from inadvertent contact with gels by wearing spectacles and setting up a sealed operating area using a rubber dam. Microabrasion will then be performed, light or intense, depending on the type of staining, using either a high- or low-concentration gel. After thorough washing with water, the teeth are cleaned, using chloroform or ether. Bleaching gel is applied to the labial/buccal and lingual surfaces, then activated under a lamp for 5–6 minutes. The solution is renewed several times, ideally 4–6 times per session. With Starbrite, the mixture is left on for longer (about 15 minutes) and renewed once per session. After thorough washing, the rubber dam is removed and a sodium bicarbonate neutralizing gel applied for a few minutes. The session can be repeated several times. The number of sessions will vary as the case requires.

Each treatment is followed by polishing and then fluoride treatment for several days.

Summary

The three chemical whitening techniques have different actions:

- microabrasion has a specific, superficial action only;

- home bleaching acts mainly on moderate even staining for yellow or light-brown shades;

- high-concentration chemical bleaching should be confined to stronger staining, especially uniform gray or blue staining.

- combination of all three methods when staining is resistant to treatment.

All these types of treatment have their own indications as well as limitations. Some tooth stains may be resistant to any chemical treatment, even a combination of these three techniques, such as third- and fourth-degree tetracycline staining, with a non-uniform pattern of gray or dark-brown streaks.

In extreme cases it is preferable to resort to prosthetic techniques, which may sometimes be preceded by chemical whitening. Here the role of the chemical treatment will be confined to reducing the intensity of the staining – a technique sometimes employed when applying ceramic laminates. It is advisable to wait at

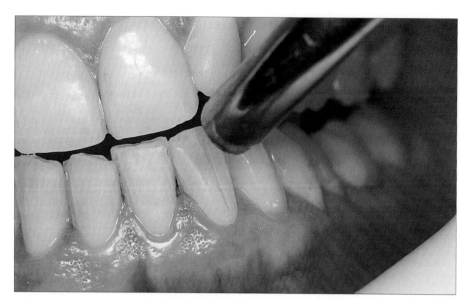

Figure 6.72 Major enamel cracks and fissures should preferably be protected before any bleaching takes place.

least 3 weeks before cementation so as to reduce interference by bleaching substances, which could affect the quality of bonding.

Biocompatability of chemical treatments

It is important to note that all these chemical tooth whitening techniques have been controversial. It should be remembered that every technique has an element of risk. One should learn how to accurately assess these risks from the various reported experiments, articles and symposia available.

All writers stress the dangerous action that hydrogen peroxide and hydrochloric acid can exert on soft tissue, and hence the need always to wash out, neutralize and, above all, to check.

Many studies have also attempted to point out the dangers of hydrogen peroxide-based techniques on the tooth and pulp. Some claim that hydrogen peroxide penetrates the enamel barrier and reaches the dentin and pulp tissues. Wainwright and Lemoine (1950) and Griffin et al (1977) have shown that the low molecular weight of hydrogen peroxide facilitates its passage through the barrier, and that it could, under certain circumstances, penetrate the enamel and dentin. However, Cohen (1976), Robertson and Melfir (1980)

and Baumgartner et al (1983) have concluded that vital bleaching may be considered free of risk for pulp tissue.

This conclusion should nonetheless be qualified, since Bowles and Thompson (1986), after examining the response of seven bovine tooth pulp enzymes under the action of hydrogen peroxide solution, heat action or a combination of these two procedures, have stated that both agents have an adverse effect on pulp enzymes. These enzymes were less damaged by heat than by the hydrogen peroxide effect, although Bowles and Thompson note that the combination of hydrogen peroxide and heat is the most dangerous. Bowles and Ugwuneri (1987) have also demonstrated that hydrogen peroxide can penetrate the pulp – an effect promoted by heating. These two alarming sets of experiments should be seen in perspective: can one extrapolate all these in vitro experiments to in vivo conditions? The amounts of hydrogen peroxide used are at the microgram level, whereas it is recognized that at least 50 µg are required to cause enzyme inhibition.

It would appear from the various sets of in vitro and in vivo experiments that when using substances at concentrations not exceeding 37% at temperatures of below 40°C, the damage induced to hard tissue and to the pulp in particular is reversible in most cases (Seale and Thrash, 1985; Arens et al, 1972).

In their clinical practices, the authors have treated several thousand teeth and have observed a few

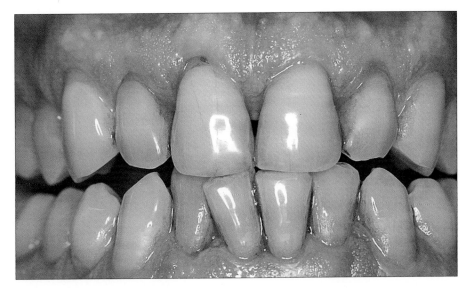

Figure 6.73 *A 55-year old patient presenting with heavy staining.*

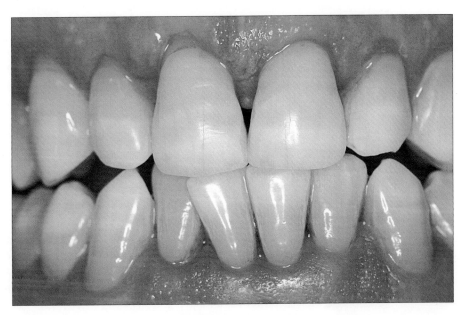

Figure 6.74 *Chemical bleaching occasionally reveals white stains, which can detract from the overall esthetic effect.*

incidents as well as two real accidents during the 1980s.

- A 20-year-old woman presented with pathological staining combined with major dysplasia of the enamel. Before producing laminate veneers, the teeth were bleached. After two chemical bleaching sessions using 70% hydrogen peroxide, major patches of demineralization accompanied by severe pain were noted. The treatment was stopped and the laminate veneers completed. This example illustrates the danger of using such products in cases of dysplasia (Figures 6.70 and 6.71).

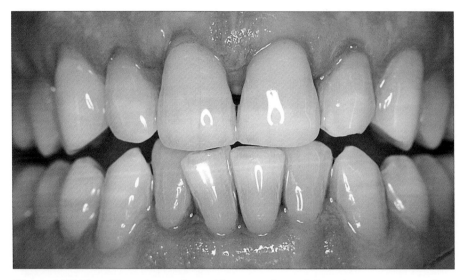

Figure 6.75 *The white stains are less evident once the teeth have been remoisturized and finely polished.*

• The second patient was aged 25 years and presented with pathological staining. A Superoxol-based treatment was prescribed. After the first session, the patient complained of pain on the lower left central incisor; the pulp of the tooth had to be removed a week later. In this specific case, a major fissure was observed in the enamel, accompanied by microscopic cracking, indicating that the product had penetrated very easily through these cracks and fissures to reach the pulp (Figure 6.72).

If the contraindications for bleaching treatment had been adhered to, these two accidents could have been avoided. However, when indications are properly established and the treatment performed properly, chemical bleaching provides an elegant and effective solution to discolouration problems in vital teeth in many cases (Figures 6.73–6.75).

Bleaching non-vital teeth

The first attempts at the internal bleaching of non-vital teeth date back almost as far as trials on vital teeth.

Garreton suggested a sodium-hypochlorite-based chemical treatment as early as 1895. Spasser (1961) introduced a mixture of sodium perborate and water, based on the work of Sylva, who first achieved clinical success with this bleaching agent in 1938. Grogan, too, was to confirm the oxidizing properties of sodium perborate in 1946. In 1958, Pearson was using heat-activated hydrogen peroxide, while Nutting and Po (1967) described their combined technique, mixing hydrogen peroxide and sodium perborate. The latter variety of ambulatory treatment was used for a long time, but many authors reported this procedure as dangerous (Rotstein et al, 1991). Under certain circumstances, which still remain unclear, cervical resorption occurs after treatment, affecting 10–15% of the teeth treated, according to these authors. The exact cause of this resorption still remains obscure, but responsibility seems to lie with the hydrogen peroxide, or rather the acid pH that it imparts to the solution. This resorption only appears 5–15 years after treatment.

In view of all these findings, and especially in the light of modern knowledge, it seems that caution should be exercised when using hydrogen peroxide. Cases treated

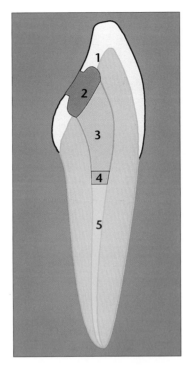

Figure 6.76 *Plan of the different stages in internal bleaching treatment:*
(1) retention;
(2) IRM temporary filling;
(3) sodium perborate–water mixture;
(4) cement base;
(5) gutta percha.

with sodium perborate alone do not appear to suffer from the same disadvantages. The authors stopped using hydrogen peroxide altogether over 5 years ago, in favor of a mixture of sodium perborate and water, as suggested by Spasser (1961). This is a simple technique involving several stages (Figure 6.76):

- Assess the quality of the endodontic treatment (retreating without hesitation if in doubt).

- Isolate the tooth, by a rubber dam for instance.

- Gain access to the pulp chamber (by removing the temporary filling), and thoroughly clean the pulp chamber, removing the gutta percha 2–3 mm below the cementoenamel junction.

- Place a cement base at the entry to the canal opening to help make this area watertight, thus preventing any infiltration of sodium perborate towards the canal.

- Once the base has set in place, insert as thick a mixture as possible of sodium perborate and distilled water into the pulp cavity. Using a cotton wool pad, the mixture should be packed down as thoroughly as

possible, leaving the edges of the cavity free, having already fashioned it into a retentive shape.

- Cover the mixture, once condensed, with temporary cement (IRM, Dentsply-Caulk).

- Seal the margins, after etching, using a light-cured resin.

- Renew this mixture once every two weeks (the number of sessions depending on the degree and type of staining).

- Once the treatment has been found satisfactory, clean the pulp cavity and remove the cement base.

- Fill the tooth with a composite resin of appropriate shade. A material that is too opaque or too white might affect the final color of the tooth.

This technique, which has become well established in clinical practice, is straightforward. Despite the often highly satisfactory results obtained overall, some staining remains wholly or partially resistant to this chemical treatment.
Figures 6.77–6.82 demonstrate six clinical cases.

CASE PRESENTATION: 1

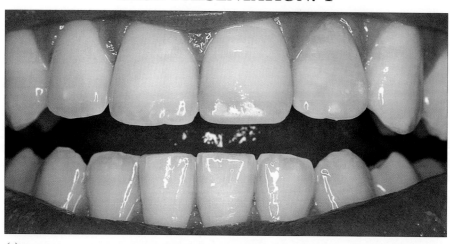

(a)

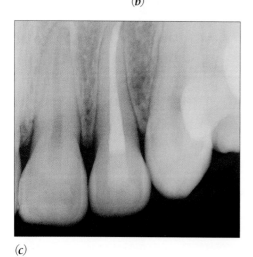

(c)

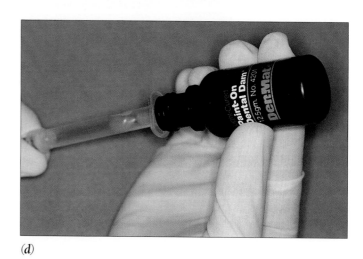

(d)

Figure 6.77 (a) *The maxillary left lateral incisor has been diagnosed with pulpal necrosis and requires endodontic treatment.* (b) *The pulp hemorrhage preceding this necrosis has discolored the tooth, and chemical treatment is planned.* (c) *It is essential to monitor the quality of the endodontic filling prior to any chemical treatment. (Courtesy of Dr P Machtou.)* (d) *Loading syringe with Paint-On Dental Dam resin.*

(contd)

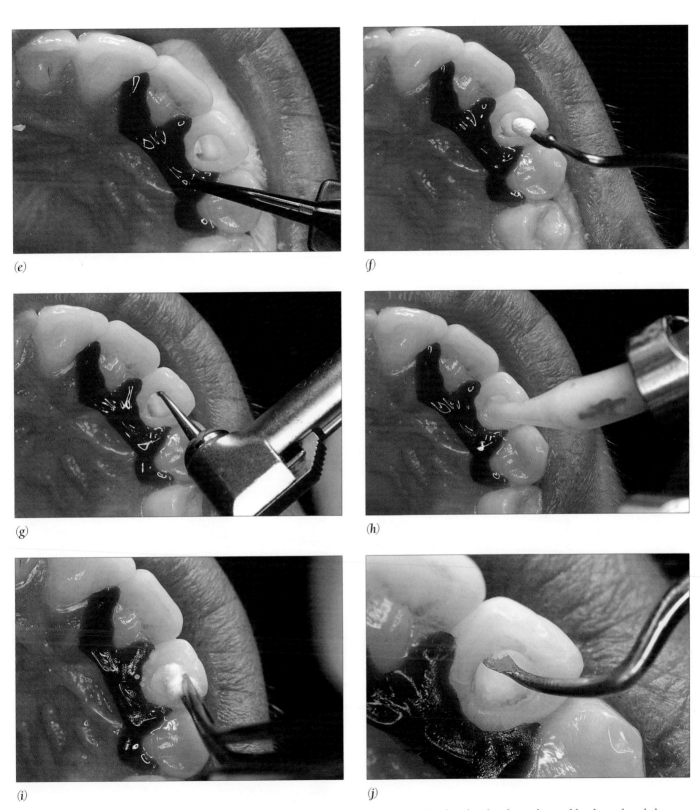

(e)

(f)

(g)

(h)

(i)

(j)

(Figure 6.77 contd) (e) This protection is fast and easy to apply. (f) Once the pulp chamber has been thoroughly cleaned and the gutta percha removed 2–3 mm below the cementoenamel boundary, a cement base is placed against the gutta percha to seal this area. (g) A retentive cavity is created using a round bur. (h) Injection of the sodium perborate–water mixture. (i) The mixture is compressed using a cotton wool ball. (j) The excess is removed in order to clear retentive features thoroughly.   (contd)

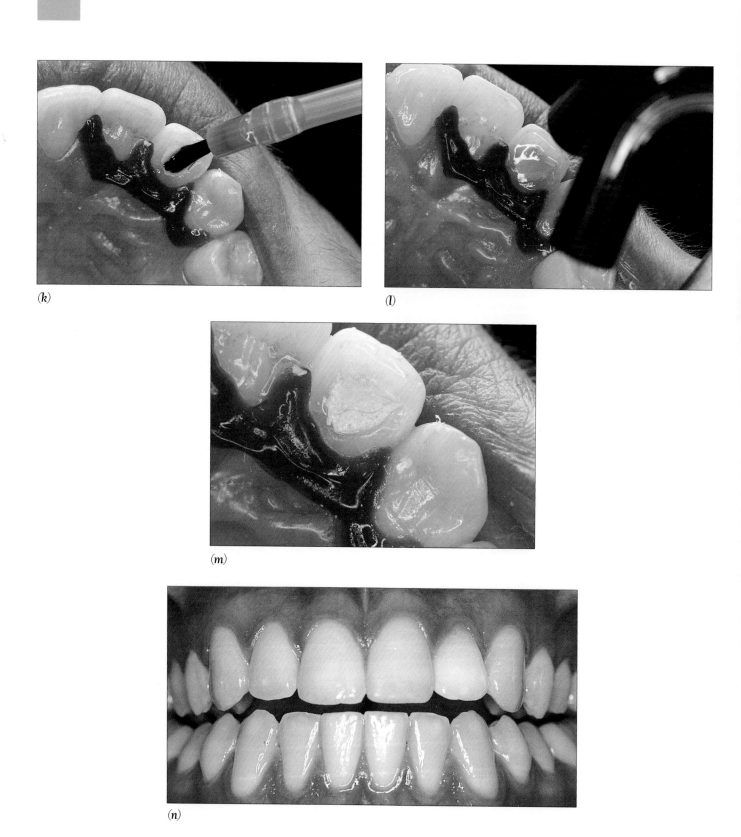

(k)

(l)

(m)

(n)

(Figure 6.77 contd) (**k**) Once the temporary restoration has hardened, unfilled resin is applied with a brush after etching. (**l**) This light resin film will ensure complete sealing of the temporary filling. (**m**) Two weeks later, the temporary restoration is intact and the margins are completely sealed. (**n**) Result after a single (2-week) treatment period reveal that the treated lateral is much lighter than the remaining teeth. Home bleaching is initiated.

(contd)

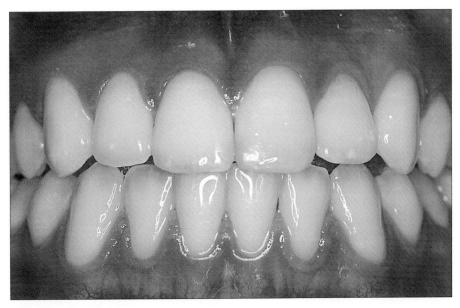

(o)

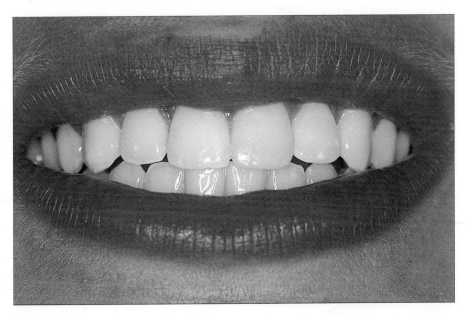

(p)

(Figure 6.77 contd)
(o) A combination of two different bleaching techniques made it possible to harmonize the final esthetic result. (p) Six-month follow-up: the color has not altered.

CASE PRESENTATION: 2

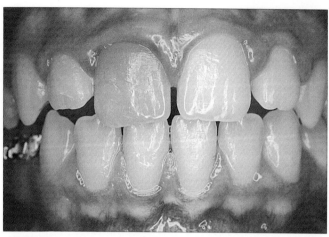

(a)

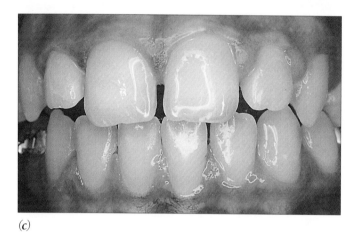

(c)

(b)

Figure 6.78 (**a**) *Discoloration of maxillary right central and lateral incisors.* (**b**) *Root canal treatment repeated so as to increase impermeability of the root canal filling. (Courtesy of Dr P Machtou.)* (**c**) *Result after two 2-week treatment periods with intracoronal bleaching.*

CASE PRESENTATION: 3

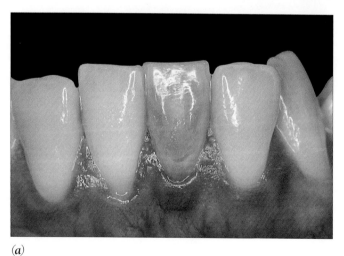

(a)

(b)

Figure 6.79 (**a**) *Endodontically treated mandibular incisor exhibiting marked discoloration.* (**b**) *Improved shade after a 2-week treatment cycle with intracoronal bleaching.*

CASE PRESENTATION: 4

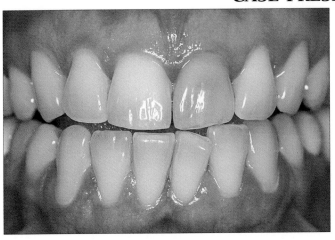
(a)

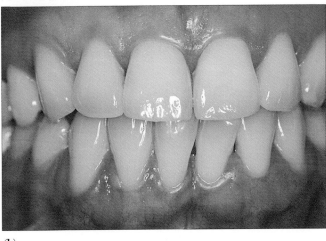
(b)

Figure 6.80 (**a**) *Devitalized maxillary left central incisor is discolored.* (**b**) *Appearance after internal non-vital bleaching coupled with vital home bleaching.*

CASE PRESENTATION: 5

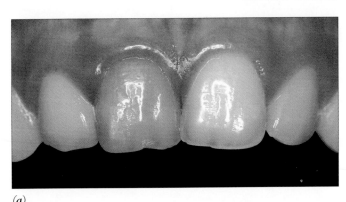
(a)

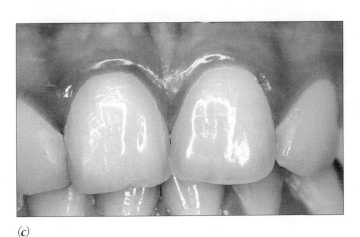
(c)

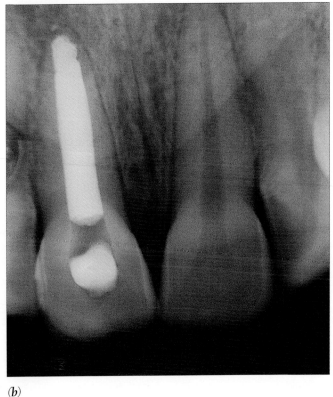
(b)

Figure 6.81 (**a**) *Traumatic impact led to devitalization of the maxillary right central incisor. In view of its extreme fragility, it was decided to restore this tooth with an all-ceramic crown.* (**b**) *Radiograph showing the endodontic treatment.* (*Courtesy of Dr P Machtou.*) ·(**c**) *Bleaching of the crown and the cervical third enables staining to be removed within a month.* (contd)

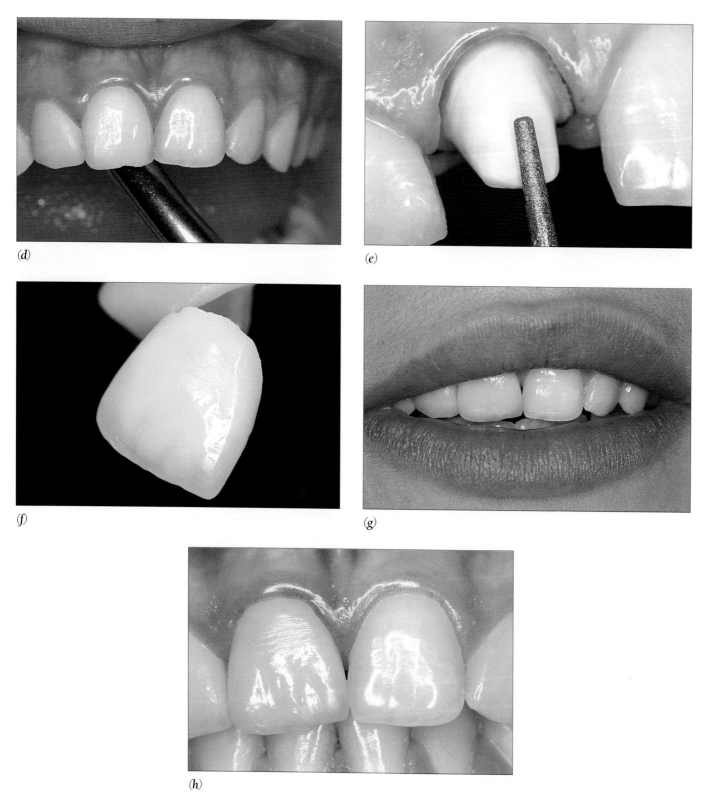

(d)

(e)

(f)

(g)

(h)

(*Figure 6.81 contd*) (**d**) *The bleached tooth is more opaque, and any translucency has vanished.* (**e**) *Bleaching of the cervical third enables performance of a tooth–ceramic shoulder preparation without endangering the final color shade (the core type used here is a composite resin).* (**f**) *LFC (Ducera) ceramic.* (**g**) *End result.* (**h**) *Good light transmission can be acquired by improving the color of the underlying tooth structure.*

CASE PRESENTATION: 6

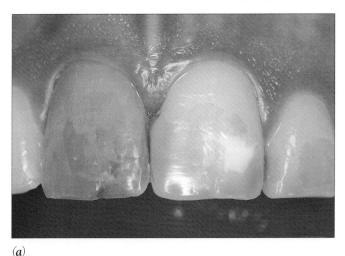

(a)

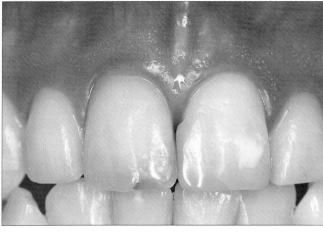

(b)

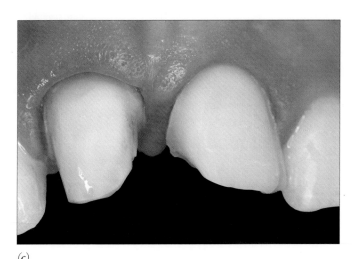

(c)

Figure 6.82 (*a*) *The right central incisor is non-vital and the left central incisor has been restored using a composite resin. A ceramic jacket is planned for the right tooth and a ceramic laminate veneer for the left.*
(*b*) *The right central has been lightened beforehand by three weeks of chemical treatment with sodium perborate (crown + cervical third).*
(*c*) *The preparations reveal uniformity of color in the supporting tooth structure, which is essential for all-ceramic restorations.*

References

Abbot C, Bleaching discolored teeth by means of 30% Perhydrol and electric light rays. *J Allied Dent Soc* 1918; **13**: 259.

Arens DE, Rich JJ, Healey HJ, A practical method of bleaching tetracycline-stained teeth. *Oral Surg Oral Med Oral Pathol* 1972; **34**: 812–17.

Baumgartner JC, Reid DE, Pickett AB, Human pulpal reaction to the modified McInnes bleaching technique. *J Endodont* 1983; **9**: 527–9.

Bowles WH, Thompson LR, Vital bleaching: the effect of heat and hydrogen peroxide on pulpal enzymes. *J Endodont* 1986; **12**: 108–10.

Bowles WH, Ugwuneri Z, Pulp chamber penetration by hydrogen peroxide following vital bleaching procedures. *J Endodont* 1987; **13**: 375–7.

Cohen SC, Human pulpal response to bleaching procedures on vital teeth. *J Endodont* 1976; **5**: 134.

Croll TP, Cavanaugh RR, Enamel color modification by controlled hydrochloric acid-pumice surface abrasion: I Techniques and examples. *Quintessence Int* 1986; **17**: 81–7.

Feinman RA, Goldstein RE, Garber DA, *Bleaching Teeth*. Chicago: Quintessence, 1989: 84–96.

Feinman RA, Madray G, Yarborough D, Chemical, optical and physiologic mechanisms of bleaching products: a review. *Pract Periodont Aesthet Dent* 1991; **3**: 32–7.

Griffin RE, Grower MF, Ayer WA, Effects of solutions used to treat dental fluorosis and permeability of teeth. *J Endodont* 1977; **3**: 139–43.

Haywood VB, Heymann HO, Nightguard vital bleaching. *Quintessence Int* 1989; **20**: 173–8.

McCloskey RJ, A technique for removal of fluorosis stains. *J Am Dent Assoc* 1984; **109**: 63–4.

McInnes J, Removing brown stain from teeth. *Ariz Dent J* 1966; **12**: 13–15.

Miara P, Touati B, Haikel Y, La microabrasion amélaire controlée. *Réal Clin* 1991; **2**: 395–407.

Nutting EB, Poe GS, Chemical bleaching of discolored endodontically treated teeth. *Dent Clin North Am* 1967; Nov.: 655.

Pearson H, Bleaching discoloured pulpless teeth. *J Am Dent Assoc* 1958; **49**: 56–64.

Robertson WD, Melfir C, Pulpal response to vital bleaching procedures. *J Endodont* 1980; **6**: 645–9.

Rotstein I, Torek Y, Misgrav R, Effects of cementum defects on radicular penetration of 30% H_2O_2 during intracoronal bleaching. *J Endodont* 1991; **17**: 230–3.

Seale NS, Thrash WJ, Systematic assessment of colour removal following vital bleaching of intrinsically stained teeth. *J Dent Res* 1985; **64**: 457–61.

Spasser HF, A simple bleaching technique using sodium perborate. *NY State Dent J* 1961; **27**: 332–4.

Wainwright WW, Lemoine FA, Rapid diffuse penetration of intact enamel and dentin by carbon-6-14 labeled urea. *J Am Dent Assoc* 1950; **41**: 135.

Zaragoza VMT, Bleaching vital teeth affected by a pathological coloration. Doctoral thesis, School of Medicine, University of Valencia, Spain, 1983.

CHAPTER 7

Transfer of Esthetic Information

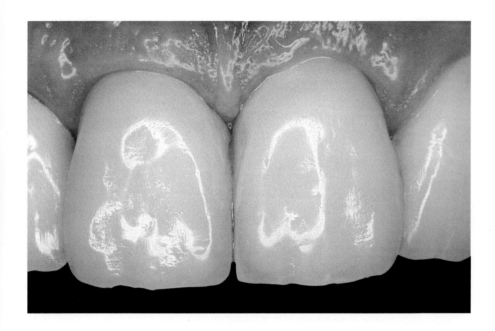

Esthetics cannot be considered an exact science, although many esthetic parameters, such as shape, color, spatial arrangement and texture, may be reproduced. In that our discipline involves a certain minimum number of individuals, if only the patient, laboratory technician and clinician, the ability to communicate all information required objectively and accurately is crucial for the success of the treatment.

Esthetic errors or failures often arise from problems in communication, which may have been inadequate, incomplete, inaccurate or, in a few cases, non-existent.

All communication must rely on tangible aids, such as

- complete or partial impressions;

- intra- or extra-oral photographs;

- study casts;

- casts modified by wax-up (using tooth-colored wax);

- silicone index (or templates);

- all types of shade guides (dental, gingival);

- intra-oral videos;
- bite registration;
- specific questionnaires;
- laboratory prescription forms;
- computer imaging systems (Dzierpak, 1991; Nathanson, 1991);
- provisional restorations.

All modern prosthetic restorations in the anterior region require at the very least photographs, casts, a questionnaire, color shade guides, an accurate laboratory prescription form, one or more satisfactory provisional prostheses, and bite registration. It is to satisfy this need for standard points of reference that this chapter has been included.

The patient

Patients do not always quite know what they want – or rather cannot always express their ideas. It is our task to help them refine these ideas and formulate their intentions: not just for the sake of ultimate patient satisfaction, but also to avoid having to make the same prosthesis over again, because of 'details' left undecided.

- Does the patient refuse to have any metal showing on the lingual surface?

- Does the patient also intend to change the position and shape of the soft tissues?

- Does the patient require a radical change in tooth color, with the other arch bleached to match?

Such examples are manifold, and hence the authors require the patient to fill in an 'esthetic questionnaire' (see page 119) when a treatment is to be initiated involving esthetic considerations. This questionnaire supplements the standard medical questionnaire, and aims to pinpoint esthetic problems and improve patient–dentist communication.

Patients may be called upon to show photographs of what they have in mind (they may arrive with pockets full of magazine photographs!), and to view photographs of similar types of treatment carried out by the dentist.

Much time will always be saved by preliminary discussion and listening to criticism – whether justified or not.

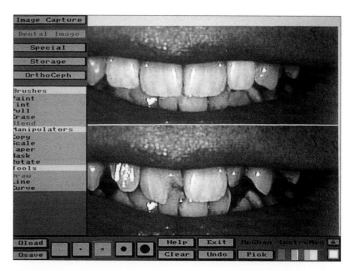

Figure 7.1 An imaging computer can help in the planning and communication of the projected esthetic changes. The system generally consists of a video camera and a digitizing pad connected to a computer. (Courtesy of Dr Michel Rogé.)

One should never forget that the patient's opinion is subjective from the outset – something that the dentist is often powerless to change. Once the treatment is under way, it can only be taken as complete (and paid for) when the patient is satisfied.

Patients should be encouraged to come to the dentist's surgery with someone close to them (and with influence over them), who will pass judgment on their teeth. The dentist should be enough of a psychologist to let this person express opinions before and during treatment so as to avoid a confrontation with the patient at the end of the day, with foreseeable consequences. Patients assume that they have every right to express an opinion where color is concerned, and will seldom yield to the dentist's superior expertise in this area. There is therefore no reason why patients should not be entrusted with shade guides, make their opinions known (if only tentatively at first), and be asked to sign the shade prescription form. The authors have learnt from experience that, unfortunately, anything can happen as far as color is concerned.

Recent advances have enabled us to turn to the computer to preview esthetic results (Figures 7.1 and 7.2). Technology can prove very useful for motivating as well as testing patients. A photograph processed by computer stands as a point of reference in its own right – but some caution is needed: can the computer not

ESTHETIC QUESTIONNAIRE

Surname:
Forename:
Age:

Pretreatment photograph, showing the smile

Main reason for seeking consultation:

Do you have reservations regarding:
– Your face?
– Your smile?
– Your lips?
– Your gums?

Previous photograph to act as reference guide

What reservations do you have about your dentition:
(please asterisk your main complaint)
– Tooth color
– Tooth shape:
   – length
   – width
   – spaces between teeth
   – position of teeth

What is your opinion of:
– Your previous treatment?
– Your previous prostheses?

Are you aiming for:
– A perfect 'media smile'
– A harmonious, natural smile
– A smile of even
   – color
   – shape
   – position

Would you rate your oral hygiene as:
– Excellent
– Satisfactory
– Unsatisfactory

Patient's signature _____

NB: In the event of treatment, the color agreed on by common consent for the prosthetic restoration is as follows:

Shade guide: Shade:

Signature _____

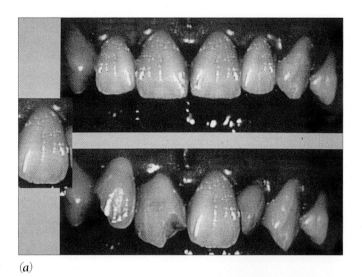

(a)

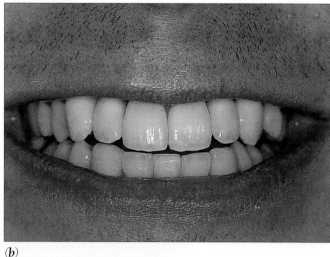

(b)

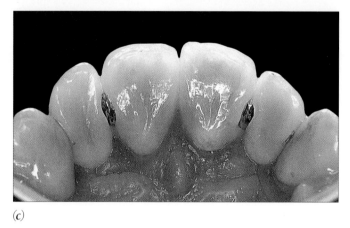

(c)

Figure 7.2 (a) The patient can pre-visualize the final prosthetic restoration before any procedure is undertaken. (b) Buccal view and (c) lingual aspect of the final ceramic restoration. (Courtesy of Dr Michel Rogé.)

manage to do things impossible to emulate? Could one, for example, produce a bridge like the one seen in a computer-generated image without wide embrasures in the presence of ridge resorption?

The first appointments are crucial for the patient: the dentist must be able to listen, record the information, and conceal nothing from the patient.

It is basically knowing how to select the right clinical cases that makes for success: knowing how to refuse can save many a sleepless night. A single setback or conflict can make the clinician forget any number of brilliant successes.

When a patient relates the unsuccessful attempts of two or three colleagues previously, one should not necessarily count on doing any better than they did, since some patients have a 'psychopathic' attitude toward their teeth.

The dentist

The dentist must collate all esthetic information and synthesize patients' wishes. The dentist has the task of analyzing them and making them cogent for the prosthetics laboratory (Brisman, 1980).

Insofar as a dentist proceeds not blindly but with the aid of objective and tangible criteria, he or she will inspire confidence in the patient, whose esthetic perception may have become distorted, perhaps, for example, by a worn-out temporary prosthesis.

The dentist has several means available for recording and communicating esthetic information.

Visual aids, such as magnifying glasses, are essential to observe teeth and to register tooth colorations and characterizations on the laboratory form (Figure 7.3).

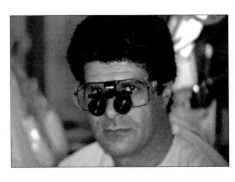

Figure 7.3 Visual aids are essential for observing tooth characteristics.

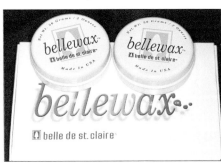
(a)

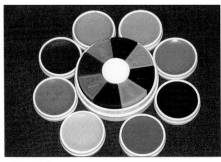
(b)

Figure 7.4 (a) Shaded wax (Bellewax, Belle de St Claire) is often used for esthetic wax-ups. (b) A wide range of colors is provided for a more realistic esthetic result.

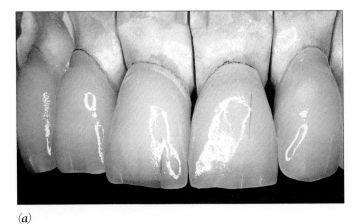
(a)

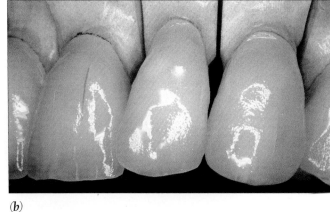
(b)

Figure 7.5 (a, b) Esthetic waxing in the case of a male heavy smoker. Some ceramic stains are also used to create deep characterizations. (Technician: Gérald Ubassy.)

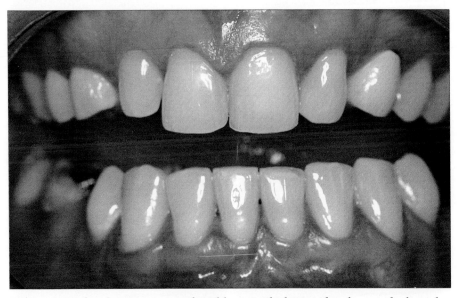

Figure 7.6 A female patient was referred by an orthodontist after the use of a lingual orthodontic appliance technique (see Chapter 8) to improve the form of the maxillary anterior teeth and their protrusion.

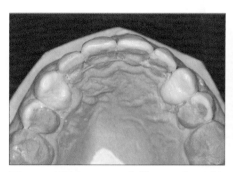 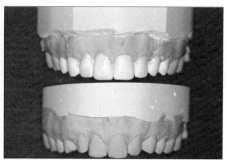

Figures 7.7 *A wax-up (left) is performed on the diagnostic models (right) to visualize the anticipated esthetic outcome and to facilitate clear communication with the patient.*

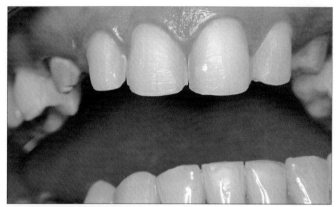

Figure 7.8 *Preparations for laminate veneers on the maxillary incisors. The premolars are prepared for crowns in order to transform them into canines.*

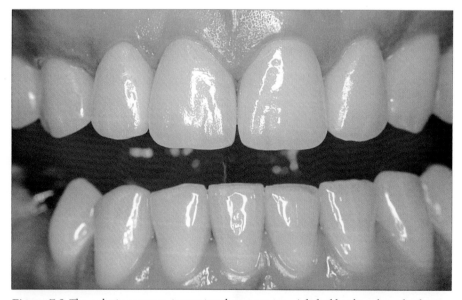

Figure 7.9 *The esthetic outcome, improving the protrusion. A light bleaching has also been performed on the lower arch. All veneers and crowns are Empress (Ivoclar) bonded restorations. Compared with the wax-up, only angles have been rounded to create a softer, more feminine smile. The patient was reluctant to undergo a gingivoplasty of the right canine.*

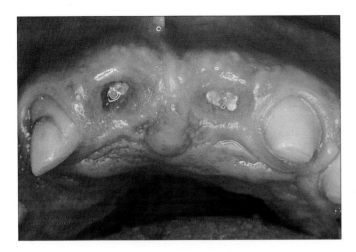

Figure 7.10 After extraction of the periodontally involved central incisors, the sockets are filled with a bone graft (HTR Polymer) and their healing is guided by the temporary bridge.

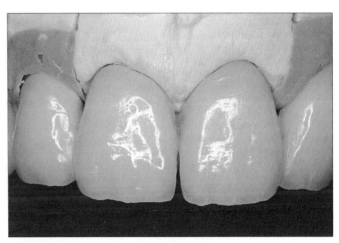

Figure 7.11 Final restoration on the soft tissue model. The silicone index is removable and helps to refine the cervical contours and embrasures. (Ceramist: Gérald Ubassy.)

Impressions

The use of study models is standard practice. The impressions are taken in alginate, and may be duplicated if a model is to be set up (wax-up) or prepared (provisional prosthesis).

Casts

These are cast in extra-hard plaster, carefully dated and mounted on an articulator.

Wax-ups

Wax-ups indicate the final result, and should preferably be produced in colored wax (Figures 7.4–7.7). They can also serve in the preparation of frameworks in heat-pressed ceramics (Empress) (Figures 7.8 and 7.9). Their shape and surface properties can eventually be previewed by coating with a metal spray, resembling gilding. It may be found practical to take an impression from these wax-ups, since plaster models are less fragile.

Silicone index (or template) and soft tissue models

Silicone indexes can often serve to ascertain tissue reduction during tooth preparation. They may not always be easy to reposition, however. They are best produced using addition silicone. Soft-tissue models, also made of silicone, are very useful for the establishment of the cervical contours, the emergence profile and the pontic/ridge interface (Figures 7.10– 7.12). Many technicians find that it is more accurate to use the 'double-model' technique, where the second master model, in plaster, is poured from a silicone impression taken during the try-in of the ceramic restorations (Touati, 1997).

Slides

Good photographic equipment is now considered essential in the dental surgery. Pre-treatment slides are not only of use once treatment has begun: they can serve to motivate patients, or be used for teaching purposes, and so on. In the event of legal action, they constitute vital exhibits in a clinician's defence, showing the initial situation unambiguously in the same way as radiographs.

Photographic images play a major role in communicating esthetic information. Although a slide cannot convey exact color, it can, by providing an image of the teeth next to the shade tab, supply much information to the technician on shape, hue, value, chroma, translucency, texture and luster.

It is always useful for the ceramist to be aware of the shape of the face and smile line. He or she can usefully employ a projector aimed at a dull (e.g. Diastar) screen

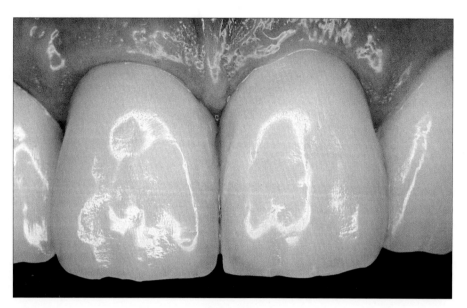

Figure 7.12 *Integration and esthetic outcome three years postoperatively. The interdental papillae are still in place around the ovate pontics, exactly as on the model, despite the fact that the patient was a heavy smoker.*

placed on the work bench. The slides should be viewed under good lighting conditions.

Dental photography

It is impossible to produce a good image without understanding the intellectual factors enabling the observer to interpret it. A photograph is a coded message conveying a visual impression (Bengel, 1990).

The system described below is flexible enough to photograph subjects ranging from the smile down to the distal surface of a single molar.

Dental photography, like photography in general, has become essential to our security as well as an indispensable means of communication (Bouhot, 1994).

Imaging techniques represent one of the major advances made at the close of this century and will certainly be dominant in the foreseeable future; with the current demand for patient awareness and involvement, imaging greatly simplifies dentist–patient relationships.

Basic techniques

Only single lens reflex cameras should be used: with these, viewing and focusing are performed through the same lens that is used for picture-taking.

A fairly long-focus (about 100 to 120 mm for a camera using 35 mm film) 'telephoto' lens is required; the normal focus, giving 'normal eye vision', is the same as the diagonal of the film frame, namely 43 mm (on a 24 mm × 36 mm frame). This focal length enables a sufficient distance to be put between the subject, the teeth and the front element of the lens.

Scales (i.e. the size of the subject as it appears on the negative) should be standardized, usually as follows: ×1/10 (base of the subject: 36 cm, close-up of the face), ×½ (7.2 cm, entire jaw with labial commissures), ×1 (real life size of subject on the negative: 2.6 cm = 4–6 teeth) and ×2 (1.8 cm = 2 teeth).

One or two Nikon 3T diopter supplementary achromatic lenses (4T, 52 mm diameter or 6T, 62 mm diameter) on a telephoto lens, or, failing that, on a standard 50 mm lens, will serve the purpose up to ×½ at relatively low cost. A macro facility on the lens (for close-ups), such as the Foca HR-7, provides an economical solution for going slightly beyond ×1, used with a standard or possibly a telephoto lens.

The specialized but costly Medical Nikkor equipment from Nikon is very easy to use and serves all the above purposes – it is the equipment used to produce the illustrations in this book (Figures 7.13–7.15).

Selecting the shutter speed (exposure time)/aperture combination regulates exposure. With Scialytic lighting, however, a faster shutter speed than 1/125 seconds is

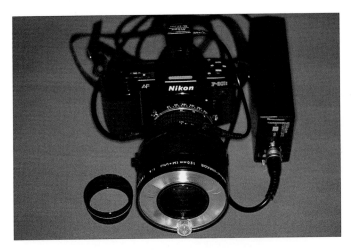

Figure 7.13 The Medical Nikkor camera and equipment.

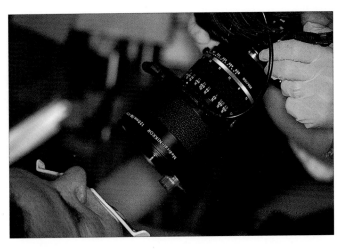

Figure 7.14 A light source may be activated during focusing to see details of the subject more clearly.

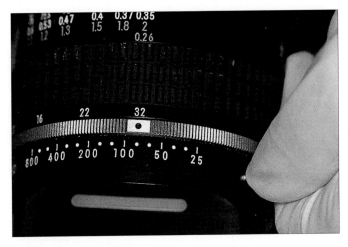

Figure 7.15 By changing the film speed displayed on the ring-flash, the exposure can be altered.

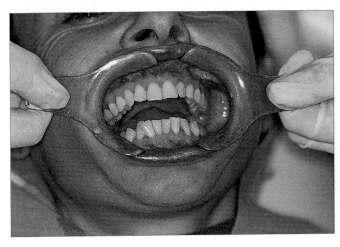

Figure 7.16 Lip retractors (automatic or manual, as shown here) must be used.

essential to avoid blurring: using flash lighting, an exposure time of about 1/1000 second is possible, thus avoiding the effects of movement.

Apart from exposure, the aperture also controls the depth of field, which is greatest when the aperture is stopped down (zone *f*/11–*f*/22).

These two settings work counter to each other, since the highest possible shutter speeds and smallest apertures are desirable, both of which reduce exposure (which is impossible when using Scialytic lighting).

If in doubt over exposure, one should bracket around an estimated value, ½ to 1 stop on either side. For example if the estimated exposure is 1/125 second at *f*/16, then also take shots at *f*/11 and *f*/22 (in practice, the sequence *f*/11, *f*/16 and *f*/22, in this case, is more convenient).

Focusing is difficult with a hand-held camera, especially for very large-scale photographic images at ×1 and ×2. Scale has to be chosen first, followed by focusing, which is controlled, using the viewfinder, by moving the camera/lens/supplementary lens/(possibly) electronic

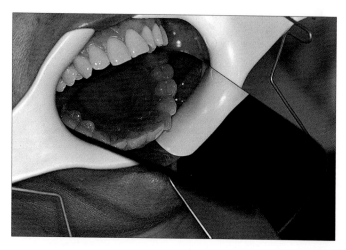

Figure 7.17 Different types of mirrors have to be used in order to see all the aspects of the teeth.

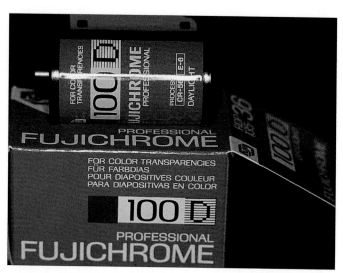

Figure 7.18 A Fuji 100 ISO film has been used to produce most of the photographs in this book.

flash assembly, without touching the focusing ring again. One should freeze as soon as the image is clear in the viewfinder, and hold one's breath when pressing the shutter; this must be done calmly but quickly to retain perfect focus – which is something very easy to lose.

To keep steady, one should stand slightly astride, left foot forward if possible, aiming to lean sideways against the seat or frame. It is advisable to use a handle, or better still a chest support or a monopod, for the camera.

It is essential to use lip retractors and mirrors to achieve the best images (Figures 7.16 and 7.17).

Lighting

Two types of lighting may be used: the customary Scialytic type or a flash. Under these circumstances, an automated system such as the Medical Nikkor best suits the purpose – provided the manufacturer's instructions are followed. The Scialytic lighting used must be a quartz halogen lamp of at least 150 W; a 1/125 second shutter speed can then be achieved at around *f*/16 with supplementary lenses, and 1/60 second at *f*/11 with a macro facility on the lens, thus remaining within the lower tolerance limits.

Exposure must be gauged against the Kodak Neutral Gray Card, placed in front of the mouth and as close as possible to it before focusing. Exposure cannot be measured correctly on a white subject such as teeth. The

Neutral Gray Card is the standard, with 18% reflectivity. Ambient lighting, whether using a flash or Scialytic lighting, has no effect.

Choice of film

For use with a flash, a slow (50 or 100 ISO) daylight-type color reversal film (giving transparencies) is recommended (Figure 7.18). Under Scialytic lighting, 'negative' film (producing prints) is not recommended, and in the case of slides, Scotch 640T film (matched for tungsten lighting) is the most sensitive of its type; 640 ISO may be used and will give total satisfaction. A photographic laboratory offering processing of the greatest possible consistency should be employed.

The use of a mirror, which reduces the amount of light falling on the subject, requires that the aperture be opened up half a stop compared with the setting for a direct shot.

The set-up recommended here is easy to master. However, it is not just the equipment that makes a good photograph.

The esthetic language of photographic images

A focal length of about 100 mm causes a foreshortening effect in the image, but this has no significance in dental photography. It likewise has only a minimal influence on the establishment of perspective.

Depth of field must be as great as possible. This requires the use of apertures of *f*/11 or, ideally, *f*/16. An aperture of *f*/22 should only be used if absolutely necessary, since diffraction problems then begin to reduce image clarity; *f*/32 is barely usable.

Focal point

One must proceed carefully as soon as the depth of the photographic subject cannot be rendered clearly, focusing on the point from which the viewer will begin to interpret the photographic image (the focal point). This would be the eye in the case of a portrait. For a complete dental arch, for example, it would be the canine and the central incisors.

Quality of lighting

The two contrasting types of lighting provide different and mutually contradictory shots of the subject.

- **Standard lighting:** this is the easiest to master, and is even and diffuse, giving flat, shallow, two-dimensional images. However, it does provide a good reconstruction of color shades and surface transparency. It can be obtained by Scialytic lighting used over a wide expanse and placed as close as possible to the focusing line. It can also be obtained using a ring flash or two identical flash units placed symmetrically on either side of the lens.

  The wider the emitting surface, the more broadly will reflection be spread over the surface (although it will be of lower intensity); unfortunately, the opposite effect is more desirable.

  For a special focus, a crossed polarizer lens and a polarized source (a ready-to-use assembly is available from Olympus) eradicate any gloss and reflection, lending images a curious matt appearance but showing up surfaces perfectly.

- **Lighting with shadows:** this requires more expertise. It provides images offering some idea of volume, because of the presence of shadows indicating hollows or adjacent points of relief. This, for example, is the only way of bringing out the minute roughnesses made by a bur. The size and distribution of shadows therefore have a great influence on indicating the subject proportions. They should not be too dense and obtrusive, otherwise they block out the subject. This problem should be dealt with by using either a light source on the left and a reflector on the right, which compensates for and fills in some of the shadows deliberately created by the light source, or two opposing light sources – stronger and fainter on the left and right respectively. The difference between the lighting of light and dark zones should not exceed 1–1½ of the aperture, especially in the case of slides.

It may be asked why one should put the powerful light source on the left. This is largely through force of habit: we write from left to right, which means that light must come from the left so that the shadow of the hand does not fall over the writing (at least in the case of right-handed writers).

The light source must also be situated above the subject, which is the prevailing natural situation, whether considering the sun, the sky, the moon, or, indeed, artificial lighting. Lighting is always located above eye level. A face lit from below will have a strange, indeed sometimes horrific, effect. Natural light comes from above, and predominantly from the left, at an angle of about 45° in northern latitudes. Any lighting other than from the upper left quadrant makes interpretation of the images of the subject very difficult.

Lighting from the left can easily be obtained using Scialytic lighting by positioning the latter to the left of the focusing line; the effect can be monitored through the viewfinder. The problem is more complicated using a flash. First, the effect has to be imagined. When using a ring-type flash made up of four lamps, one must then be able to cut out one or two of these. With a true ring flash, a translucent or opaque mask is placed over the right-hand semicircle. Alternatively, one can use a model combining ring flash and direct flash, with the latter placed to the left. With two flashes, the most powerful is placed to the left and the other, one-quarter or one-half as powerful, to the right, controlled by a remote sensor cell or synchro lead.

General advice on slides

Any important original slide should be duplicated before use. Having ascertained the importance of a subject, it

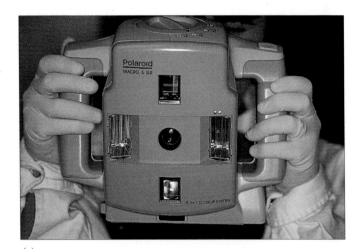

(a)

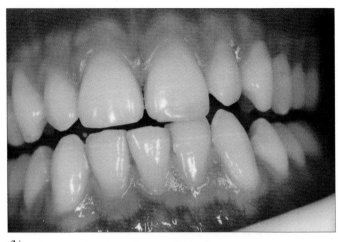

(b)

Figure 7.19 (a) The Polaroid Macro 5 SLR has recently become available, and is especially designed for macrophotography. (b) An Instant image produced by the Polaroid Macro 5 SLR.

is better to take as many shots of it as required, which will prove more economical. (This is especially important for those authors who often send articles for publication in dental journals.)

Slides should subsequently be protected by glass mounting (placing the slide between two thin sheets of glass). The slide must be mounted when it is completely dry, otherwise residual moisture will evaporate as soon as projection begins and condense on the cold glass, making the image dark and diffuse. The slide should be entirely free of dust, otherwise colored interference rings may appear around it. Anti-Newton glass mounts may be used to counteract this, although care must be taken because the special processing of this glass can occasionally result in opacity and diffusion of light, leading to reduced definition when the slides are projected.

For projection using equipment with xenon lamps, it is especially important that slides be mounted in glass, preferably using special protective mounts, since the high temperatures generated by these lamps can cause damage by discoloration, melting of emulsion and so on.

White headings on a blue background can be obtained fairly easily from black typewriter print on white paper, using Polaroid AutoProcess 35 mm PolaBlue film. The same applies to black-on-white diagrams.

Instant photographs

Instant photographs have also been found extremely useful, especially during try-in (Figure 7.19). When passed to the laboratory with felt-tip annotations written directly on the photograph, they promote clear and rapid communication between the dentist and the laboratory. These photographic images can be produced by a Polaroid or intra-oral video camera connected to a video printer (Figures 7.20–7.22).

Shade guides and laboratory prescription forms

Shade guides, although not perfect, remain the most widely used reference point for communicating tooth color between clinicians and ceramists (Figures 7.23 and 7.24). Two types of shade guide exist for every brand of ceramic:

• hue–chroma shade guides;

• mass shade guides (e.g. Chromascop, Ivoclar).

Hue–chroma shade guides, the most widely used of which is the Vita Lumin Vacuum, which includes 15 shades, enable an approximate color shade to be given. For greater accuracy (setting out the color pattern of the tooth to be copied, for example) a mass shade guide system should be employed. Since they are more complete, mass shade guide systems enable the hue, value and chroma to be more accurately measured over all areas of the tooth to be copied. Whereas the method of handling of conven-

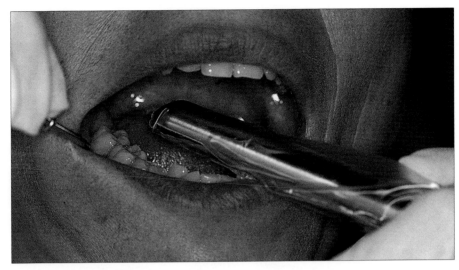

Figure 7.20 *Intra-oral placement of the video camera.*

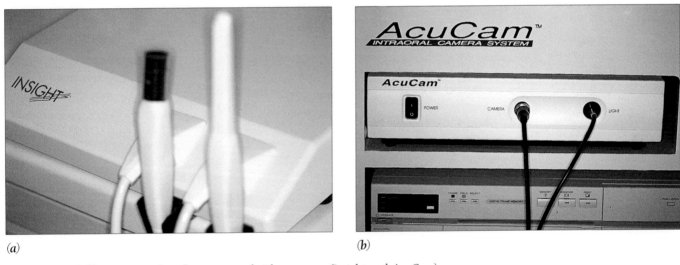

(a)   (b)

Figure 7.21 *(a,b) Two examples of an intra-oral video camera (Insight and AcuCam).*

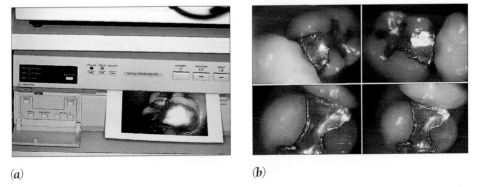

(a)   (b)

Figure 7.22 *(a) The video-printer releasing the instant photographs. (b) Instant photographs taken using an intra-oral camera.*

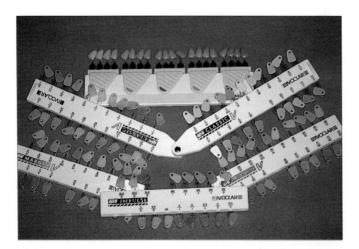

Figure 7.23 Different types of shade guides (e.g. Chromascop, Ivoclar) and mass shade guides.

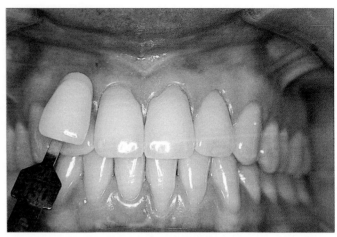

Figure 7.24 Shade guides are the most widely used reference point for communicating tooth color.

tional shade guides is fairly well known, working with a mass shade guide system requires some training on the part of the clinician, who should be particularly well versed in techniques of building up ceramic powders.

The laboratory prescription form should be scrupulously filled out, avoiding unnecessary details. Any references to hue, value and chroma should be noted. Other information regarding surface texture, luster, position of transition angles, and the presence of cracks, fissures and discoloration should also be recorded, to give the ceramist as accurate a guide as possible to the building up of powders. Ideally, this basic means of communication should be drawn up with the ceramist in attendance.

Impression of lips

A recording and silicone reproduction, mounted on an articulator, of the lower face and the patient's lips in particular can be made using the Kalco system (Zermack) (Figure 7.25). This relatively easy-to-use technique serves to convey the patient's smile in a three-dimensional form. It may be likened to that used by ceramists to make silicone copies of the patient's gums on a plaster cast.

The fact that hard and soft tissue and occlusion can now be reproduced on the laboratory model enables the ceramist to work under optimum conditions and, most importantly, to keep a true image of the actual clinical presentation.

Bite registration

This final aspect does not appear to have a direct bearing on the communication of esthetic information. Occlusal relationships do have a decisive effect on esthetic considerations, however, ranging from occlusal measurements to facial symmetry.

As far as the subject of this book and single ceramic restorations are concerned, registration can generally be taken quite simply, using Moyco waxes. For static occlusal relationships, conditioned low-viscosity silicones in cartridges (Memosil, Heraeus-Kulzer or Regisil, Dentsply-Caulk) are particularly useful (Figure 7.26).

Speaking the same language as the ceramist, based on experience of shared successes and failures, is even more important than means of communication.

While certain objective factors can be conveyed clearly and accurately, subjective concepts require dialogue, consensus, trust, and even complicity between the patient and dentist.

The laboratory technician

Difficulties arise initially from the lack of sustained contact between the technician and the patient, whom he or she never sees in many cases. Hence there is a need for excellent communication between the dental surgery and the prosthetics laboratory: the ceramist

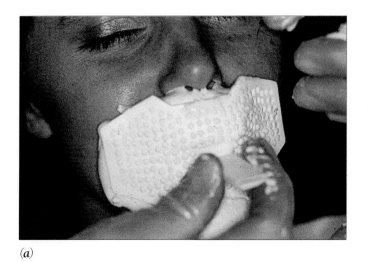

(a)

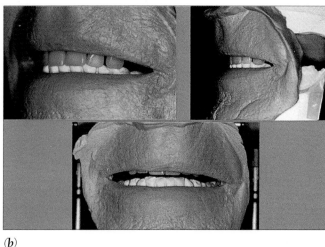

(b)

Figure 7.25 *(**a**) An impression of the lips can re-create the patient's smile three-dimensionally. (**b**) The Kalco system enables the technician to make a realistic molding in silicone of the patient's lips and lower face. (Courtesy of Zermack.)*

should regularly be called to the chairside. This frequently occurs when difficulties arise, so one should not hesitate to introduce the technician to the patient before problems arise. Several top ceramists are accustomed to seeing patients and communicating with them. They tend to make good 'psychologists', and can greatly assist dentist–patient relationships, thus easing the problems of three-way communication. However, it should be borne in mind that most ceramists have now become accustomed to working in isolation, and occasionally find it unsettling to be introduced to the patient. Individual psychological factors need to be taken into account in deciding whether it is right to introduce a third person into the 'special dialogue' between the patient and dentist (Shelby, 1977).

Since the best relationship is one built on trust, the authors do not necessarily consider it a bad thing for the clinician and his or her assistant to be the only ones in direct contact with the patient.

Under these circumstances, the ceramist must have all the information required for each piece of work:

- photographs prior to treatment;

- photographs with shade guide;

- photographs and casts of provisional restorations (even if they are not perfect, at least the ceramist will know what to improve upon);

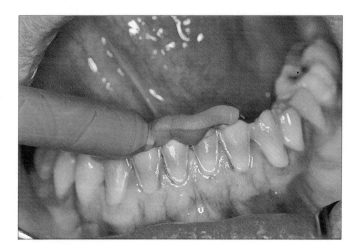

Figure 7.26 *Special low-viscosity, fast-setting silicones are formulated for registration of static interocclusal relationships (Regisil, Dentsply-Caulk is shown here).*

- casts of dental arches prior to preparation;

- casts with tooth-colored wax-up;

- color prescription (hue, value, chroma, etc.);

- indication of translucency and texture;

- accurate bite registration.

The technician often needs to be supplied with one or several 'reference' teeth (see page 137) produced directly in the mouth during the preparation session. These 'provisional references' are produced by the clinician before suppression of the information provided by the adjoining teeth, such as length, position and occlusion, enabling the technician to formulate accurately and effectively

• the new incisal length;

• the new anterior position;

• a bite stop;

• the vertical axial guide line.

These spatial and chromatic points of reference will simplify the ceramist's work considerably. It should be added that one can also use a reference album (Figure 7.27). This is a catalogue consisting of dental photographs with teeth of varying ages, arrangement, shape and distribution of enamel/dentin/cement tissue, etc. Each photograph is given a reference number, so that the dentist can refer the ceramist to that most closely resembling the desired attributes of the prospective prosthesis:

• incisal pattern;

• appearance of cracks;

• general arrangement;

• existence of a 'false root', etc.

This reference album can be put together by the dentist and ceramist for their own internal communication. It will be of considerable help to the technician, giving an example of natural teeth that may serve as an inspiration during work on the ceramic.

The authors have learnt from experience that every great ceramist is above all an excellent 'observer'.

Understanding the problem and visualizing the solution

Communication between the clinician and the patient is a vital element in the esthetic success of prosthetic treat-

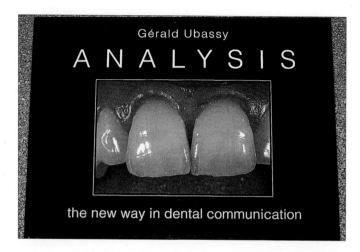

Figure 7.27 *'Analysis', a comprehensive catalogue from Gérald Ubassy, is an excellent source of various shapes, arrangements and characterizations, and serves as a useful reference text for the dentist and ceramist.*

ment. The clinician must understand the aspirations of the patient, who, in turn, has to envisage a technically feasible outcome.

The age of plain oral communication has passed, although it remains a starting point for any prosthetic measures. Computer imaging helps to facilitate the choice of an ideal esthetic solution from a number of alternatives, and serves to guide subsequent wax-ups and temporary prostheses. This computerized process promotes better appraisal of the patient's expectations on the one hand, and a better assessment of technical and therapeutic options on the other.

This process results in informed consent that will be fairer and better balanced. The dentist can always show the patient examples of similar cases, but patients tend to be most concerned with their own individual case, and the computer imaging process refines their esthetic perception of this. Moreover, this technique can also be helpful to the dentist seeking to persuade the patient about alterations in tooth color, shape or position, or in coronal length, bleaching of the opposite arch, etc.

Although of major assistance, this technique does not serve as a three-dimensional prototype. It shows a silhouette of teeth and gingivae, a two-dimensional visualizing of the final image, not of the final prosthesis. For this reason, colored waxes, used for esthetic wax-up (diagnostic or treatment wax-ups), are essential for refining esthetic perceptions. They can subsequently be shot in a position identical to that photographed in the

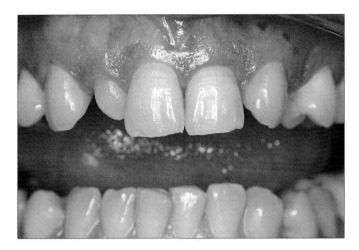

Figure 7.28 *A female patient, in her late 30s, presented with several esthetic problems: a congenitally missing left lateral incisor, a peg-shaped right lateral incisor, and a somewhat dark appearance to the teeth (A3.5 Vita).*

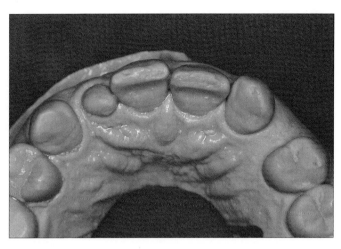

Figure 7.29 *The study model shows the malalignment of the central incisors, and the wide diastema between the left canine and the first bicuspid.*

surgery, then superimposed by computer on intra- and extra-oral clinical images. The image so obtained will replicate options for ceramic prostheses fairly accurately.

It is important at this stage to plan the preparation of provisional restorations. It is only these prostheses that will enable the patient to test the function, phonation, position of the lips and vertical dimension. Esthetic results are inextricably bound up with these other (functional and phonetic) parameters. Longer, shorter, more protruding and more receding teeth, and other similar factors must be tried out in real-life conditions, otherwise ceramic preparations may be jeopardized:

• A metal–ceramic prosthesis built up by segmentation and layering can be neither thinned down nor shortened without severely affecting its esthetic properties, by eliminating effects of the incisal edge or of the enamel surface, for example.

• An entirely ceramic restoration may be difficult to alter, except for minor corrections.

Certain systems, such as IPS Empress, In-Ceram and Duceram-LFC, do, in fact, allow for modification of the surface cosmetic ceramic in theory, but the additional firings rarely give satisfactory results in practice.

Preparation of the final prosthesis without a temporary prosthesis to serve as guide is often fraught with risks.

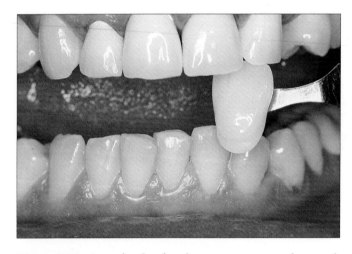

Figure 7.30 *Immediately after the temporization, a photograph of the selected shade guide (A2 Vita) is taken for the technician's use. Home bleaching was administered to maxillary teeth only, hence the darker appearance of mandibular teeth.*

Figures 7.28–7.40 set out a plan for anterior esthetic treatment:

1 Questioning to establish the patient's esthetic aspirations and requirements.

2 Tooth-colored diagnostic waxes set up on study casts.

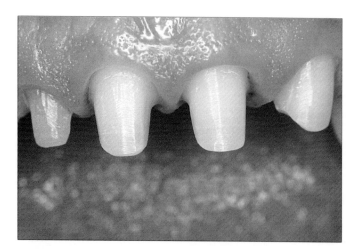

Figure 7.31 *A view of the preparations for the incisors for bonded all-ceramic jacket crowns. Note the rounded angles to minimize the fragility of the ceramic material.*

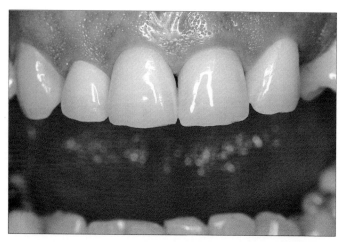

Figure 7.32 *The immediate temporary crowns, showing good healing of the soft tissue. At this stage, the patient was unhappy with the form of the teeth (there was not enough space between them, and the incisors were too square), so a second set of provisional crowns was made.*

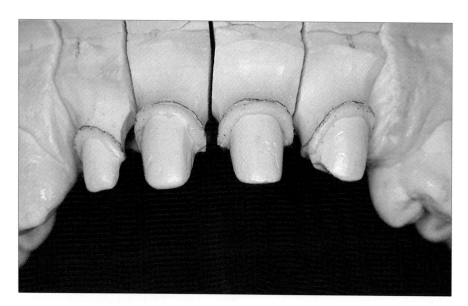

Figure 7.33 *After the impressions are made, an accurate master model is fabricated with well-defined dies.*

3 Computer imaging (Rogé, 1989).

4 Provisional prostheses to test function, phonation and esthetic effect. If the patient is satisfied at this stage, or after a few minor modifications, the final restoration can be fabricated once the ceramicist has been supplied with an impression, and sometimes photographs of the temporary prosthesis.

5 If the patient is in any doubt at all about the provisional prostheses, tooth-colored treatment waxes are set on the master cast (i.e. after taking the definitive

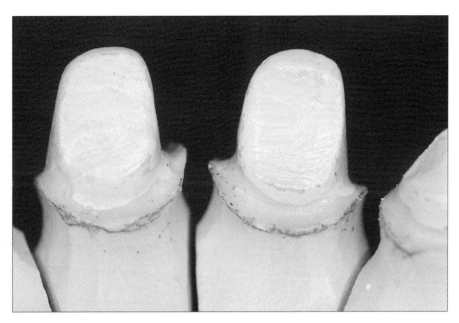

Figure 7.34 *The lingual view of the dies: note the form and width of the deep chamfers (1.3 mm).*

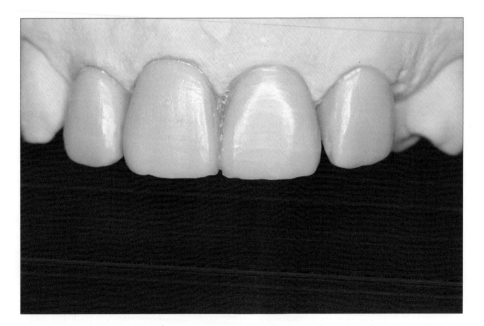

Figure 7.35 *A treatment wax-up (fabricated onto the dies) is altered and carved in the operatory with the patient's input.*

impression), bearing in mind the patient's comments and suggestions.

6 A second set of temporary prostheses is then produced and fixed in place in the mouth for a minimum of 8–15 days to dispel any remaining doubts on behalf of the patient and ensure that his or her family approve of the esthetic design – a factor that should never be underestimated. Acceptance of temporary prostheses is the key to success for esthetic treatment. It gives the patient confidence, and supplies the necessary information to the

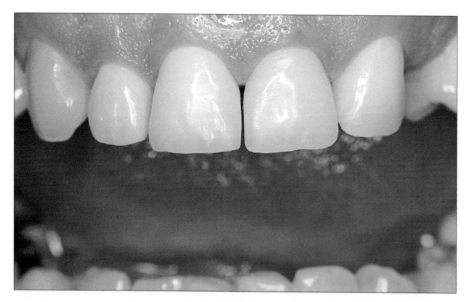

Figure 7.36 *The second temporization: only when the patient is fully satisfied with the esthetic (form, position, color, lip support) and phonetic aspects of the provisional restorations, will the technician fabricate the final restorations.*

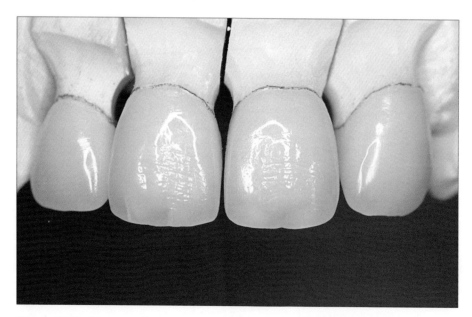

Figure 7.37 *Empress all-ceramic crowns (stratification technique) with excellent surface texture and good opalescence – they fulfilled the patient's requirements. (Ceramist: Gérald Ubassy.)*

ceramist, who can also feel confident about the options adopted. Finally, it relieves the clinician's anxiety at the point of try-in. Our trio is now embarked on the road to success, with a positive attitude and only a shadow of doubt.

7 The definitive prosthesis is prepared. The results will have been revisualized, ensuring a predictable outcome.

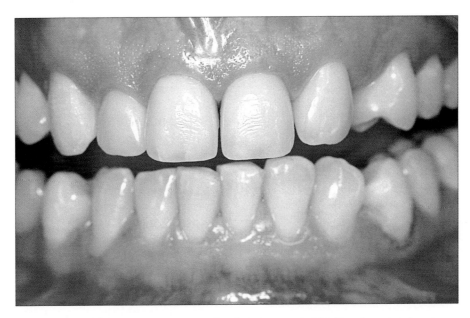

Figure 7.38 *The ceramic crowns are bonded. A ceramic 'chip' has been luted on to the mesial aspect of the left bicuspid to reduce the space. Mandibular teeth have been bleached.*

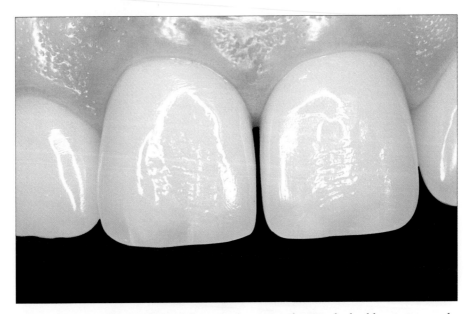

Figure 7.39 *A close-up view of the central incisors, showing the healthy gingivae and the pleasing translucency of the ceramic restorations.*

Temporary 'reference' teeth

For communication and confidence-building, the authors often include a 'temporary reference restoration' technique (see also pages 228–30). A patient

may, for example, require alteration of the front teeth (e.g. worn natural teeth or old prostheses considered esthetically unsatisfactory). Before preparing all teeth of the anterior area according to the indications received from the esthetic questionnaire and/or

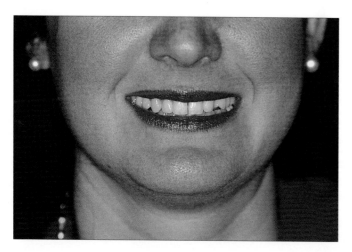

Figure 7.40 *The patient's smile after treatment: despite the absence of the left lateral and the peg-shaped right lateral incisor, the esthetic effect is harmonious and pleasing.*

colored waxes and/or computer imaging, a single, central incisor is prepared. A temporary crown is then fabricated using the adjoining teeth as points of reference to lengthen it, produce some degree of protrusion, alter the color, shape, and so on. The patient can then see these changes, some of which can be measured, such as tooth length. Having been approved, the temporary tooth (or teeth) is sent to the prosthetics laboratory. As well as serving as an accurate bite stop, this tooth will convey invaluable information on the vertical axis, length, width and protrusion (and hence labial support); the additional information from this temporary reference restoration, which is easy to prepare, will boost the patient's confidence, since all the data are accurate and visually controlled by the patient.

References

Bengel W, Modern dental photosysteme mit autofocus funktion. *Quintessenz* 1990; **41**: 1319–20.

Bouhot G, Surprise ... à la lacture d'images photo. *Argus* 1994; No. 198: 51–6.

Brisman AS, Aesthetics: a comparison of dentists' and patients' concepts. *J Am Dent Assoc* 1980; **100**: 345–52.

Dzierpak J, Computer imaging: its practical application. *J Am Dent Assoc* 1991; **122**: 41–4.

Nathanson D, Dental imaging by computer: A look to the future. *J Am Dent Assoc* 1991; **122**: 45–6.

Rogé M, Prévisualisation et esthétique dentaire. *Inf Dent* 1989; **33**: 2951–61.

Shelby DS, Communication with the laboratory technician. In Yamada HN, Grenoble PB (eds) *Dental Porcelain: The State of the Art.* Los Angeles: University of Southern California School of Dentistry, 1977: 269.

Touati B, Excellence with simplicity in aesthetic dentistry. *Pract Periodont Aesthet Dent* 1997; **9**: 806–12.

CHAPTER 8

Shape and Position of Teeth

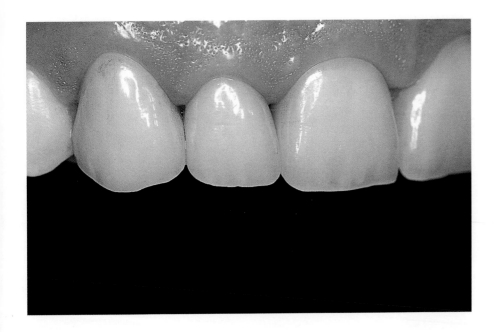

It is frequently easier to visualize and plan the shape and position of teeth to make them appear quite natural than it is to recreate the hue, value, chroma and translucency of live teeth (House, 1939; Hall, 1987). This could be due partly to the inadequacy of speech to express and convey color and partly to the blocking of light transmission by metal frameworks and layers of opaque ceramics – or traditional cements in the case of jacket crowns. Dental morphology should not be relegated to second place, however, and is often prioritized by clinicians.

Tooth shape and position make a major contribution to the smile and the balance and harmony of the face, complying with certain esthetic criteria, which are open to interpretation: a pleasing smile cannot be expressed as an equation! The pursuit of beauty is beset by numerous subjective factors, concepts of which arise from the customs, education and culture of civilizations, races and individuals. However, a pleasing and attractive smile need not comply with the rules of symmetry or any golden proportion. It can combine harmony with asymmetry or balance with irregularity of shape. Above all, it must evoke a feeling of beauty or harmony that helps to bring out the subject's personality as well as looking natural and attractive (Figures 8.1–8.11).

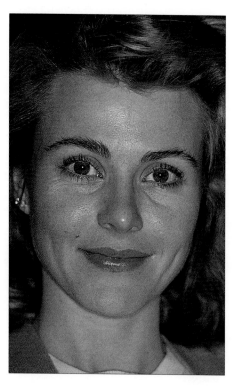

Figure 8.1 *In a certain way a face can seem 'incomplete' without a smile, and this shows how important the teeth are in the perception of the personality of an individual.*

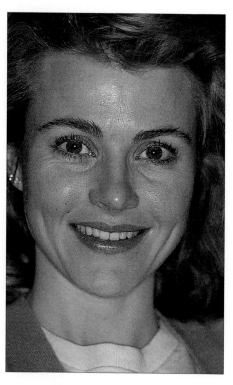

Figure 8.2 *An example of a harmonious teeth arrangement that fully complements the shape of the face.*

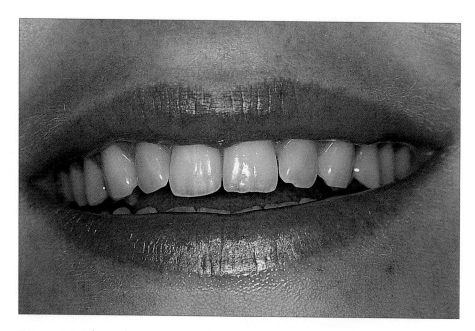

Figure 8.3 *Balance does not necessarily mean symmetry: here the chroma and value change from one tooth to another, and yet the teeth arrangement is pleasing and natural.*

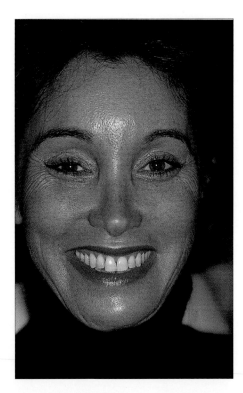

While some constraints do apply to the choice of both tooth shape and spatial arrangement, and certain esthetic laws exist that should be roughly followed, exceptions commonly account for the success of the esthetic effect achieved. The aim must be to achieve an overall pleasing effect, rather than seek 'perfection' in symmetry.

One tooth may well survive intact, and this can serve as a point of reference for the anterior region – or, at least, there may be old casts or photographs to go by. Should these not exist, or should a patient object to the shape of his or her own teeth, the dentist will be obliged to balance the patient's aspirations with the practicalities of occlusal function.

Figure 8.4 A very pleasing smile: the teeth form a natural balance with the lips and the face.

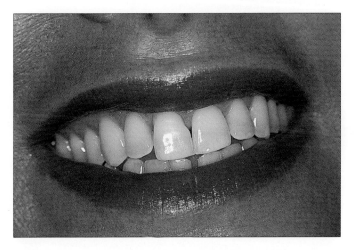

Figure 8.5 The arrangement of teeth looks natural and balanced.

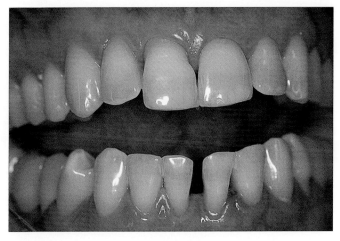

Figure 8.6 In this case a large diastema still existed between the lower central incisors, but the patient was used to it and was insistent upon keeping it.

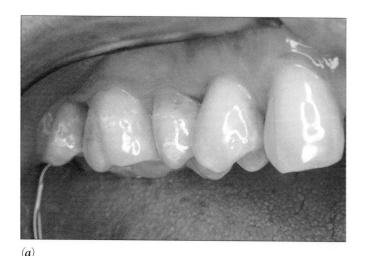

(a)

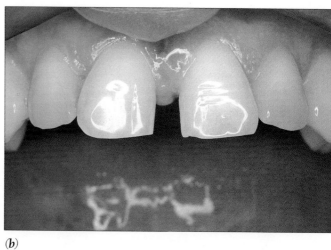

(b)

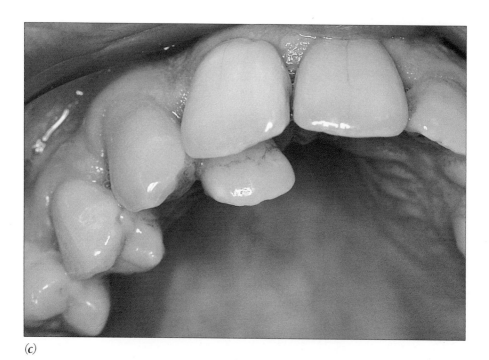

(c)

Figure 8.7 *The diversity of tooth positioning: none of these patients came to the office for a problem related to the shape or position of their teeth.* (**a**) *Second bicuspid is rotated 180°.* (**b**) *Wide diastema between centrals.* (**c**) *Lateral incisor is located in the palate, behind the central incisor.*

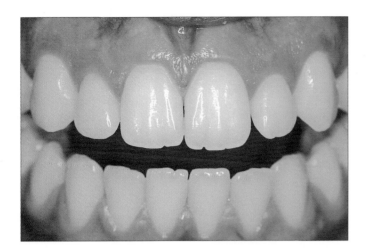

Figure 8.8 *Natural dentition with harmonious form and position of the teeth. Note the higher value and the dominance of the centrals. While the chroma is increasing from the central to the canine, the opalescence effect is decreasing. The position of the teeth is not symmetrical, yet it is pleasing.*

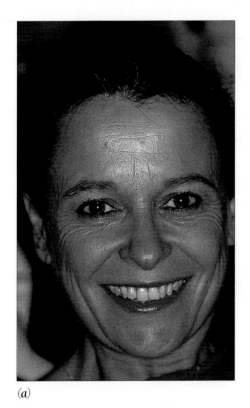

(*a*)

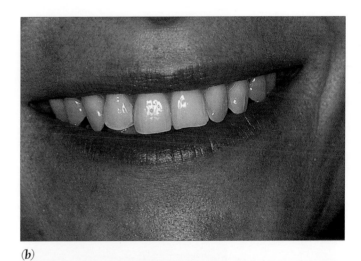

(*b*)

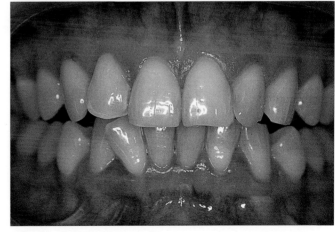

(*c*)

Figure 8.9 (*a–c*) *Another case where the position of the teeth is pleasing and harmonious, yet asymmetrical, with rotations and even malpositions. The smile is natural, however, and reflects well the personality of the patient.*

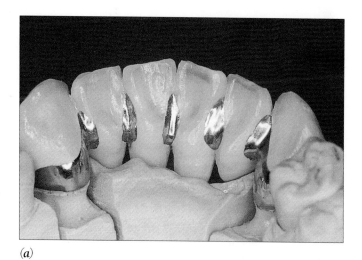

(a)

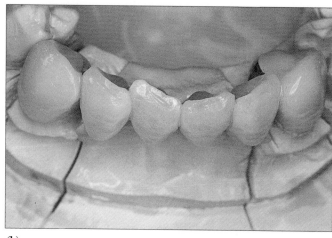

(b)

(c)

Figure 8.10 (**a**) A six-unit bridge on the lower arch to replace the missing incisors. (**a**) Lingual view. (**b**) Incisal view. The span is not long enough to accommodate the incisors, of a normal width, in a good alignment. Modest rotation of the teeth gives a pleasing and natural illusion. (**c**) In the mouth, the metal–ceramic bridge produces an esthetically pleasing result. (Ceramist: Gérald Ubassy.)

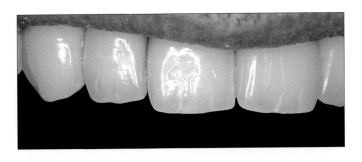

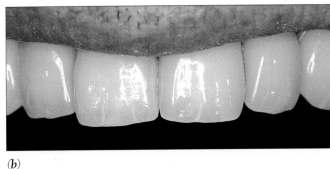

(a)   *(b)*

Figure 8.11 *(a) Full arch rehabilitation by ceramic crowns in a patient with a low lip line. (b) The central incisors are very dominant, and strengthen the smile. Generally speaking, the central incisor represents the personality, the lateral incisor, charm, and the canine, strength. Note the subtle texture and the natural appearance of the incisal edges. (Ceramist: Gérald Ubassy.)*

The proportion and dominance of teeth

First, the dentist must establish the size of the central incisor, which acts as the keystone of the smile line; its measurements will be in proportion to facial width, width of the dental arch, interpupillary distance, and volume of the lips, and hence to the face as a whole. Pre-teenagers who have their permanent incisors but a childish face serve as a good example of the esthetic mismatches encountered. Although many publications on complete dentures are filled with mathematical formulae, the authors advocate determining harmony and balance by eye (Rufenacht, 1990). This sometimes involves relying on one or more temporary prostheses and getting to know the patient. The incisor, in fact, often reflects the patient's true self and expresses his or her personality. Its shape – whether square, triangular or oval – is often related to that of the face seen upside down (chin uppermost), although in the West slim, feminine women with square, masculine teeth can be seen in many a modern magazine. In general, those with thick or thin cortical bones have convex or flat teeth respectively.

The authors share the opinion of Chiche and Pinault (1994) that the central incisor should be predominant. It should be considered perfectly proportioned when its maximum width is roughly 75% of its maximum length (this relationship applies solely to the clinical crown).

The size of lateral incisors and canines will follow from that of the central incisor in view of the fact that an ideal ratio, varying from one school of thought to another, exists between these various types of teeth as viewed from the front. This is the famous 'golden proportion',

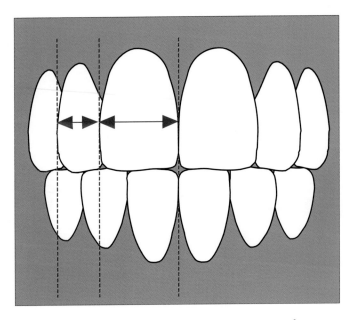

Figure 8.12 *The golden proportion 1.618:1 represents the ratio of the visible part of the central incisor to the visible part of the lateral incisor. This theoretical approach merely represents the dominance of the central over the lateral. The same ratio also applies to the visible part of the lateral to the visible part of the canine.*

which goes back to the architects of Ancient Egypt and their pyramids and to Greek temples such as the Parthenon. It was expressed in numerical form and applied by classical mathematicians such as Euclid and Pythagoras in pursuit of universal divine harmony and balance.

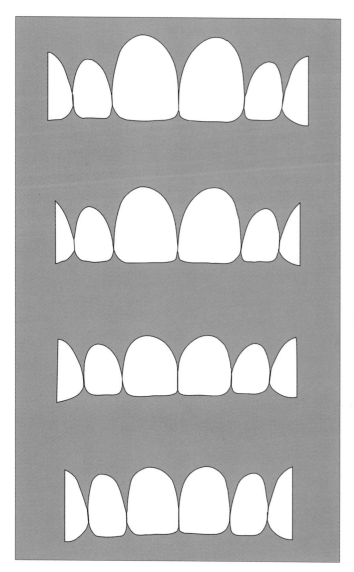

Figure 8.13 As the 'golden proportion' is varied as shown in the diagrams, the ratios between the teeth are changed, thus increasing or decreasing the overall dominance.

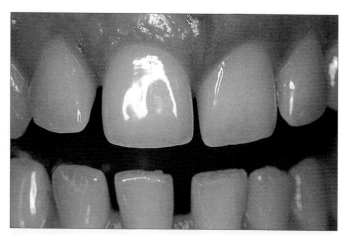

(a)

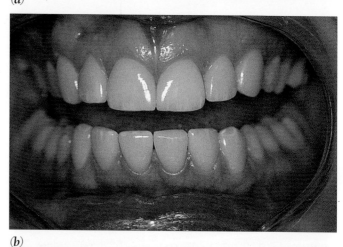

(b)

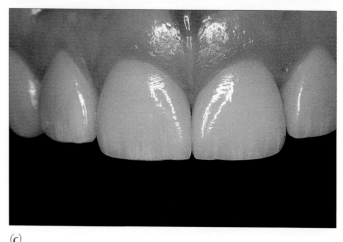

(c)

These laws of proportion have been applied to teeth for very many years in attempts to restore dental harmony and balance to the smile as viewed from the front (central incisors, lateral incisors and the visible portion of canines).

The golden proportion may be expressed as the ratio 1.618:1 (Figure 8.12). If this ratio is applied to the smile made up of the central incisor, lateral incisor and the visible portion of the canine (i.e. about half of the tooth), it will be seen that the central incisor is 62% wider than

Figure 8.14 (a) An example of numerous diastemata. (b) The patient is treated with six upper and six lower ceramic laminate veneers. A few days after the proximal contacts have been re-established, the interdental papillae are reformed. (c) There is a close interaction between teeth and soft-tissues: good proximal surfaces are indispensable to the natural shape of the gingiva.

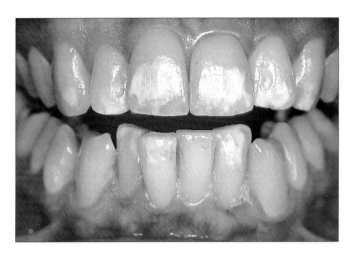

Figure 8.15 *A female patient in her mid-20s has been referred by the endodontist for root resorption of the central incisors that were reimplanted when she was 12: at present these incisors appear slightly too short.*

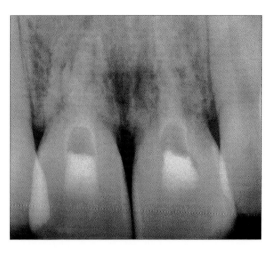

Figure 8.16 *Radiograph of central incisors showing severe root resorption.*

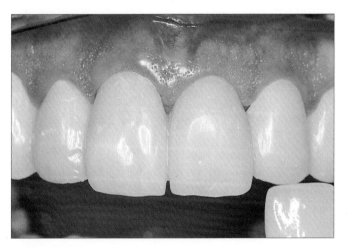

Figure 8.17 *The provisional bridge after extraction of the centrals. Immediate temporization has guided the healing and maturation of the tissue. On the right is the A2 shade tab, for the technician's information. The length of the centrals has been increased.*

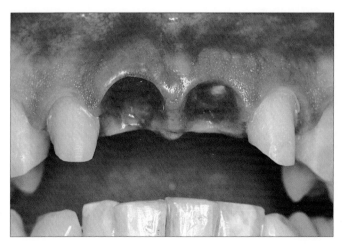

Figure 8.18 *Close-up view of the sockets of the centrals. The interdental papillae are guided and maintained by the morphology of the prosthesis and the excellent oral hygiene (dental floss and chlorhexidine gel).*

the lateral incisor, which in turn is 62% wider than the visible portion of the canine, viewed from the front.

Albers (1992) describes several other 'golden proportions' (Figure 8.13).

that of Plato		1.733	(proportion: 57%)
the 'esthetic norm'	7:5	1.408	(proportion: 71%)
the 'quarter'	4:3	1.333	(proportion: 75%)
the 'human norm'	6:5	1.2	(proportion: 80%)

For the present purposes, it is ratios of 71–75% that best fit the dominant role ascribed here to the central incisor that shapes the central array, backed up by lateral incisors and canines, which add a touch of masculinity or femininity.

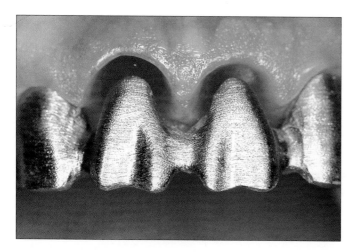

Figure 8.19 *Try-in of the framework. The sockets will be filled with well-polished ceramic. The papillae are three-dimensionally well formed and recaptured.*

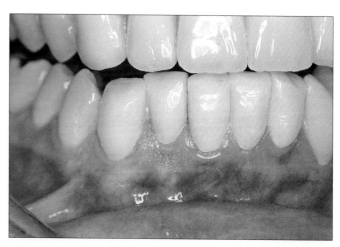

Figure 8.20 *After preparation for the lower laminate veneers, temporary resin restorations are cemented with a non-eugenol cement.*

While serving as a basis for the pursuit of cosmetic success, these values cannot disguise the fact that dental anatomy is three-dimensional, and morphology cannot be reduced to an equation relating height and width. It is only by viewing natural teeth from the front, side and lingual aspects that we can extend our own experience and that of the ceramist and create pleasing teeth.

Teeth form a whole: they do not merely consist of four different surfaces; factors such as transition angles, the shape of the incisal edges (whether straight or curved), the aspect of labial–buccal and lingual surfaces (whether flat, convex or concave), the shape of the neck, rotation or attrition, etc., should also be taken into account when shaping ceramic restorations.

No formula for a successful outcome can be offered in a brief paragraph or two, in view of the high degree of subjectivity and the many interrelated considerations involved.

Failure can be due to a variety of factors: arrangement, shape, volume, texture, hue, value, chroma and translucency. It may thus be claimed that ceramic prosthetics is an area where beauty is indeed sought by applying scientific knowledge but that artistic qualities and a great deal of psychology are also required, both of which must be developed through observation and experience.

While predominance of the central incisors remains one of the prevailing rules for an esthetically pleasing smile, it should nonetheless be viewed with caution, since observation has shown that natural dentitions of this kind are most commonly found in young female patients: increasing the gap between the proportions of the central and lateral incisors and selecting a 75% ratio between the width and length of the central incisor helps to make the smile look younger and more feminine. Therefore we cannot apply this rule to all our patients (Figure 8.14), since the proportions between the general shape of the face, size, sex and teeth have to be maintained (Figures 8.15–8.21).

It is found that pre-teenagers generally tend to have attrition-free central incisors with lily-shaped incisal edge and lobes. The central incisor will characteristically be highly dominant in these subjects irrespective of sex, with the much discussed ratio of 75% or even higher.

Abrasion will occur with age in the following two ways:

- lengthwise initially: the incisal edge wears at varying rates, according to occlusion, acquired habits, diet and parafunction activities; the relationship between width and length alters, with the tooth becoming stubbier;

- wear to the labial–buccal surface, with slight flattening; convexity is toned down and transition angles grow further apart towards proximal surfaces; this attrition will also depend on numerous parameters (Figures 8.22 and 8.23).

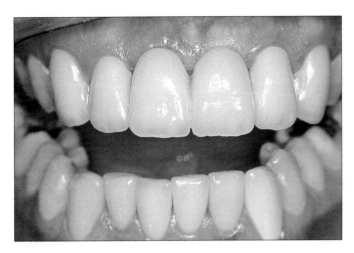

Figure 8.21 *The metal–ceramic maxillary bridge one year post-operatively. Note the harmonious balance between the teeth and the gingivae. There are feldspathic ceramic laminates on the lower anterior teeth, except for a Captek crown on the mandibular left canine. (Ceramist: Serge Tissier.)*

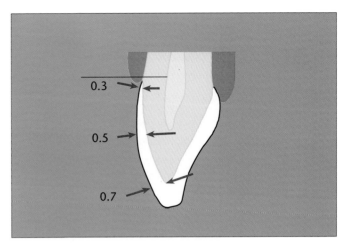

Figure 8.22 *Enamel thickness varies from the CEJ to the incisal edge, and decreases with age. This is an important consideration in the preparation of laminate veneers.*

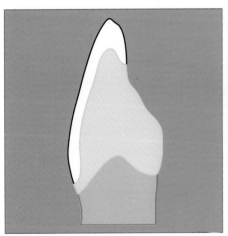

(a)

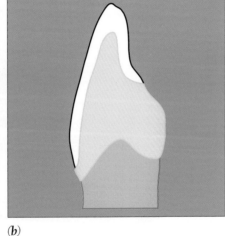

(b)

Figure 8.23 *Before preparing the tooth, the thickness of the enamel must be assessed. Where a ceramic laminate (**a**) or a three-quarters ceramic crown (**b**) is to be prepared, it is crucial that the margin be located in the enamel and, if possible, enamel should remain on most of the surface, so that the bond will be strong and reliable.*

It is interesting to note that the proportions of clinical crowns change completely when one is dealing with those over 50 years old.

The following conclusions may be drawn from this set of considerations.

1 The drop in volume between the central and lateral incisors should be increased and the width-to-length ratio of the central incisor should be roughly 75% when one is seeking to promote a youthful smile; this arrangement will lead to a child-like and rather feminine appearance.

2 Proportions should be reviewed according to the effect desired in the case of mature male patients. The role played by the position of convexities and

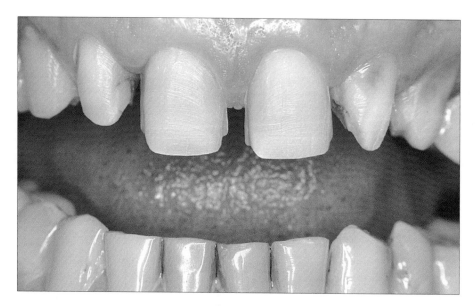

Figure 8.24 *A male patient in his 40s, with diastemata between his incisors and with severe abfractions on the left lateral and canine. Teeth were prepared for ceramic laminate veneers at the patient's request.*

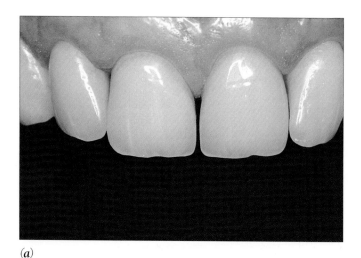

(a)

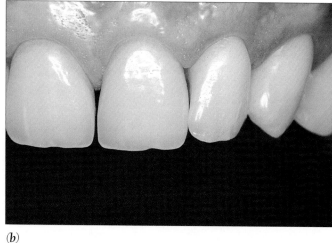

(b)

Figure 8.25 *(a,b) The natural esthetic result, with Empress (Ivoclar) ceramic laminates, exhibiting good opalescence and a natural position of the laterals. The patient requested to retain a small diastema between the centrals to avoid a sudden dramatic change in his smile.*

transition angles should be stressed at this point, since a tooth can be made to appear finer or, conversely, wider while still maintaining the same proportions (Figures 8.24–8.27).

3 The shape, length and volume of lips when active and at rest also play an important part in assessing tooth shape and spatial arrangement. Occlusion permitting, it is occasionally necessary to lengthen clinical crowns considerably so that the teeth can be seen. A balance has to be established between the length of the lipline when smiling and when at rest, which could mean a fundamental alteration in proportions.

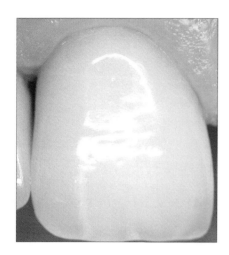

Figure 8.26 Close-up of the right central incisor.

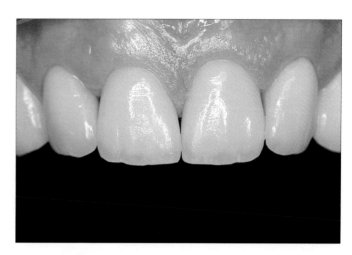

Figure 8.27 After 18 months, the patient asked for central incisors without any space once his acquaintances became used to the reduced diastema.

4 Occlusal analysis must inevitably precede any attempt to alter the length or anatomy of lingual surfaces or the incisal edge.

5 Elsewhere, as in the case of a gummy smile, other steps need to be taken; this time the relationship between the gingival line, smile line and that of the incisal edges needs to be considered.

For the purposes of everyday practice, esthetics are not necessarily synonymous with either youthfulness or rejuvenation.

Finally, the influence of teeth on phonation should not be underestimated; in the absence of any guides as to tooth shape, pronunciation of certain syllables also gives valuable hints as to the furthermost point of the free edge of the upper central incisors. Thus the incisal edge of the central incisor rests on the lower lip, which it brushes, in pronouncing the letter 'F'. Excessive protrusion of the incisal edge of the upper incisors will be deduced if the letter 'S' is pronounced with a lisp.

In practice, tooth shape and position will be planned on colored diagnostic waxes or composite mock-ups after discussion with the patient and analysis of his or her personality and physical characteristics (Portalier, 1996).

These wax-ups are first set up on study casts. However, it is via temporary prostheses that the cosmetic concept is put to the test for a number of days or weeks. The temporary prosthesis, which may be altered by the addition of resin or composite, will act as a pilot model, and its importance should never be underestimated.

All the care devoted to determining the shape and position of teeth will be rewarded in terms of successful prosthetic treatment, good periodontal condition and normal phonation.

> 'Golden rules' are only rough guides, and should never be applied without taking account of the subject's sex, gingival line, lip shape and position, as well as general physical type and age group (Levine, 1978).

CASE PRESENTATION: 1

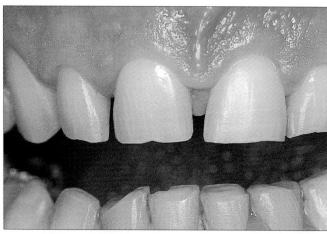

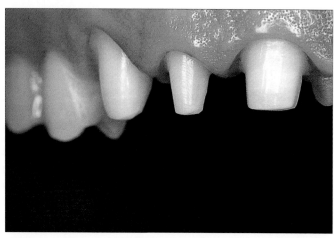

Figure 8.28 (*a*) *A male in his 50s presents after orthodontic treatment for restoration of the upper incisors and canines – the teeth have to be lengthened and brightened, and the diastemata slightly closed.*

(*b*) *Preparations for crowns.*

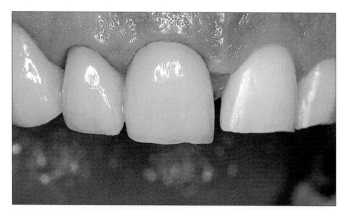

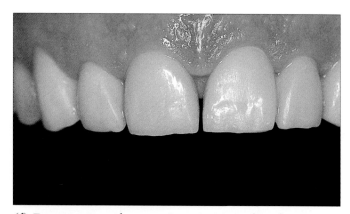

(*c*) *Only one side is prepared and temporized in order to assess precisely the amount of lengthening required, and the position of the incisal edge: the left side is the reference.*

(*d*) *Temporization – the composite resin crowns show the new shape derived from the wax-up.*

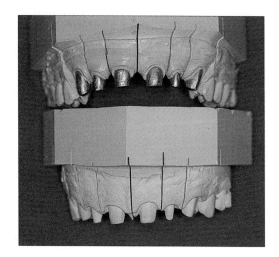

(*e*) *Two laboratory models will be fabricated. The first one is for the fabrication of the frameworks and biscuit ceramic: the plaster is ground around the dies to facilitate the waxing. The second model is poured from one impression taken after the try-in of the frame and biscuit porcelain: it will allow fabrication of an ideal emergence profile. No soft-tissue silicone is used in this technique.*

(contd)

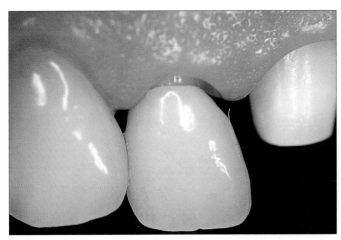

(f) *The emergence profile is carefully recreated thanks to the second plaster model.*

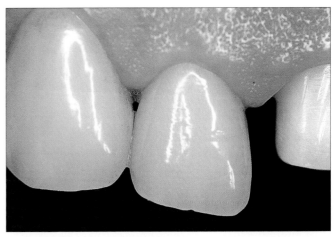

(g) *The proximal surfaces appear natural, and offer excellent support to soft tissues and papillae.*

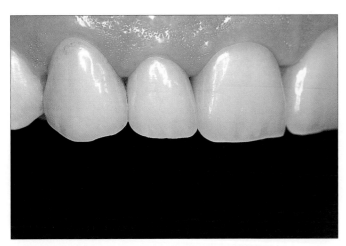

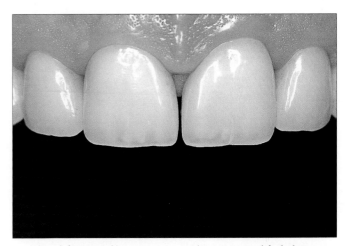

(h,i) *The esthetic outcome after bonding the metal–ceramic (with vertically reduced framework) restorations with a resin-modified glass-ionomer cement. There is good gingival integration, and harmonious shapes.*

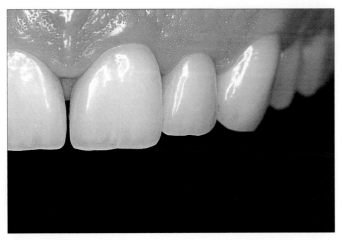

(j) *The esthetic outcome.*

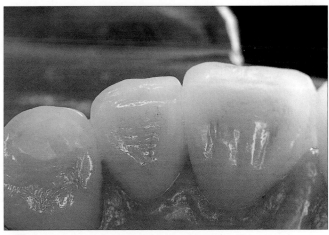

(k) *No metal framework is visible on the lingual aspect thanks to the peripheral ceramic butt-joint margin. (Ceramist: JM Etienne.)*

Esthetics and orthodontics

Prosthetic techniques varying in complexity and involving one or more specialists are usually required to correct the shape, color and position of the teeth. Of these, orthodontics remains the chosen technique when esthetic and functional inadequacies arise from tooth position or intermaxillary relationships. Both function and a harmonious smile can be restored and the profile transformed without tissue damage using these techniques. The application of these non-invasive and conservative types of treatment has become widespread because of their suitability for adults of all ages as well as children.

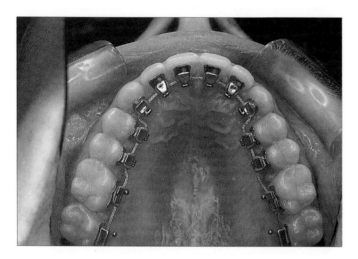

Figure 8.29 *The placing of orthodontic brackets on the inner tooth surfaces meant that they were virtually out of sight – this technique became known as 'lingual orthodontics'.*

Thus, in a book on current methods of recreating a pleasing smile, it is hardly possible not to mention the latest developments in adult orthodontics, especially those involving lingual techniques. The clinical details of pre-prosthetic orthodontics could easily fill an entire chapter. Instead, the following section is a brief summary of the principal benefits and potential of lingual orthodontics for adults.

Lingual orthodontics

The decision to have teeth straightened is a major one for any adult patient aware of the benefits to be had from a pleasing smile in everyday life. But how many adults have felt unable to satisfy this deep desire for fear of displaying an unattractive-looking device for a number of months?

In the mid-1970s, following developments in bonding techniques, the American orthodontist Craven Kurz had the idea of placing the orthodontic brackets on the inner tooth surfaces (those in contact with the tongue). The appliances were virtually invisible. This technique came to be known as lingual orthodontics (Figure 8.29). Just as in fixed labiobuccal techniques, the appliance is basically made up of bonded metal brackets and a wire passing through the slot of the brackets, held in place by ligatures. Lingual orthodontics has not been widely practised, and remains difficult to perform, although introduced over 15 years ago.

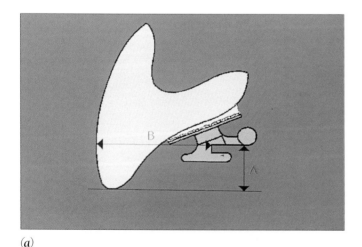

(a)

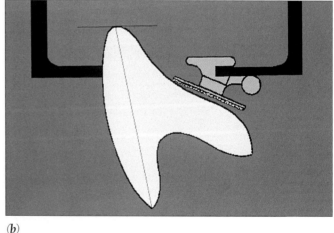

(b)

Figure 8.30 (a) *The tooth is directed into the space, and the bracket is bonded by taking into account the height from the edge and the distance from the labial surface, as measured by callipers* (b).

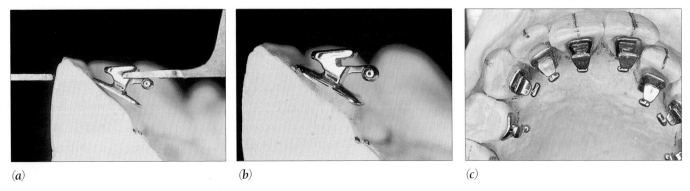

(a)   (b)   (c)

Figure 8.31 (a,b) *The gap between the lingual surface and the bracket base is filled with composite.* *(c)* *The composite pads vary in thickness according to lingual anatomic variations. (Courtesy of Dr D Fillion.)*

Difficulties encountered

Access and visibility are limited, and unusual operating positions are required, although all the skill associated with traditional labiobuccal techniques can be acquired by proper training. The main difficulty lies in positioning the brackets accurately. Two factors have a direct influence on the eventual tooth position in fixed orthodontics.

1 *The archwire*, owing to its elastic properties, will encompass the teeth and bring them into the best position; the eventual shape of the dental arch will match that of the archwire.

2 *The brackets* serve as a link between the archwire and the tooth. The position of the slot through which the archwire passes, its height in relation to the vertical axis of the crown, and its curvature in relation to the tangent of the labiobuccal surface (the principle of torque) are all set individually by the practitioner to optimize the final position of each tooth (Figure 8.30).

Correct placement of brackets on the lingual surfaces (Figures 8.30 and 8.31)

Using indirect bonding techniques, with a plaster cast and an orthodontic orientation device (TARG-ORMCO-USA), each tooth is directed into the space it is to occupy by the end of the treatment. A bracket is then temporarily bonded onto the plaster at a given height as measured from the occlusal edge. In view of the anatomical variations of lingual surfaces and the discrepancies in vestibulolingual volume in the front teeth, it is necessary to make up for such differences in shape and width by adapting the depth of composite used to bond the brackets so as to obtain a perfectly smooth progression of the labiobuccal surfaces of the front teeth without having to add numerous horizontal bends on the arch. Bends will still remain between the canine and the first premolar as well as the second premolar and molar. A silicone transfer agent is then used to bond all these to the patient's teeth in one sitting, in the same position as the plaster cast. The quality of the end result largely depends on how accurately this stage of the work has been carried out.

From the patient's point of view, the indisputable advantage of lingual orthodontics is that the appliance remains concealed. The presence of brackets in the oral cavity requires a 15–30-day adaptation period, however, marked by temporary irritation of the tongue, difficulties in masticating (depending on the degree of overbite) and a slight alteration in the speech. Studies have shown that the patient could lose weight over the first few weeks, but would regain normal weight during the second month of treatment.

Methods of treatment

As far as treatment programmes are concerned, these do not differ from those of traditional fixed orthodontic techniques – although they are adapted to the fact that lingual orthodontics involves mainly adult patients, implying a lower incidence of extraction, an increase in treatment with interproximal enamel reduction and, occasionally, the need for corrective surgery to the jaws.

The following three clinical cases illustrate the three types of treatment most frequently applied in adults (Figures 8.32–8.34).

CASE PRESENTATION: 2

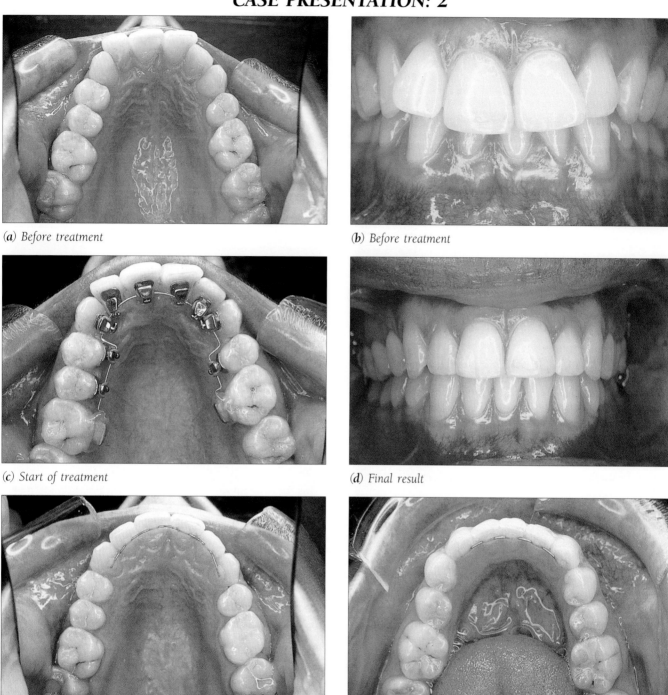

(**a**) Before treatment

(**b**) Before treatment

(**c**) Start of treatment

(**d**) Final result

(**e,f**) Archwires bonded to the lingual surfaces of the canine and incisors provide stabilization

Figure 8.32 (**a–f**) In this young female patient, the position of the four upper incisors was not esthetically pleasing, with considerable overlapping of the lower teeth. The lower incisor region was crowded, despite a missing incisor. The upper incisors could be straightened and the discrepancy in volume due to the missing lower incisor could be reduced by interproximal enamel reduction, thus producing class I canine and molar occlusion without any overjet of the dental arches. Treatment was of 12 months duration. Archwires bonded to the lingual surfaces of canines and incisors provided stabilization. (Case courtesy of Dr D Fillion.)

CASE PRESENTATION: 3

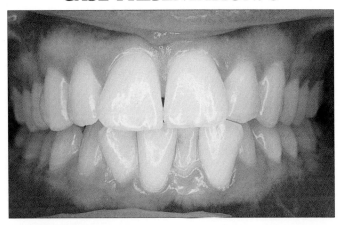

(**a**) Before treatment

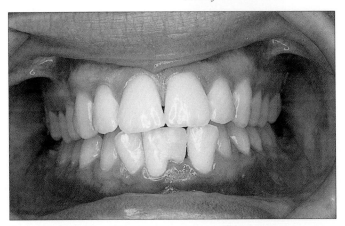

(**b**) Post extraction of lower incisor

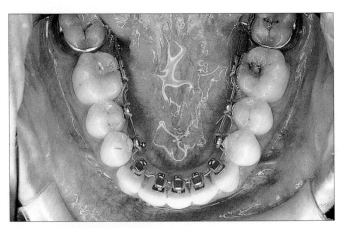

(**c**) Reduction of upper central incisors

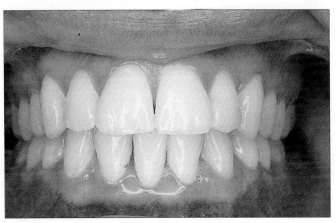

(**d**) Final result

Figure 8.33 (a–d) *The front view of a young female patient shows pronounced crowding of the lower incisors and very bulky upper central incisors. The patient exhibited slight protrusion of the lower jaw and a slightly protruding chin. To avoid any risk of aggravating this tendency (class III) when straightening the lower incisors, even after enamel reduction, the treatment program included extraction of a lower incisor. The upper central incisors were reduced to make up for this loss in tooth volume, which served to make the width of the four upper incisors match. Treatment was of 15 months duration. (Case courtesy of Dr D Fillion.)*

CASE PRESENTATION: 4

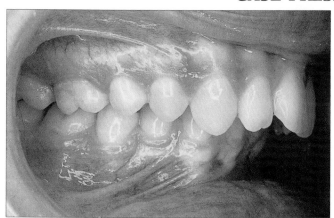

(**a**) Before treatment

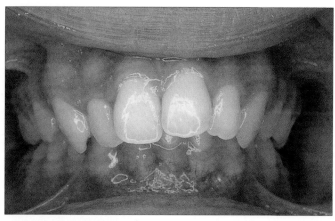

(**b**) Before treatment

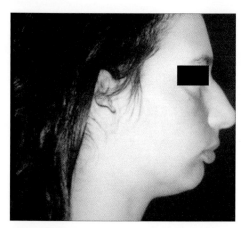

(**c**) Profile before treatment

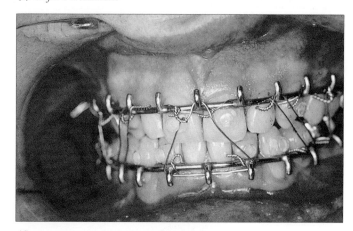

(**d**) During surgery: setting of surgical wires

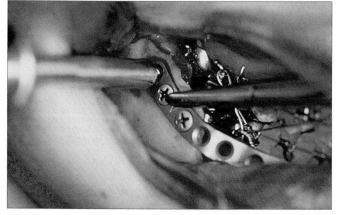

(**e**) During surgery: setting of rigid fixations

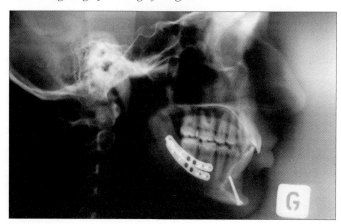

(**f**) Radiograph after treatment

Figure 8.34 (**a–i**) This female patient could no longer accept the major discrepancy between the two dental arches due to inadequate development of the lower jaw. Pronounced overjet and deepbite could be observed. The unsatisfactory position of the lower lip with the upper incisors resting on it could also be seen on the profile. Orthodontics alone could not correct the orthopedic discrepancy in this case, and so surgery to the lower jaw was required. Straightening of the arches and postoperative coordination was achieved by a stage of orthodontic treatment prior to surgery. Surgical procedures involved advancing and

(contd)

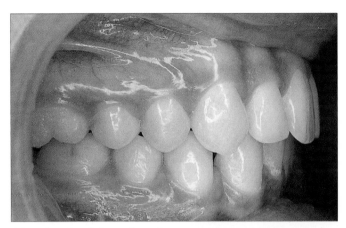

(**g**) *Right side of the arches after treatment*

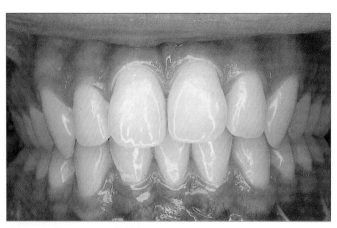

(**h**) *Outcome after treatment*

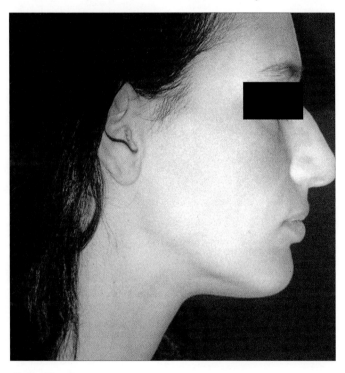

(**i**) *Profile after treatment*

lowering the mandible and genioplasty. There was no rigid, postoperative intermaxillary fixation. The surgeon (JJ Tulasne, Paris) used miniature stabilization devices, enabling the bone segments to be fixed so that intermaxillary fixation by surgical archwires applied during surgery to ensure that occlusion relationships were accurate could be disposed of once the operation was over. The postoperative period was then simpler and the patient's comfort greatly improved. She was able to communicate and eat almost normally. After surgery, occlusion was dealt with by a 4–6-month stage of orthodontic treatment, making the total duration of treatment 18 months. (Case courtesy of Dr D Fillion.)

Summary

Because of lingual orthodontics, adults no longer have any reason to fear the ugly look of orthodontic appliances: any adult patient can be treated, even those whose careers bring them face to face with the public. With the use of lingual orthodontic and miniature stabilization devices, orthodontic surgery is better adapted to patients, and it fits in perfectly with their social life. Lingual brackets remain the only completely esthetically acceptable solution for adult patients anxious to enhance their looks and occlusal function. They help in the pursuit of a pleasant smile and hence of a greater sense of well-being.

References

Albers H, Esthetic treatment planning. *Adept Report* 1992; **3**:45–52.

Chiche G, Pinault A, *Esthetics of Anterior Fixed Prosthodontics.* Chicago:Quintessence, 1994.

Hall WR, *Shapes and Sizes of Teeth from American System of Dentistry.* Philadelphia: Lea Brothers, 1987: 971.

House MM, Loop JL, *Form and Color Harmony in the Dental Art.* Whittier, CN: MM House, 1939.

Levine EL, Aesthetics and the golden proportion. *J Prosthet Dent* 1973; **29**:358.

Portalier L, Diagnostic use of composite in anterior aesthetics. *Pract Periodont Aesthet Dent* 1996; **8**:643–52.

Rufenacht C, *Morphopsychology and Aesthetics: Fundamentals of Aesthetics.* Chicago: Quintessence, 1990: 59.

Touati B, Etienne J-M, Improved shape and emergence profile in an extensive ceramic rehabilitation. *Pract Periodont Aesthet Dent* 1998; **10**:129–35.

CHAPTER 9

Ceramic Laminate Veneers

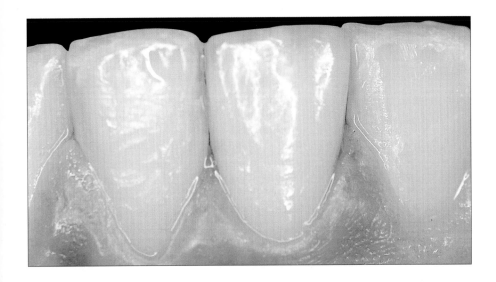

The advent of new tooth-colored restorative materials within the last three decades has caused a stronger customer orientation towards esthetic dentistry. The 1980s have witnessed a surge in various modern techniques to make the smile more esthetically pleasing. A study of the earlier literature will reveal, however, that as early as 1886 Land had produced an all-ceramic jacket crown over a platinum foil. A few years later, the first ceramic inlays and onlays were developed. In 1877, Chapple introduced a bleaching technique for discolored teeth. In the 1930s, Charles Pincus used a unique procedure to improve the smile of certain Hollywood actors without being invasive (Pincus, 1938). He was able to enhance or actually transform their dental appearance for filming purposes by applying fine temporary resin facings; later on he used ceramic facings fired in air and applied to teeth without prior preparation. Although esthetically pleasing, this cosmetic technique had many limitations, primarily the lack of permanent retention. It gradually fell into disuse, like other similar techniques around the same time.

It was only through a combination of the following three discoveries that the concept of modern ceramic laminate veneers has evolved:

* etching of the enamel by Buonocore (1955);

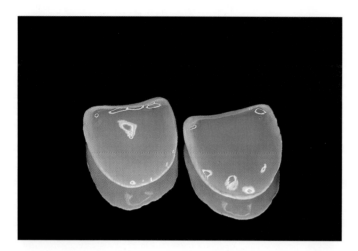

Figure 9.1 Etching the inner surface of ceramic veneers using hydrofluoric acid.

• introduction of BIS-GMA resins by Bowen in the 1960s, and the subsequent development of dental composites;

• ceramic surface treatment and bonding conceived by Rochette in 1973 and fully documented by Horn (1983) and Calamia and Simonsen (1984).

Apart from these three main discoveries, other equally important advances were made, enabling these fine ceramic structures to be luted over the dental enamel:

• the continuous evolution of laboratory techniques, including:

  – the documentation by Greggs (1984) of the build-up of ceramic laminate veneers on a platinum matrix;
  – the development of refractory investments for ceramics, allowing a higher degree of precision;
  – the creation of new ceramics with ever-improving mechanical, optical and esthetic properties;

• improvement of the ceramic surface treatment with the development of acid gels suited to the ceramics used (Figure 9.1) and more effective, stable silane coupling agents that were easier to use;

• improvement of adhesion to tooth structure with the advances made in enamel and dentin bonding systems;

• improvement of composites, used for veneer bonding:
  – the first light-cured composites, which, since the 1980s, have helped simplify bonding procedures;
  – use of the first dual-cure composite resin during the 1980s;
  – the current availability of composite cements, uniquely suitable for bonding fine restorations;

• the evolution of clinical procedures, with:
  – the introduction of the concept of preparation for veneers and special diamond instrument kits (the shape and grain of these facilitate veneer preparations);
  – establishment of preparation procedures (general design, position and configuration of margins, minimum occlusal clearance allowable, etc.): these have now been properly established for different clinical circumstances and for the ceramic material selected;
  – establishment of procedures for optimal bonding.

All these advances and improvements in technology, occuring in rapid succession, have contributed to making the use of laminate veneers a reliable modern technique. According to a statistical study drawn up by Peter Schärer (personal communication) of Zürich University, the failure rate is not more than 5% in 5 years, i.e. very similar to that of highly popular metal–ceramics. Clinical experience obtained in the field of ceramic laminate veneers over the past 10 years confirms this low failure rate. However, were esthetic shortcomings to be included in the figures, the rate would certainly be higher.

The ceramic laminate veneer is without a doubt the ceramic restoration that best serves to reproduce the capacity for light transmission of natural teeth, although this can be altered by such factors as the color of the underlying structure, choice of cement, and depth of preparation. The choice of ceramic preparation and bonding composites is governed by the following objectives:

• enhancing mechanical properties;

• improving biocompatibility;

• maximizing optical properties;

• improving longevity.

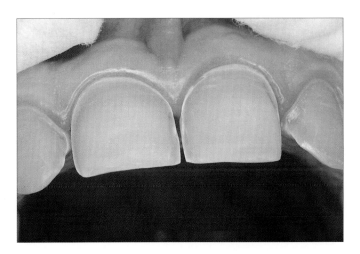

Figure 9.2 Very fine veneer preparations without overlaying the incisal edge. All margins are kept within the enamel. This is a 'contact lens' type of preparation.

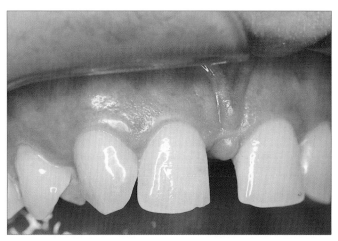

Figure 9.3 In this patient, with a congenitally missing lateral, the canine can be converted into a lateral incisor by means of a ceramic laminate veneer.

Benefits and shortcomings of ceramic laminate veneers

For the most part, this prosthetic treatment consists of replacing the visible portion of the dental enamel with a ceramic substitute, intimately bonded to the tooth surface, yielding optical, mechanical and biological properties closely resembling those of the natural enamel. This 'substitute enamel' now brings us closer to achieving the goal of prosthodontics – to replace defective human enamel with bonded artificial enamel.

Benefits

Minimally invasive treatment method
This treatment method utilizes minimal tooth preparation, keeping clear of the gingival margins, mainly confined within the dental enamel, thus respecting mechanical, periodontal, functional and esthetic principles. It preserves soft tissue integrity, which constitutes one of the main advantages of this technique (Figure 9.2).

Shape, position and surface appearance
The shape or position of natural teeth can be afflicted with functional or esthetic problems. However, with ceramic laminate veneers, one can, for example, change a canine into a lateral incisor (Figures 9.3–9.5). One can also adjust tooth length, seeking to observe the laws of proportion

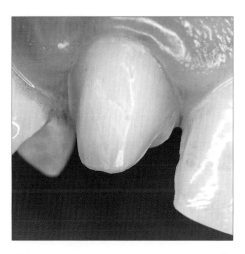

Figure 9.4 A more extensive preparation is required in this case, approaching that for a ceramic three-quarters crown.

(while respecting the requirements of occlusion), which will often indicate a lengthening of the two central incisors. Correct alignment can easily be obtained by well-designed preparation in cases of slight malposition. One of the major advantages of ceramic laminate veneers is that the surface texture can be transformed permanently and elegantly, eliminating any dysplasia or dystrophy of the enamel. It is here, above all, that use of 'substitute enamel' is the best technique, since an unhealthy tissue is

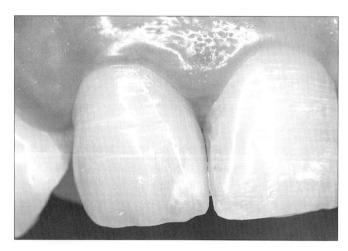

Figure 9.5 A ceramic veneer bonded to the canine shown in Figure 9.4. Mastering the skill of lamination and faithful reproduction of surface properties can lend a highly natural look. (Ceramist: JP Levot.)

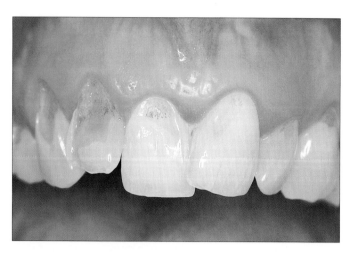

Figure 9.6 Considerable loss of enamel has occurred in this female patient suffering from anorexia nervosa.

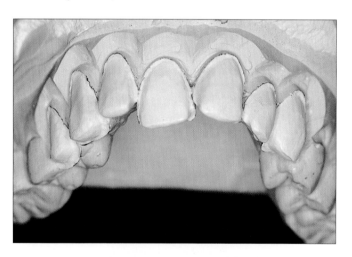

Figure 9.7 View of veneer preparations on the cast.

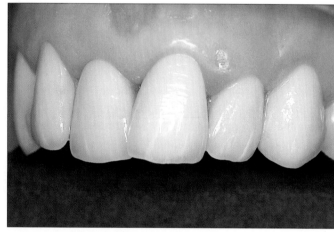

Figure 9.8 The ceramic veneers serve as an enamel substitute and an elegant means of rectifying many instances of dystrophy of the enamel (Empress cosmetic veneer). (Ceramist: Laboratory GH.)

being replaced by an artificial one, but without damaging the healthy underlying tissue (Figures 9.6–9.8).

Color

When bleaching techniques become ineffective, laminate veneers may be the treatment of choice for improving or changing natural tooth color. However, these changes do have their limits, depending on the color of the underlying tooth, the choice of ceramic, the

bonding cement used, and the depth of preparation (Figures 9.9 and 9.10).

Durability

Ceramic laminate veneers stand up extremely well to biological, chemical and mechanical action. However, certain ceramic systems, such as Dicor and Empress, which use surface staining, may deteriorate eventually owing to mechanical abrasion of the outer layer. This surface degra-

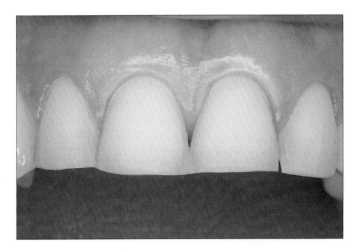

Figure 9.9 *Maxillary anterior teeth treatment planned for veneers. In this instance the excellent color of the dental tissue will provide good-quality light transmission in the bonded veneers.*

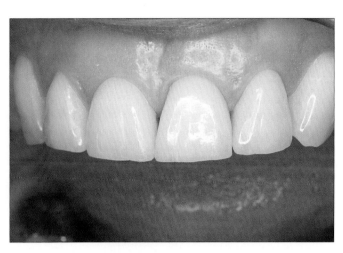

Figure 9.10 *Despite the minimal thickness of the veneers, all features of natural enamel can be reproduced in ceramic. This is more difficult to achieve with heavily stained teeth. (Ceramist: Serge Tissier.)*

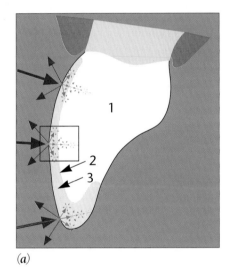

(a)

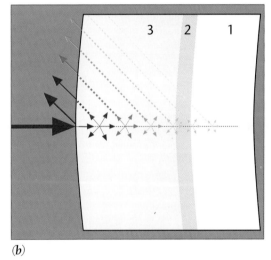

(b)

Figure 9.11 (*a*, *b*) *If the tooth is not stained, the laminate veneer should transmit light progressively through its thickness. Stratification and the choice of different ceramic layers should allow for some light radiation by the underlying tooth. Selecting a translucent adhesive favors reflection. (1) Normal dental structure; (2) fine translucent resin film; (3) stratification of the ceramic material, allowing light rays to pass through.*

dation can be more pronounced with patients' use of acidic fluoride preparations. Even fluoridated toothpastes may enhance this adverse surface effect.

Light transmission

Using dentin porcelain of varying chromas, as well as transparent, translucent or opalescent (but not opaque) porcelain, it is possible to achieve moderately thick build-ups by a layering technique or lateral segmenta- tion that reproduce all the characteristics of natural enamel, such as cracks, fissures and opalescence.

To use the optical properties of this 'substitute enamel' effectively, one must be aware of the influence of the tooth substrate and of the bonding material on the final appearance. Ideally, the bonding material should bring out the color of the underlying dentin and not serve as an opaque screen to mask this tissue. The laminate veneer should transmit light progressively

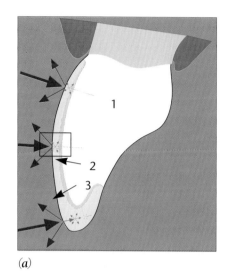
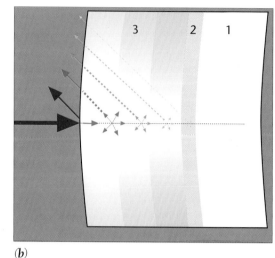

(a)   (b)

Figure 9.12 (a, b) If the tooth structure is discolored, the ceramic veneer should reflect or absorb light rays in their entirety so as to avoid any reflection from the underlying tooth. Laminating by means of layers of decreasing chroma and the choice of a less-translucent ceramic should serve to suppress any

light radiation by the tooth. Selection of a composite cement with low translucency can sometimes help. (1) Stained dental substructure. (2) Thick composite cement film. (3) Stratification of the ceramic material, letting no light rays through.

throughout its thickness (Figure 9.11). The eventual color will then be the result of the number of rays reflected and absorbed overall by the ceramic, the composite cement and the tooth.

It must be understood that the curbing of light rays should be progressive, proceeding from the surface to the underlying tooth structure. An unsuitable texture, too opaque a ceramic, or insufficiently translucent bonding composite, will inevitably lead to a sudden halt in light transmission, resulting in greater reflection than required, manifesting as a rather unnatural opaque white or gray appearance (Figure 9.12). The same effect may be noted in defective ceramic jacket crowns, despite their increased thickness.

Tissue response

The minor degree of tissue damage sustained in preparation or making an impression, the position of margins (usually supragingival), the ease and accuracy of control over adjustment, and ease of access to margins for a toothbrush or dental floss are factors promoting excellent prognosis for periodontal tissues with veneering procedures.

Whatever the technique or ceramic used, most authors report excellent tissue response with the use of ceramic laminate veneers, especially when compared with traditional prosthetic restorations applied under the

same conditions of hygiene and maintenance (Figures 9.13–9.15).

Speed and simplicity

Laminate veneer treatment procedures are usually carried out under light anesthetic, often without gingival retraction, with minimal tooth reduction, and at greater speed than other techniques. Moreover, impressions are easier to make, because of the accessible position of the margins.

What patients particularly appreciate is being able to remodel their smile very rapidly. Whatever the number of laminate veneers required, they can be prepared and luted over two sessions, generally separated by a few days.

This technique does not routinely require application of provisional prostheses, which often accounts for significant loss of time and requires the most skill.

Disadvantages

Preparation

Veneer preparation is not a simple procedure, nor does it deserve a 'simplistic' approach. Preparations for laminate veneers do, in fact, require great stringency and a great deal of training, since no rectification can be made subsequently. The finer the preparation is, the

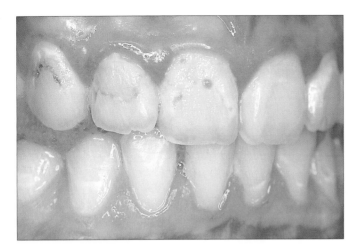

Figure 9.13 *Female patient with localized gingival inflammation associated with faulty composite resin restorations.*

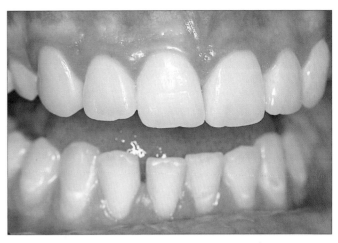

Figure 9.14 *Six maxillary anterior teeth restored with ceramic veneers. Note the improvement in gingival tissue. (Ceramist: Serge Tissier.)*

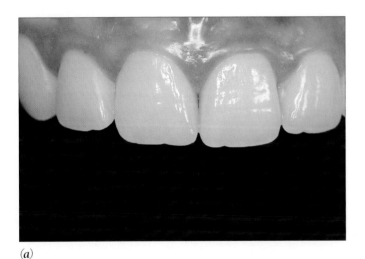

(*a*)

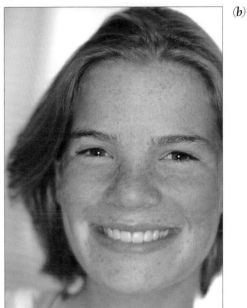

(*b*)

Figure 9.15 (*a*) *Ceramic veneers of patient from Figure 9.14 shown at one week postoperatively. Note that gingival inflammation has not recurred and there is no accumulation of dental plaque.* (*b*) *Full face view. (Ceramist: Serge Tissier.)*

more it requires special instrumentation, with specific profiles, diameters and coarseness. This, more than any other type of preparation, requires experience for mastery of 0.3–0.5 mm reductions.

Esthetic results

When dealing with light transmission, the laminate veneer can, under certain circumstances, be a good indicator of where one can play with effects of light and

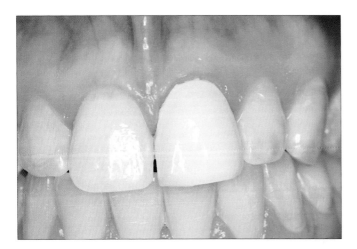

Figure 9.16 Inadequate preparation, too opaque a ceramic and use of an opaque composite cement have contributed to the esthetic failure of this ceramic veneer.

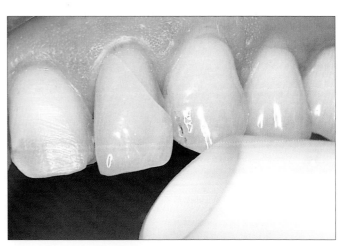

Figure 9.17 Veneers should be handled carefully at try-in. This example shows a fracture in the ceramic, a fragment of which was drawn into the high-volume aspirator.

hence with color at every stage of its production. In other cases, it can be fraught with problems, especially when the underlying tooth is heavily discolored, the laminate veneer thin (Figure 9.16) or the restored teeth crowded.

Bonding procedures

At the bonding stage, the slightest error can mean failure – either immediately or later on. This is a major disadvantage of laminate veneers, where strict bonding procedures are of vital importance.

Whereas about 90 minutes may be required to prepare and take an impression for six laminate veneers at the initial session, double that time will be needed for placement.

Try-in, surface conditioning, cleaning, bonding, finishing and adjustment of occlusion are all crucial and demanding procedures, which will have to be repeated for each laminate veneer.

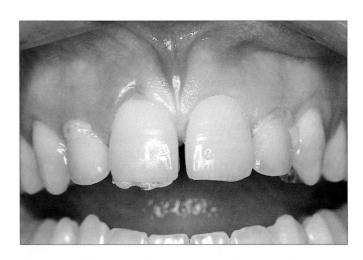

Figure 9.18 Veneers and crowns are tried-in using Memosil (Heraeus-Kulzer), a transparent silicone.

Fractures

Handling of such fine ceramics requires very special precautions. Prior to bonding, they are extremely fragile, and the slightest irregularity could produce fracturing (Figure 9.17). The ceramic veneer should always be handled over a surface that would not damage it if it happened to fall.

Try-in procedures require special care. The angle of introduction should be gauged, and this often requires

rotation: no pressure should be exerted at this stage. Generally speaking, feldspathic ceramics are more fragile, requiring more precautions than reinforced ceramics, such as Optec or Empress. Always try-in the laminate when damp or loaded with a colorless silicone, such as Memosil (Heraeus-Kulzer) (Figures 9.18–9.20). After cementing each of the laminate veneers, the next one must be tried in again, since too cramped a contact

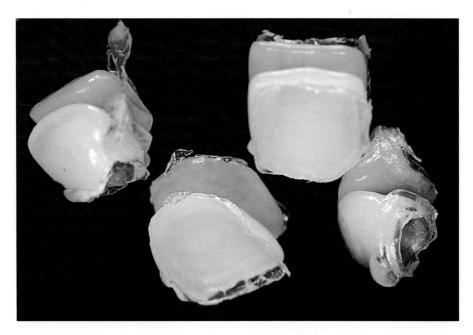

Figure 9.19 After try-in, the silicone film is easily removed.

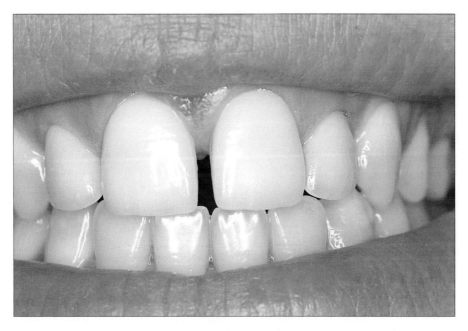

Figure 9.20 The end result – here, a combination of ceramic veneers, metal ceramic crowns and bleaching was used. (Ceramist: Serge Tissier.)

or any surplus hardened composite will risk malpositioning and could produce fracturing during bonding.

Despite delicate handling, these fine structures are still liable to fracture after bonding during function.

Over 90% of fractures affect the occlusal edge or angles. It is rare to see cervical fractures or fracturing of the labial–buccal surface.

Most fracturing is due to inadequate depth (thickness)

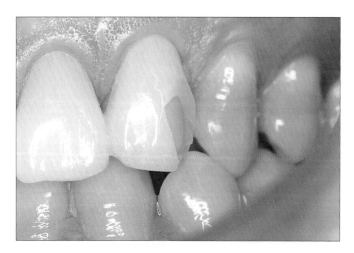

Figure 9.21 *Mesial angle fracture of a ceramic veneer due to insufficient depth and unsuitable location of the lingual margin.*

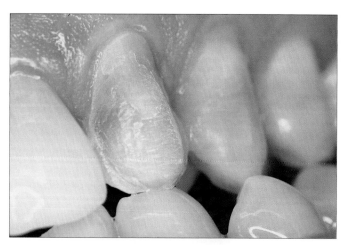

Figure 9.22 *Once the ceramic material of the fractured veneer has been removed, the lack of depth can be better seen during lateral movements.*

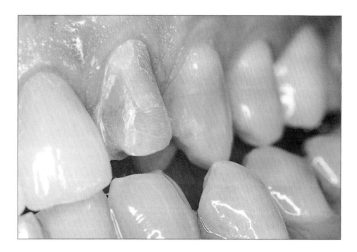

Figure 9.23 *Occlusal reduction has been increased to approximately 1.2 mm.*

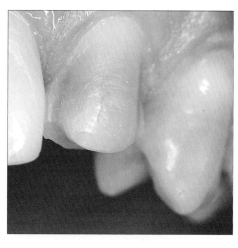

Figure 9.24 *The preparation provides much greater coverage for the lingual surface and better maintains occlusal contact areas and depth.*

(Figures 9.21–9.24), maladjusted occlusion, or parafunction activity. All these fractures are of a cohesive nature. It is very unusual to find fractures of an adhesive nature, and complete debonding of the veneer is even rarer. This occurrence is mostly due to a serious shortcoming at the time of bonding, or, most commonly, to the use of products that have passed their expiry date.

It is important to design the preparation so as to restrict flexural stresses (Figures 9.25 and 9.26). Increasing thickness and covering the incisal edge, allowing for generous lingual clearance, allow the ceramic restoration to work in compression – an important consideration for limiting fractures, since ceramics have better resistance to compressive than to shear stress.

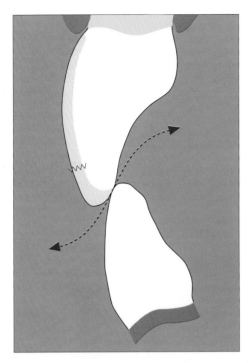

Figure 9.25 Faulty occlusal stop: flexural forces prevail during protrusion, and can bring about fracturing.

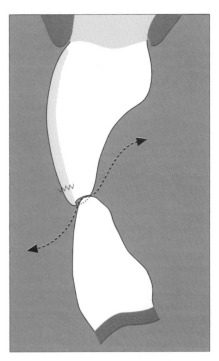

Figure 9.27 Faulty occlusal stop, especially in patients with bruxism. The tooth, which wears faster than the ceramic, leaves a very fragile and unsupported ceramic edge.

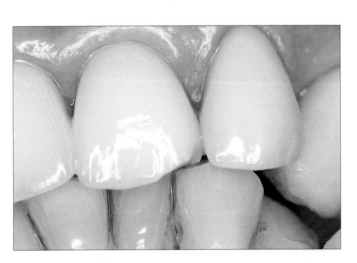

Figure 9.26 Faulty lingual stop leading to a fracture in the ceramic veneer due to flexural forces during protrusion.

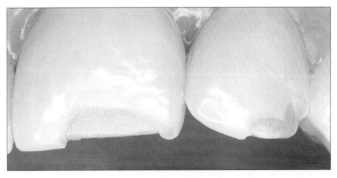

Figure 9.28 Fracture of the occlusal edges in a patient with bruxism.

The fracture rate is highest for laminate veneers with no incisal coverage (Figures 9.27 and 9.28), especially in canines or premolars, where peak shear force has been noted. This is why many authors now recommend that the incisal edge be overlaid in most cases.

Although repairs are technically feasible using composites, it is often preferable to make the laminate veneers over again. This can actually be a constructive exercise, since it brings out the quality of the tooth–ceramic–composite bonding!

Problems in the laboratory
Techniques are becoming simpler, especially with the progress made in phosphate investment, but the

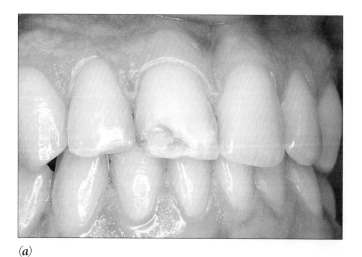

(a)

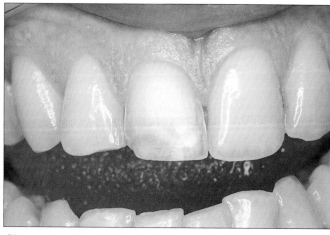

(b)

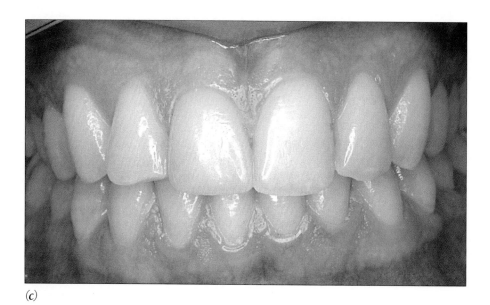

(c)

Figure 9.29 (a) Structural irregularities are among the most common indications for ceramic laminate veneers. (b) Preparation of the right central incisor for a ceramic veneer restoration is minimal. (c) Appearance of the cemented veneer in the mouth. (Ceramist: Serge Tissier.)

creation of fine natural ceramic veneer restorations remains a difficult and highly skilled task, the two main drawbacks being:

- stability during different types of handling;
- the difficulty of getting the right balance of powders for layering or segmental build-up with a thickness ranging from 0.7 to 0.3 mm.

Post-firing modifications

There is practically no possibility of touching up feldspathic porcelain veneers processed over investment or even using platinum foil, because the ceramic cannot be re-fired once removed from its support. Neither the IPS Empress ceramic (Ivoclar) nor the Duceram-LFC low-fusing ceramic (Ducera) has this disadvantage, and may be touched up at any time.

Temporization

The fabrication of temporary restorations is not mandatory. Nevertheless, they are often necessary in the case of an individual tooth or of a major overlay of the occlusal edge (lower incisor, angle fractures, etc.).

This temporary restoration remains a skilled process. It is difficult to adjust the margins, and provisional cementation is particularly complicated since it has to be carried out without any risk of mechanical or chemical damage to the supporting tissues (eugenol cements must not be used).

Indications and contraindications

The main indications and contraindications for ceramic laminate veneers are summarized in Table 9.1, and a common indication is illustrated in Figure 9.29. It must be stressed that contraindications should not be too rigidly set for a technique now still evolving.

The best example of this ongoing evolution is related to dentin adhesion, which is now more reliable and may obviate the 'classical' limitations of bonding onto dentin surfaces. The incontrovertible rule prevailing over the past decade required the positioning of the veneer margins in enamel, and ensuring that at least 50% of the prepared surface remained in the enamel (Garber, 1991). Although this recommendation still applies at the time of writing, it is evident that dentin adhesion is becoming as reliable as adhesion to enamel; this will require that we review our preparations and extend the terms of our indications again. Perhaps the term 'current contraindications' should be preferred.

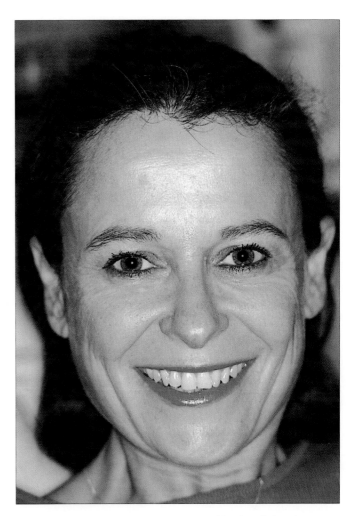

Figure 9.30 Appraisal of the smile should take all facial qualities into account: shape of the face, size of lips, etc.

Clinical examination

All prosthetic interventions require preliminary clinical examination.

It is of utmost importance to create a climate of confidence with the patient so as to establish as clearly as possible the motives for his or her visit; the dentist should understand accurately the patient's disatisfaction with the existing dentition and the exact type of change he or she would like to have made. The nature of this first, decisive contact generally depends on whether the dental practitioner and the assistant are 'good listeners'.

This 'one-way dialogue' enables the patient's aspirations to be made known and the dental practitioner to obtain guidance in his or her choice of treatment.

It is also useful to back up this initial contact by a medical and esthetic questionnaire that the patient is requested to sign. The questionnaire can help pinpoint the exact reason for the patient's visit (whether esthetic or functional, for example) as well as his or her wishes regarding any changes in shade of color, shape, position, and so on.

Once this information has been noted, the examination itself can proceed.

Procedures

The coronal, as well as the periodontal, condition of the teeth to be overlaid must be assessed. A healthy periodontium is imperative for successful results.

Table 9.1 *Indications and contraindications for the use of ceramic laminate veneers*

INDICATIONS

Color defects or abnormalities	Defective amelogenesis, medication (such as tetracycline), fluorosis, physiological aging, trauma, extrinsic staining with infiltration of the tissues (by tea, coffee or tobacco)
Abnormalities of shape	Microdontia, atypical tooth shape: malformed incisor, retained deciduous teeth (bonding onto deciduous teeth never performs as well as onto the enamel of the permanent teeth)
Abnormal structure or texture	Dysplasia, dystrophy, erosion, attrition, mechanical or chemical abrasion, and coronal fractures
Malpositioning	Correction of minor malposition: rotated tooth, change of angulation
Individual cases	
Diastemata	Any closing of diastemata must take the overhanging porcelain into consideration, since this involves risk of fracturing
Missing lateral with canine in lateral position	Usually requires a partial crown preparation
Lingual laminate veneer	Useful for creating canine function or correcting anterior guidance
Ceramic laminate veneer over ceramic crown	The ideal treatment in cases of partial fracture
Lengthening	Lengthening will be in proportion to the volume of non-supported ceramics and occlusion

CONTRAINDICATIONS

Insufficient surface enamel	Laminate veneers are contraindicated if preparation does not provide for preserving at least 50% of enamel and if the margins are not located within the enamel
Pulpless teeth	In addition to being fragile, these teeth are liable to change color in time
Unsuitable occlusion	Pronounced overbite, etc.
Parafunction	Bruxism and other ingrained habits
Unsuitable anatomical presentation	Clinical crown too small (frequently found with the lower incisors, i.e. slender or outstandingly triangular teeth)
Single laminate veneers	A typical example of 'relative contraindication'. These may be used if the tooth to be veneered resembles neighboring teeth in color, but is very hard to accomplish if the tooth to be treated is very discolored
Caries and fillings	Ideally, laminate veneers are intended for either healthy or slightly defective teeth. It is always preferable to replace defective fillings using glass ionomer or composites before placing veneers
Poor dental care and hygiene	Any bonded restorative prosthesis should be avoided in cases where the basic rules of dental care and hygiene are not respected

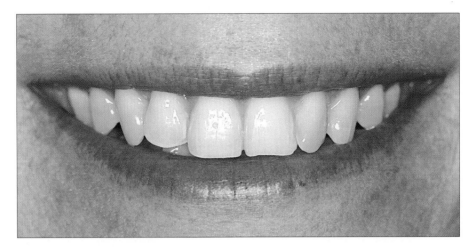

Figure 9.31 A pleasing smile depends on the ratios between three lines composed of the upper edge of the lower lip, the incisal edges and the lower edge of the upper lip.

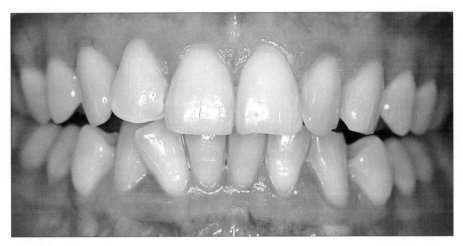

Figure 9.32 Although the teeth are not straight, an even balance exists which gives the smile a pleasing look.

Examining occlusion

The relative fragility of ceramic veneer restorations requires an accurate analysis of the patient's occlusion, to ensure that the restorations are not extended into areas of occlusal stress. The results of this analysis may limit the opportunities for remodelling. There is no point in aiming to increase the incisor group in height, for example, without dealing with canine malocclusion when present. Any attempt to establish a different height clinically, in cases of attrition or bruxism, carries its share of risks and should be approached with caution.

Occlusal factors should be considered even with veneer restorations that do not involve the lingual surfaces (i.e. when the incisal edge is preserved). In fact, it is in this situation that the risks are greater, especially when canines and posterior teeth are involved.

Examining a single tooth

Once again, shape, position, available enamel and occlusion are all factors to be considered. A tooth that is outstandingly triangular or very slender raises difficulties, which will all have to be appraised and dealt with accordingly.

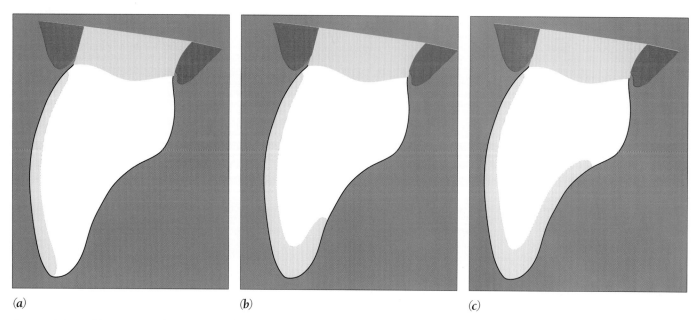

(a) (b) (c)

Figure 9.33 *Different types of preparation for veneers. (**a**) Preparation without overlaying the incisal edge (contact lens type). (**b**) Preparation with overlay of the incisal edge (classic type). (**c**) Preparation with major overlay of the incisal edge (three-quarters type).*

Examining the gingival tissue

Although the margins of laminate veneers are often located away from the gingivae, the condition of the latter must always be appraised before deciding on any treatment. Poor dental hygiene, gingival inflammation as well as one or more gingival recession sites should all be treated before applying ceramic laminate veneers.

Appraising the smile

Clinical examination should focus not just on the teeth to be restored (their color, shape, etc.) but also on the shape of the face, size of the lip, and the lip-to-tooth relationship during various movements (Figures 9.30–9.32). All these inspections should be carried out both frontally and from the side. The dental practitioner must also use other methods of visualization, such as the following, which are discussed in more depth in Chapter 7:

- diagnostic wax-ups;

- photographs – full face and profile;

- cast models;

- computer imaging analysis.

Table 9.2 lists the main considerations when appraising the smile.

Table 9.2 The main considerations for analyzing the smile

The smile must be viewed from the front and sides (both left and right).

• Shape of the face	
• Size of the lips	
• Visible coronal and gingival levels	– At rest – When talking – Broadest smile
• Harmony and proportion	– Of the cervical line – Of the line of the incisal edges – Of the lip line
• Tooth color	– Hue – Value – Chroma – Translucency – Texture and luster
• Tooth shape	– Size of tooth (height : width ratio) – Incisal edge – Contour – Assessing triangular tooth shape – Analysis of static and dynamic occlusion – Spatial arrangement of teeth

Tooth preparation for ceramic laminate veneers

Principles

The preparations must fulfil the following four basic principles if perfect, functional, biological and esthetic integration is to be achieved: stabilization, reinforcement, retention and adhesion. Relying on adhesion without taking the other three factors into account generally leads to immediate or ultimate failure.

Preserving as much of the natural enamel as possible, although desirable, must never jeopardize the planned restoration by minimizing the preparation (Figure 9.33).

A stage-by-stage description of a standard preparation involving major or minor overlays of the incisal edge will be given below, followed by other clinical situations.

Enamel reduction requires special instrumentation and involves the four surfaces of the teeth.

Instrumentation

The concept of ceramic laminate veneers has become inseparable from that of controlled enamel preparation, finally resulting in a prosthetic substitute enamel with optical, mechanical and biological properties closely resembling those of natural enamel.

It is the shape of the instrument that determines the profile of the preparation. Many authors, including Garber (1991) and Lustig (1976), have concentrated on the rationalization of instrumentation in fixed prosthetics. The present authors, too, contributed to this field, having suggested TPS (Touati) Brasseler kits in 1985. This instrument kit consists of eight burs, enabling veneer preparations to be accomplished in total safety (Figure 9.34). The laminate veneer preparation kit comprises:

- two instruments (gauges TFC1 and TFC2) to monitor labial reduction;

- two instruments (TFC3 and TFC4) for reduction of enamel and margins;

- two instruments (TFC5 and TFC6) for occlusal reduction;

- two finishing instruments (TFC7 and TFC8).

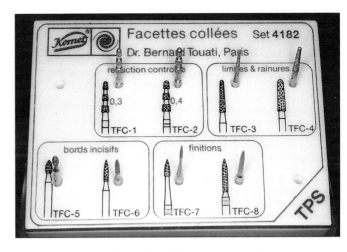

Figure 9.34 *Brasseler TPS tool kit: instruments for preparation and finish of ceramic veneers.*

The advantage of this kit lies in simplifying preparation by plain codifying and offering a limited number of instruments.

The two 'depth-cutter' instruments (TFC1, TFC2) serve to guide, visualize and, in particular, quantify enamel reduction. In addition, margins can be plotted, owing to the rounded tip. The authors consider it dangerous to gauge reduction in enamel depth of between 0.3 and 0.5 mm without some type of depth guide (Figure 9.35). Goldstein (1984), who also recommends two instruments based on the same principle in his laminate veneer preparation kit (Brasseler, LVS), obviously shares the same concern.

Other techniques exist for monitoring depth, such as those advocated before the introduction of penetration gauges. A spherical diamond bur (Komet H01 314 009) traces out a 0.4–0.5 mm groove as a guide in the same way as Lusco's 'enamel depth cutter' (a small diamond disc with a smooth stop).

Labial preparation

Uniform enamel preparation must result in an average tissue reduction of 0.5 mm. One may, in cases of extreme discoloration, be inclined to increase the depth to 0.7–0.8 mm. A depth below 0.3 mm is not recommended.

A chart devised by Crispin (1993) that indicates depths of enamel, broken down by dental aspect and tooth type, can be used to stay within the rule of thumb of conserving at least 50% of the enamel.

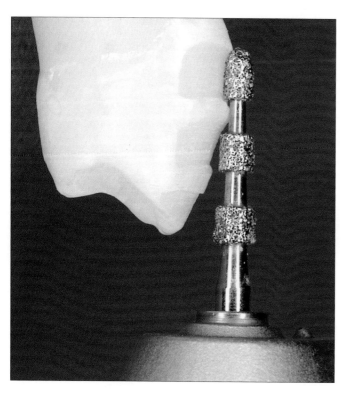

Figure 9.35 Gauge TFC1 and TFC2 instruments to monitor enamel reduction. Depth of grooves ranges between 0.3 and 0.4 mm. The rounded tip enables the cervical margin to be plotted.

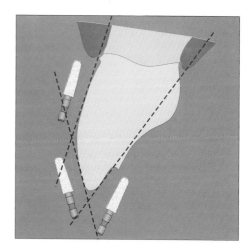

Figure 9.36 Dual convergence of the labial reduction so as to preserve the anatomical form of the labial surface.

Generally speaking, depths of 0.7–0.8 mm and 0.6–0.7 mm for the incisal and medial areas respectively preserve an enamel layer in most cases. In the cervical area, on the other hand, depths of 0.3 mm can often expose patches of dentin, especially on the lower incisors.

Two instruments, TFC1 and TFC2, tracing grooves of 0.3 and 0.4 mm respectively, are available for producing these penetration guides.

Preparation always begins with the tracing of horizontal grooves. These striations, on the labial surface, must remain apart from the margin. The natural curve of the facial surface rarely allows the three striations to be traced simultaneously, especially in the case of the lower premolars or canines. It is therefore recommended to begin with the cervical and medial striations, followed by adjusting the angle of the instrument and tracing the occlusal striation, with the medial one as a guide.

Because of the rounded tip of the diamond instrument, the cervical margin can be initiated slightly above the gingival level. Instrument TFC1, for a depth of 0.3 mm, serves to create the cervical and medial grooves, and TFC2, for a depth of 0.4 mm, serves to create the occlusal and deepen the medial grooves.

After completing the depth cuts, the remaining areas of enamel will be removed by grinding, using a coarse conical instrument with a rounded tip. Two different diamond instruments, TFC3 and TFC4, with different diameters, are available to fit different clinical situations. Systematic facial reduction must always be carried out in two stages, with the instrument inclined at two different angles so as to preserve the double convergence of the labial–buccal surface (Figure 9.36).

This double convergence can only be obtained by working with the lower third of the diamond instrument. Axial reduction begins with the cervical portion, creating a gingival chamfer at the same time. Proximal reduction should be initiated keeping clear of these set margins and without destroying the contact areas.

Preparation then proceeds in the axial and occlusal portion, adhering to the principle of double convergence. An accurate profile of the preparation will be obtained once the 'pilot' grooves have been eliminated, which will have to be modified on a case-by-case basis.

Cervical margins

The final cervical margin will take on the profile of a mini chamfer measuring an average of 0.3 mm, matching the tip of diamond instrument TFC3 or TFC4 in shape. This margin will be juxtagingival or very slightly subgingival as a general rule (0.5 mm at most in cases of severe discoloration).

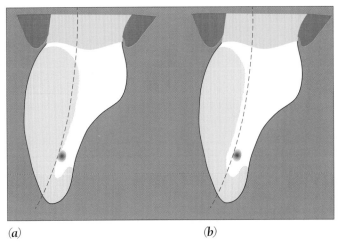

(a)   (b)

Figure 9.37 (a) Correct preparation of the proximal surface, where the margin cannot be seen and the contact area still maintained. In (b) the proximal margin will be visible and therefore unesthetic.

It is highly inadvisable to sink the margin deep into the gingival sulcus, as is the norm for certain circumferencial preparations, such as jacket and metal–ceramic crowns. Ceramic laminate veneers generally allow the supragingival margin to remain invisible (because of their optical properties) and maintain a good emergence profile.

This less invasive approach (as compared with crowns) is one of the advantages of these fine restorations; the benefit is that many drawbacks of traditional prostheses can be eliminated.

For bonding, supragingival or juxtapositioned margins should always be preferred, for the following reasons:

- increased areas of enamel in the preparation;

- simplified moisture control;

- visual confirmation of the marginal fit;

- margins that can be accessible for finishing and polishing;

- access to margins for routine maintenance and dental hygiene procedures.

A rounded 0.3 mm chamfer serves as an ideal margin for either a ceramic laminate veneer or a partial crown. It enables:

- the natural visible tooth profile to be reproduced;

- avoidance of overcontouring in the cervical zone;

- an accurate finish line to be determined, which should be easy to record, easy to identify and reproducable in the laboratory;

- margins of higher fracture resistance, and avoidance of fractures to the edges of the laminate veneer in the course of construction, try-in and final placement;

- the laminate veneer to be more easily inserted at try-in and during the final placement.

Proximal surfaces

The preparation of proximal surfaces will have already been plotted during labial preparation and creation of the cervical margin. Two major principles should be observed in preparing the surfaces (Figure 9.37):

- preserving the contact area;

- placing margins beyond the visible area.

The preparation of the proximal surfaces is carried out with instruments TFC3 and TFC4, often at the same time as axial labial preparation.

Here, too, minimum depths should be adhered to in the interest of allowing sufficient thickness for strength of the ceramic laminate veneer. Depths can often be as great as 0.8–1 mm, since the enamel layer is very thick towards the occlusal third of the tooth.

The proximal 'stop' will be plotted as a miniature rounded channel, thus preventing the contact area from being destroyed, always preserving a buccolingual slope.

These interproximal extensions will create a true interlock, which will improve the stability and mechanical properties of the bonded veneer.

Location of margins

Providing that the tooth is free of proximal restorations, placing of the proximal 'stop line' should always be guided by esthetic considerations. It is imperative to go beyond the visible area, which should be determined from both the front and the side view – an especially important rule when the color of the tooth differs greatly from that of the laminate veneer.

In creating the proximal margins, it is not usually necessary to destroy the contact area. However, it is important to extend the cervical margin back in a lingual

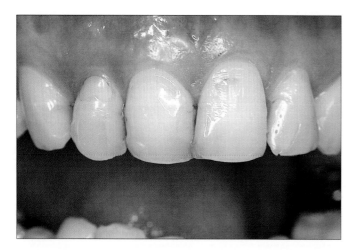

Figure 9.38 The four maxillary incisors have composite resin restorations on the proximal surfaces.

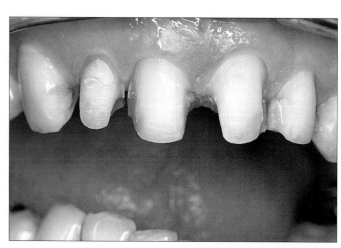

Figure 9.39 The extent of the composite restorations and the need to cover them completely in the preparation necessitated the removal of contact areas in this instance.

direction to displace it from what is often the most highly visible area. In cases where the natural contact area is lost, e.g. to encompass a proximal composite, close up a diastema or restore a broken angle, the margin should be drawn back even further in a lingual direction.

The more the proximal aspects are extended, the more they will have to be increased in thickness (depth), since the ratio has to be maintained between the depth and the length of proximal curve.

Contact area

The use of the platinum foil technique has been gradually declining owing to the progress made in investments and new systems such as Empress and In-Ceram, where the ceramic build-up is achieved on a ceramic core.

The platinum foil technique involves splitting the working model in order to obtain individual dies onto which the foil may be burnished. This would require that the contact area be opened. With modern techniques, it is no longer necessary to split the models. Therefore the question of whether or not to prepare the contact area depends on clinical factors alone.

Why preserve the contact area? It is always preferable to preserve the contact area, if the clinical circumstances allow it, because:

- it is an anatomical feature that is extremely difficult to reproduce;

- it prevents displacement of the tooth between the preparation and placement sessions when no provisional restorations are used;

- it simplifies try-in procedures;

- it saves clinical adjustment of contact areas, which are particularly intricate with such fine ceramics;

- it simplifies bonding and finishing procedures;

- it allows better access for home care techniques (toothbrush and dental floss).

However, as previously noted, certain circumstances occur where the contact area has to be prepared, such as with small proximal caries lesions, old composite restorations and angle fractures (Figures 9.38 and 9.39). Other clinical circumstances, such as closing a diastema or changing the shape or position of a group of teeth, may require some specific preparation of the contact area.

Lingual surfaces

The question of whether or not to preserve incisal edges has provoked a wide range of interpretation on the part of various writers. In the 1980s the common trend was to preserve the incisal edge under appropriate circumstances in the interests of tissue conservation. The margin was located at the incisal edge when

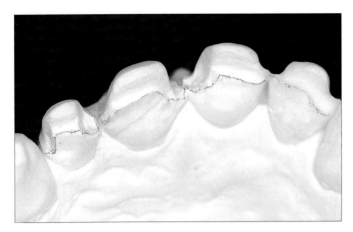

Figure 9.40 *Degree of overlay illustrated in lingual view. These preparations are three-quarters type.*

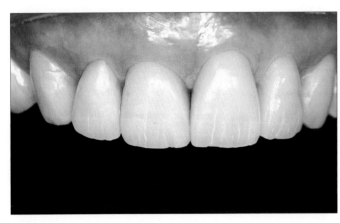

(a)

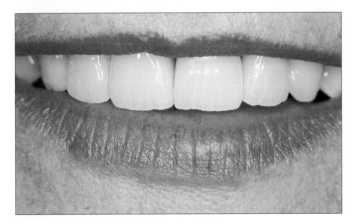

(b)

Figure 9.41 (*a*, *b*) *Final esthetic effect. (Ceramist: GH Laboratory.)*

sufficiently thick. Although we were confining this type of preparation to the upper anterior region at that time, through the years a higher number of fractures have been observed with this preparation technique than in cases where the edge had just been simply overlaid. This observation, confirmed by numerous clinicians, has made complete coverage of the incisal edge (Figures 9.40–9.42) in almost all cases the procedure of choice. This offers numerous advantages, as follows:

- It restricts angle fractures. Where the free edge is not overlaid, the occlusal third of the laminate veneer is often very thin (less than 0.3 mm). When the teeth are very slender, the difference in resilience between the prepared natural tooth and the laminate veneer can, under certain occlusal constraints, lead to cracking or fracturing of the ceramic.

- It enhances the esthetic properties of laminate veneers.

- It allows latitude for altering tooth shape.

- It facilitates changes in tooth position.

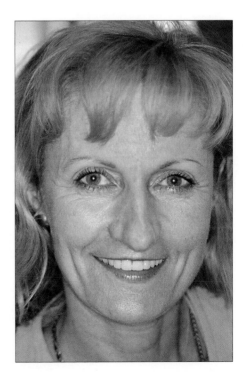

Figure 9.42 *Ceramic veneer restoration – full face view.*

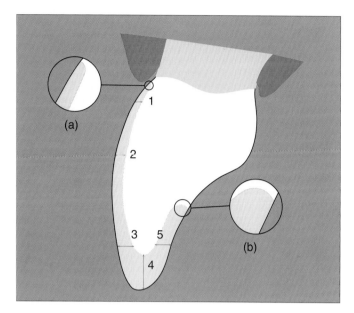

Figure 9.43 *Scale of average depths to be maintained in preparing ceramic veneers for overlaying.* (**a**) *Margin in the form of a rounded chamfer: 0.2–3 mm.* (**b**) *Rounded lingual margin: 0.4–0.6 mm.* (1) *depth of 0.2–0.4 mm;* (2) *depth of 0.3–0.5 mm;* (3) *depth of 0.5-0.7 mm;* (4) *depth of 1–1.5 mm;* (5) *Depth of 0.5–0.7 mm.*

- It enables occlusion to be adjusted.

- It facilitates handling and positioning of the laminate veneer at try-in and, in particular, during bonding.

- It enables the margin to be placed outside the area of occlusal impact.

Incisal reduction must provide for a ceramic layer of at least 1 mm in thickness. A thicker layer of 1.5–2 mm should be used for canines and lower incisors.

Reduction of the occlusal edge is imperative for preparation of the lingual surface (Figure 9.43).

The degree of lingual preparation will depend on the particular clinical situation. The lingual margin, wherever possible, should be located away from the area of occlusal impact. This finish line is traced using a spherically shaped diamond instrument, to create a slightly concave margin.

Once the four tooth surfaces have been prepared, examination of thicknesses, occlusion, path of insertion, shape and position of margins (Figure 9.44) must be repeated before proceeding to make an impression.

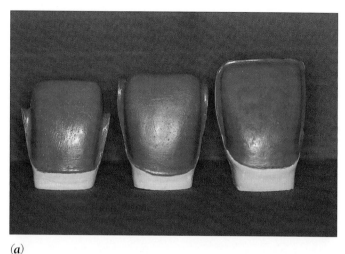

(a)

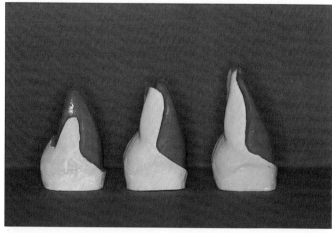

(b)

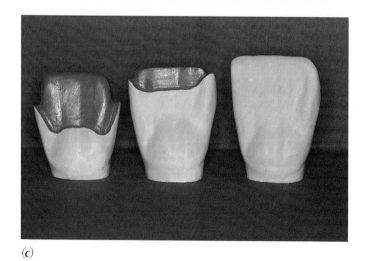

(c)

Figure 9.44 *Models of maxillary anterior teeth showing the three possible preparations for ceramic veneers:* (**a**) *facial view;* (**b**) *lateral view;* (**c**) *lingual view.*

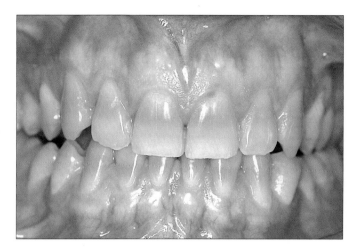

Figure 9.45 *Severe discoloration requiring the fitting of 12 veneers to correct tooth color.*

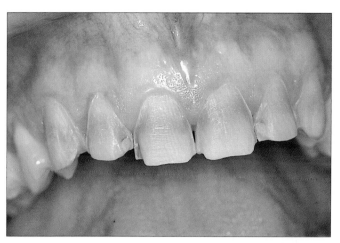

Figure 9.46 *Two alterations should be made to traditional preparation for severely discolored teeth: location of margins in slightly subgingival position; preparations are more extensive, and incisal overlay is introduced routinely.*

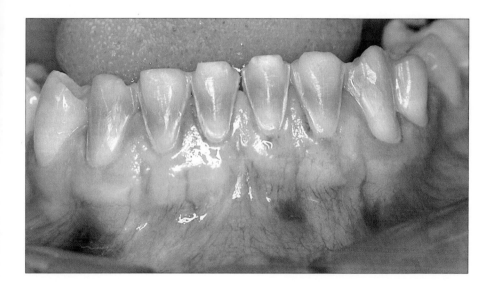

Figure 9.47 *Preparation of the lower teeth follows the same principle: note the 1.5 mm reduction of the incisal edge.*

Clinical presentation

Severe discoloration

Any major change in tooth color due to intake of antibiotics or to diseases such as fluorosis or dentinogenesis imperfecta requires special considerations with regard to preparation (Figures 9.45–9.52).

Two modifications should be made to the standard preparation techniques that have been described.

Location of the cervical margin

This is the only indication for placing the cervical margins in a slightly subgingival position. The margin should not be placed more than 0.5 mm subgingivally, since beyond this depth bonding becomes extremely challenging, if not impossible.

More extensive preparation

To tone down the darkening effect that the underlying tooth might have on the veneer, the depth of the preparation should be increased, enabling:

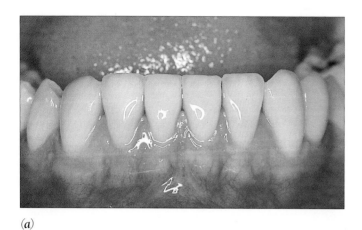

(a)

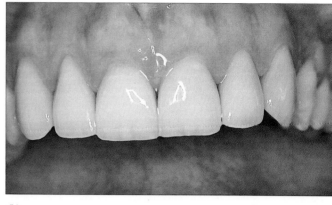

(b)

Figure 9.48 (*a, b*) *Despite the very dark color of the underlying tooth, the ceramic (Empress, stratified) retains its esthetic properties.* (*Ceramist: JP Levot.*)

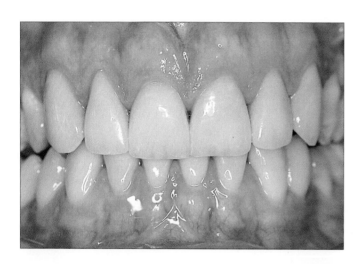

Figure 9.49 *Correct location of margins and mastery of stratification techniques remain the key elements of successful esthetics in clinically difficult cases.*

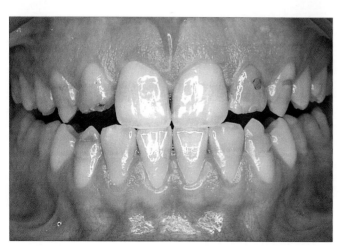

Figure 9.50 *Pronounced staining associated with enamel hypoplasia treatment planned for correction with 10 maxillary and 10 mandibular veneers.*

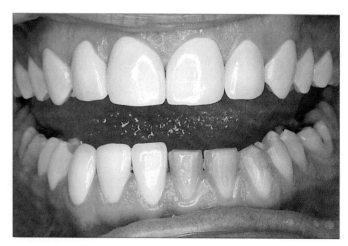

Figure 9.51 *This earlier case was carried out in Dicor ceramics: note the powerful effect of these ceramics, despite their relative thinness.*

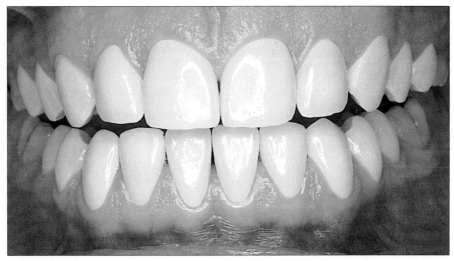

Figure 9.52 *The Dicor ceramic is more opaque, but does give esthetically acceptable results in cases of this severity.*

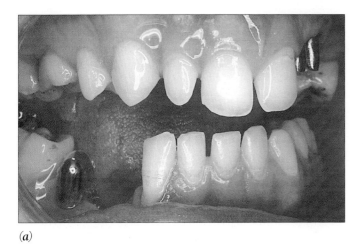

(a)

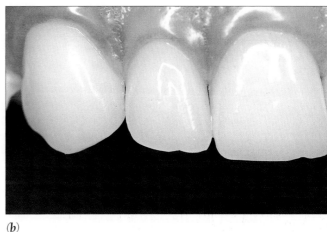

(b)

Figure 9.53 *(a, b) Closure of diastema by ceramic laminate veneers.*

- plaster or investment dies (Nixon, 1994) to be spaced out by 6–8 layers of die spacer (i.e. 50–80 µm);

- the ceramic technician to produce, by means of a layered build-up and the use of opaque dentin, a porcelain veneer that can mask the discolored tooth.

In such an event, the labial surface should be reduced by 0.7–0.8 mm in depth, with a cervical chamfer 0.4–0.5 mm deep. The combination of a skillful layering technique and cementing with a relatively thick, slightly opaque film of composite cement can often produce satisfactory results.

Exposure of patches of dentin, which is expected in these circumstances, is compensated for by more extensive (three-quarter type) preparation and use of a strong dentin–enamel adhesive.

Diastemata (Figure 9.53)

Proximal preparation will be more comprehensive, since retaining ridges have to be unambiguously sloped off in

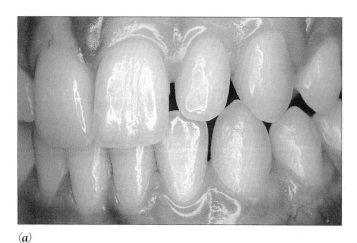
(a)

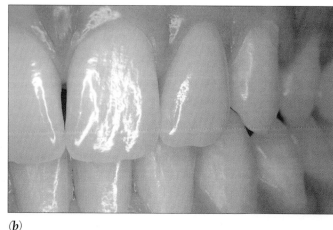
(b)

Figure 9.54 (a,b) Microdontia is one of the strongest indications for ceramic laminate veneers. (Ceramist: Serge Tissier.)

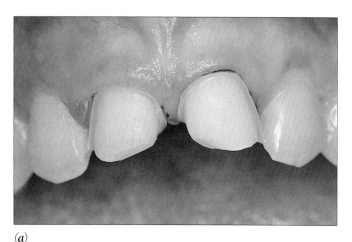
(a)

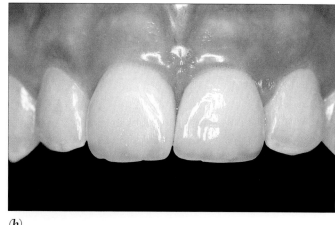
(b)

Figure 9.55 (a) A young female patient with two major mesial angle fractures of the central incisors. Fairly extensive preparation was required in this case. (b) This type of fracture, very common in children, is harmoniously restored with two bonded Empress laminate veneers. (Ceramist: Jacques Diligeart.)

a lingual direction. However, proximal preparation can occasionally be reduced to a simple 'slice'. These special procedures should prevent the proximal margins of the laminate veneer from being visible from the front and, more particularly, from the side.

Lingual laminate veneers

Lingual addition of 'artificial enamel' by means of ceramic laminate veneers, although less common, may still be utilized. These additions can be configured in various shapes, depending on their purpose. With canines, for example, it seems particularly appropriate to re-establish canine disclusion. Here, preparation may be reduced to simple resurfacing.

Atypical teeth

Lateral incisors, where very pronounced microdontia sometimes occurs, are those most frequently encountered in this category (Figure 9.54). With these teeth, preparation will be very limited in depth and will encompass virtually the entire available surface. This is the only type of case requiring fine, knife-edge margins.

Angle fractures

Angle or edge fractures of the maxillary incisors are certainly the most common accidents involving teeth among adolescents (Figures 9.55–9.61). Although direct application of composites provides an excellent short-

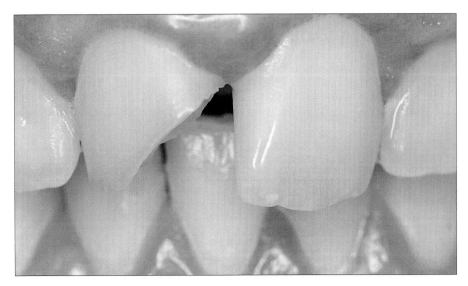

Figure 9.56 *Extensive fracture of a maxillary central incisor, induced by accident.*

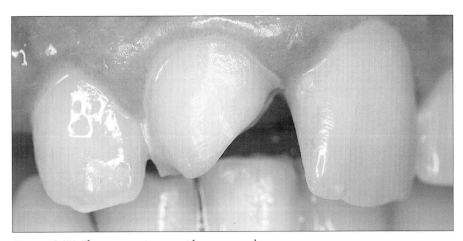

Figure 9.57 *The preparation provides very good coverage.*

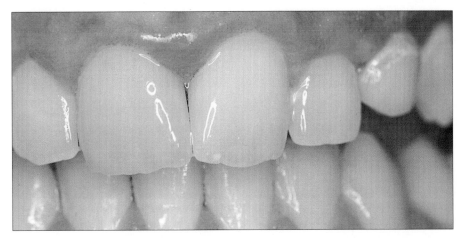

Figure 9.58 *The esthetic challenge consists of achieving the same light transmission in the thinner and thicker parts of the ceramic veneer. (Ceramist: Jacques Diligeart.)*

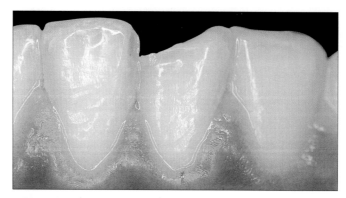

Figure 9.59 *Fracture of the incisal edge of a mandibular anterior tooth.*

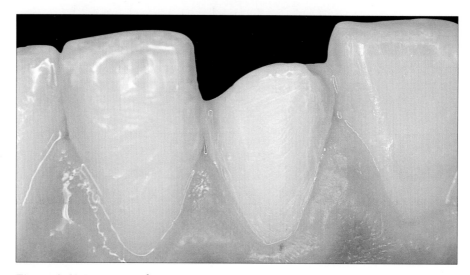

Figure 9.60 *Preparation for ceramic veneer.*

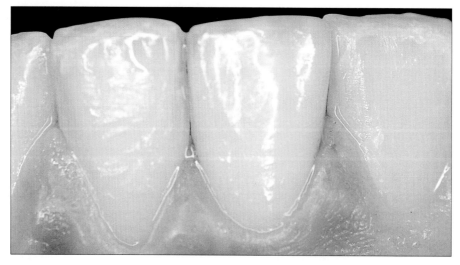

Figure 9.61 *Laminated Empress ceramic allows for accuracy of margins, and visual properties lend a natural look to these delicate restorations. (Ceramist: Jacques Diligeart.)*

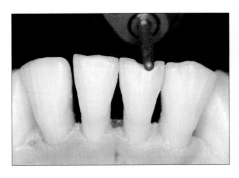

Figure 9.62 Preparation of lower incisor veneers starts with horizontal reduction of the incisal edge.

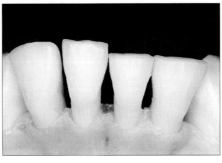

Figure 9.63 The incisal reduction is about 1.5 mm.

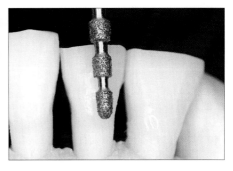

Figure 9.64 TFC1 or TFC2 diamond burs serve to guide labial reduction.

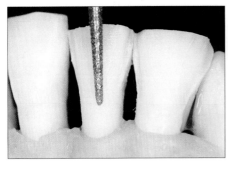

Figure 9.65 TFC3 or TFC4 diamond burs are used to complete labial preparation and plot cervical and proximal margins.

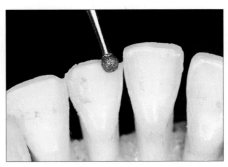

Figure 9.66 A round diamond bur serves to plot the lingual margin.

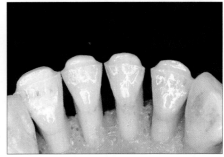

Figure 9.67 Lingual view of preparation.

term alternative, one often has to produce a more permanent restoration as adulthood approaches. Restoration with a ceramic laminate veneer may be considered if the fracture is not too extensive. Two types of difficulty may be encountered:

- shade matching with a single ceramic laminate veneer is always a challenge;

- the variation in thickness due to the missing angle presents the ceramic technician with a difficult exercise, since the same optical effect will have to be recreated in both fine and thicker areas by judicious build-up of ceramic.

Lower incisors (Figures 9.62–9.69)

Occlusal reduction of 1.5–2 mm is accomplished by flattening off the incisal edge. The ridge between the labial surface and the incisal edge should be rounded off, checking on static and dynamic occlusal relationships in maximal intercuspation and excursions. The lingual margin may be extended one-third of the way down the lingual surface, transforming the laminate veneer in effect into a partial crown. With this type of preparation, the ceramic restoration will be exposed mostly to compressive stresses and less to flexural stresses. Despite the small surface area, in comparison with an upper incisor or a canine, the failure rate is relatively low.

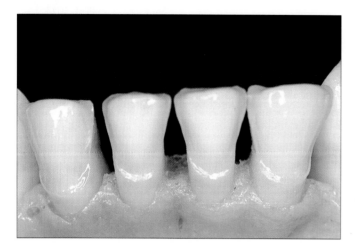

Figure 9.68 Labial view of preparations.

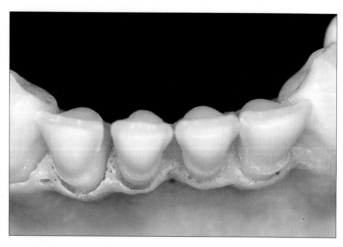

Figure 9.69 Occlusal view of preparations.

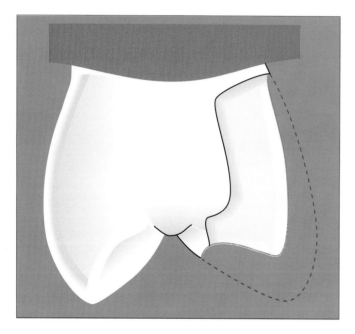

Figure 9.70 Laminate veneer preparation for premolars.

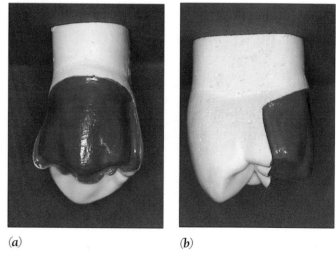

(a)   (b)

Figure 9.71 Front (a) and side (b) views of preparation for a laminate veneer over a maxillary premolar.

Premolars (Figures 9.70–9.72)

The labial cusp, whether maxillary or mandibular, should be reduced by at least 1 mm, placing the occlusal margin away from the occlusal contact and grooves.

The overlay extends to the occlusal three-quarters of the labial cusp, the margin being produced with a spherical bur and connected with the proximal margins by a rounded angle.

Dentin zones and caries

Many clinical situations require extension of the veneer preparation into dentin. If the extension into dentin does not go too deep, the tubules can be sealed effectively by using a new-generation adhesive. With deeper pitting of the dentin, however, which often occurs in the case of cervical erosion, cavities can be restored

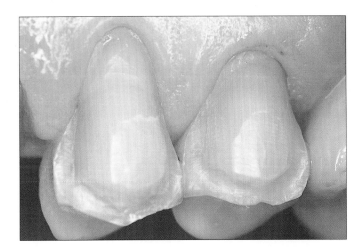

Figure 9.72 *Veneer preparations for maxillary premolars. Occlusal reduction should measure 1–1.5 mm.*

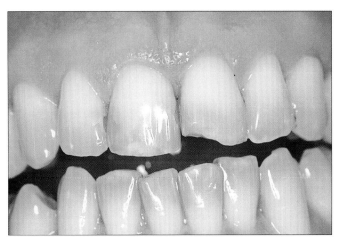

Figure 9.73 *Preoperative view showing a fracture of the incisal edge of a maxillary central and staining of the four maxillary incisors.*

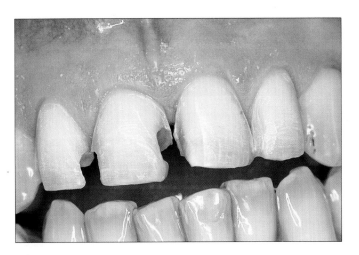

Figure 9.74 *Once the teeth have been prepared, the old composite resins are removed and the cavities cleaned out.*

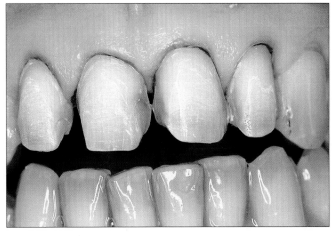

Figure 9.75 *The cavities are filled using a light-cured resin-modified glass ionomer.*

with a modified glass ionomer, such as Fuji II LC (GC) or Vitremer (3M), prior to veneer preparation. These materials, obtainable in various shades, make it possible to match the color of the underlying tooth structure.

Light-cured resin-modified glass ionomers are most suitable because of their advantageous mechanical properties, bonding capability with dentin and high fluoride release. These materials must be handled as suggested by the manufacturer.

When the teeth to be veneered have small proximal or cervical caries or old restorations, caries must always be treated and old restorations removed. These cavities should then be filled using a light-cured resin-modified glass ionomer, rather than composites (Figures 9.74 and 9.75).

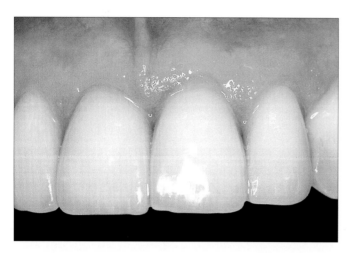

Figure 9.76 *Proximal margins have been positioned lingually enough to avoid any labial appearance of filling material. (Ceramist: JP Levot.)*

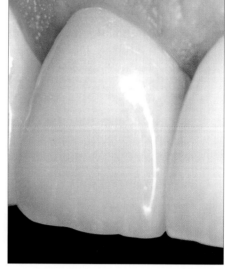

Figure 9.77 *Note the high-quality fit and excellent tissue response.*

The final preparation for the veneers should include and cover these restorations as fully as possible (Figures 9.76 and 9.77).

Impressions

Any indirect technique requires making an impression, enabling as accurate a master cast as possible to be obtained, on which restorations can be built up. The choice of material and impression technique used will be guided by:

• clinical requirements;

• laboratory requirements.

Clinical requirements

Gingival retraction may be considered necessary, according to the position of the margins in the sulcus. Also, special attention should be paid to the undercut areas very often found at embrasures. Where these exist, materials with significant mechanical properties should be preferred to avoid any deformation or tearing when withdrawing the tray.

Laboratory requirements

Should laboratory dies be separated? Should they be duplicated? Should a refractory investment be cast directly in the impression? These questions must be answered before determining the type of material to be used for impressions, as well as which technique to apply.

The impression should normally be made with a standard fixed prosthodontic impression material such as polyether, polysulfide or polyvinyl siloxane. Hydrophilic polyvinyl siloxanes are most suitable, and seem to be the materials of choice for their excellent accuracy and detail reproduction, remarkable mechanical properties and excellent stability. Neither reversible nor irreversible hydrocolloids are well suited for this type of impression, since their lack of tear resistance often poses insurmountable problems over recording of proximal margins. Hydrocolloids also do not allow a plaster duplicate to be obtained from the same impression. Nor is it possible, when using refractory material, to cast a phosphate investment directly into a hydrocolloid impression, since the hydrophilic properties of the impression material, combined with the exothermic reaction of the investment procedure, would culminate in quite irretrievable deformation.

In view of the delicacy of preparation involved and the existence of undercut areas, the use of the 'wash' technique is generally not recommended.

Easy access to all margins further contribute to a simple one-stage, dual-viscosity impression technique (double-mix technique).

Gingival displacement

Laminate veneers are most commonly juxta- or even supragingival, and require no special preparation of the

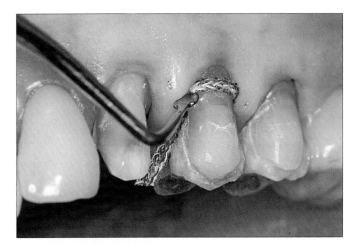

Figure 9.78 Placing of a braided cord (Ultrapak No. 2).

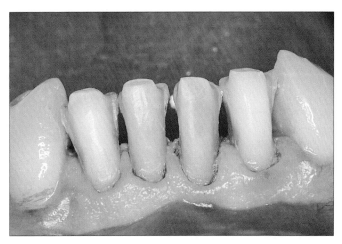

Figure 9.79 Preparation for four mandibular veneers involving major embrasure areas, rendering impressions very difficult.

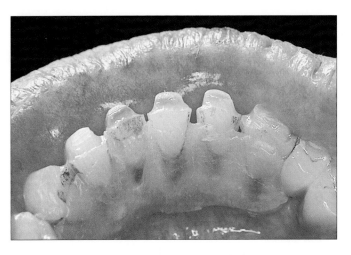

Figure 9.80 Softened wax is spread lingually between proximal surfaces to avoid tearing the impression during removal.

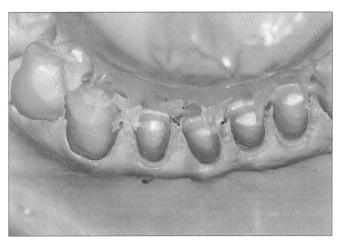

Figure 9.81 Impression made using an addition silicone and double-mix technique.

soft tissues. However, gingival displacement, enabling the root emergence profile to be recorded, is required when the cervical margin is subgingival. This displacement is obtained by inserting into the sulcus surgical suturing threads or small braided cords (Ultrapak No. 1 or 2, Ultradent), handled with care so as to avoid any bleeding (Figure 9.78). It is preferable to use non-medicated retraction cords, since astringent, vasoconstrictor, hemostatic action sometimes brings about secondary gingival recession.

Any undercut areas created by the embrasures can be lingually filled in (without impinging on the preparation) using softened wax to avoid any tearing of the impression (Figures 9.79 and 9.80).

Impression

Preparation sites are cleaned using a disinfectant–surface-tension reducer. After cleaning the surface, any threads

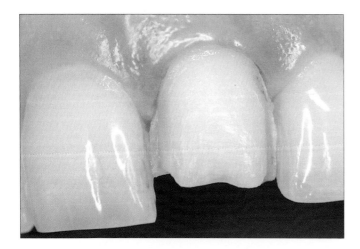

Figure 9.82 A single laminate veneer preparation.

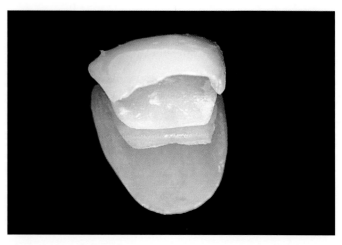

Figure 9.83 Temporary veneer produced at chairside using light-cured composite resin.

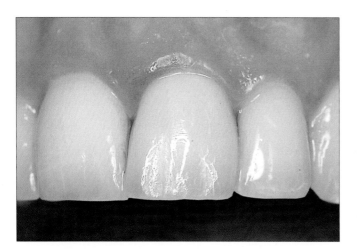

Figure 9.84 Temporary veneer bonded over left central incisor with zinc oxyphosphate cement.

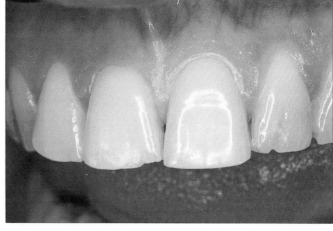

Figure 9.85 Prior to each preparation, an impression is taken so that the laboratory can fabricate the provisional veneers – in this case, four upper incisors and two canines.

are removed and preparation sites dried. Low-viscosity silicone is injected by syringe or brushed on, and is immediately covered over with a high-viscosity silicone.

Upon setting, the impression is removed, checked (Figure 9.81) and disinfected, before being processed or sent to the prosthetic laboratory.

Provisional restorations

Despite the minor degree of tissue reduction required, and the relatively low incidence of postoperative sensi-

tivity, the authors have begun increasingly to resort to provisional restorations because of patients' esthetic demands. The current trend toward converting laminate veneers into partial crowns likewise increases the number of cases where temporary coverings must be considered.

Fabricating provisional veneer restorations is considered a most delicate stage, since the minimal tissue reduction gives the preparation poor retention properties. Special considerations are therefore required in fabricating the provisional restorations and with the temporary luting procedures.

Numerous techniques have been introduced.

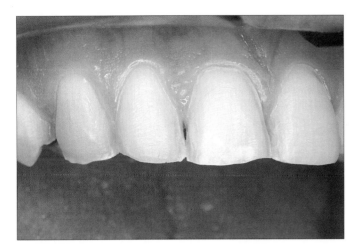

Figure 9.86 Classic preparation for incisor and canine veneers.

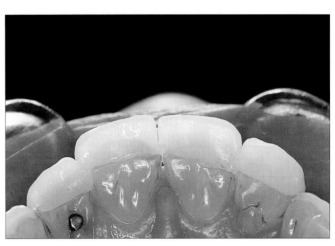

Figure 9.87 Temporary veneers are relined with resin and the surplus is removed, except at the embrasures, so as to enhance retention.

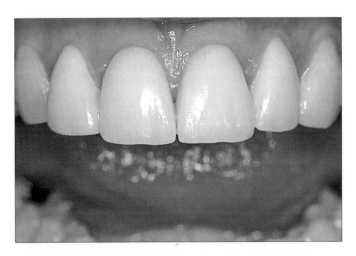

Figure 9.88 The provisional veneers have been luted with a zinc oxyphosphate cement.

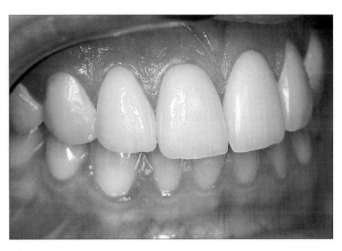

Figure 9.89 Permanent veneers bonded with a resin cement.

Direct methods

Direct methods generally use restorative composites, and are only applied to a single preparation at a time (Figures 9.82–9.84).

Once the tooth concerned has been coated with a layer of water-soluble separator, the composite is applied with a spatula, taking care to free the interproximal spaces of excess material before any curing takes place. After the material has been hardened by light curing, it is removed, adjusted, shaped and polished. All these delicate steps have to be carried out with care, since the temporary restoration is very thin. Particular attention should be paid to the margins, which may need to be relined once or even twice.

Indirect methods

Indirect methods use composites or chemically cured resins (Figures 9.85–9.89). They are particularly well suited to groups of several laminate veneers. Here, too, a number of procedures exist for the creation of temporary coverings. The most practical of these involves clinical and laboratory stages, as described below.

A complete upper and lower impression is made before preparing the teeth, followed by mounting the models on an articulator and making any corrections desired, such as lengthening or closing up diastemata using either light-cured resin or wax.

A transparent plastic mold is then produced in a vacuum so as to give an exact replica of the teeth to be treated.

Once preparation has ended, a water-soluble separator is spread over prepared and non-prepared teeth alike in fine layers, and the plastic mould is loaded with a light-cured resin (e.g. Triad light-cured resin VLC, Dentsply–DeTrey).

The mold loaded with resin is applied to the prepared teeth and light-cured. Once removed, it is placed in a laboratory resin-curing unit to complete the polymerization process.

After trimming and adjusting, the temporary coverings often need to be relined in order to improve the fit of the margins. These temporary prostheses are generally not separated, but used in one piece.

When the margins are correct and occlusion perfectly adjusted, the internal and external surfaces of the resin provisional veneers are sandblasted very lightly with 50 µm aluminum oxide.

Once sandblasted, the labial surface can be treated using ceramic stains mixed with a transparent light-cured resin to obtain the desired shade. Shade adjustment, final characterization and an excellent luster can be achieved by this simple procedure.

The provisional restorations are then luted with a temporary cement not containing eugenol or with zinc phosphate cement.

It is also possible to prepare the teeth to be covered on plaster casts, and then to have temporary coverings made over these preparations in the laboratory. Once the teeth have been prepared in the mouth, it will suffice to adjust these coverings and reline them. This rapid technique gives excellent results where the temporary devices are fused in pairs.

In the case of single-laminate veneers, one may resort to prefabricated temporary polycarbonate teeth, trimmed round and adjusted over the preparation. These coverings are often confined to the lingual–buccal surface only, and will be relined once or twice, using a resin, then cemented on temporarily.

Provisional restorations also make it possible to vizualize the intended changes, as well as serving as a reference point on which to base permanent laminate veneers.

Clinical procedures for bonding laminate veneers

The bonding of laminate veneers can often be the most challenging step in the execution of these fine ceramic restorations. This procedure usually includes three main stages (Figures 9.90–9.110):

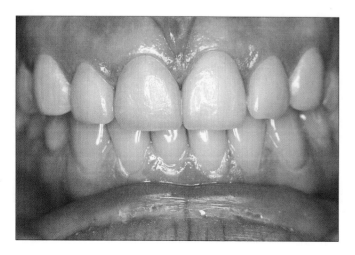

Figure 9.90 Six ceramic laminate veneers were applied to the maxillary anterior teeth of this young female patient ten years ago; she now requires a lighter color and longer incisors.

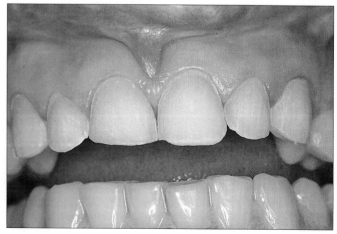

Figure 9.91 Preparation involving overlay of the incisal edge after removal of the old laminates.

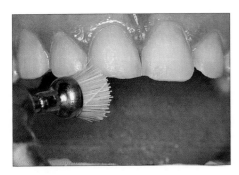

Figure 9.92 *Teeth are cleaned with pumice, and rotatory brushes.*

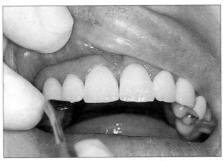

Figure 9.93 *The veneers are tried-in one by one.*

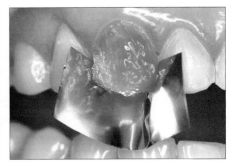

Figure 9.94 *Once the tooth has been isolated by a fine soft metal matrix, a 37% phosphoric acid gel is applied to the site for 15 seconds.*

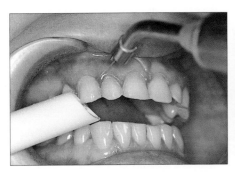

Figure 9.95 *The tooth is well rinsed for 30 seconds; any major drying off should be avoided prior to bonding. The surface should be kept slightly moist at all times.*

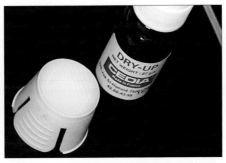

Figure 9.96 *The previously etched laminate veneer is submerged in a volatile solvent for 3 minutes.*

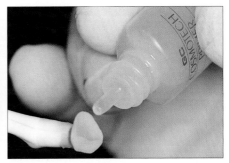

Figure 9.97 *A silane coupling agent is painted onto the inner surface of the veneer once it is completely clean and dry; 2 minutes later, the silane is dried-off using a warm air jet.*

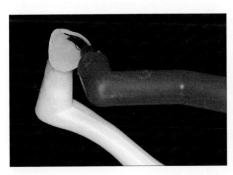

Figure 9.98 *Application of adhesive resins to inner aspect of veneer.*

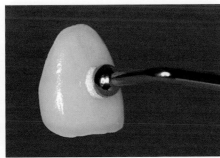

Figure 9.99 *This type of instrument (Accu-Placer, Hu-Friedy) can be used to handle the laminate veneer.*

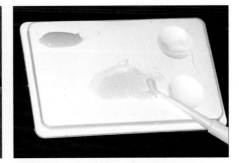

Figure 9.100 *The composite cement coloring is prepared. A light-cured composite resin is used for the veneers; a dual catalyst is added if they are thick or very opaque.*

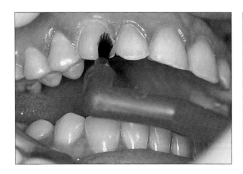

Figure 9.101 *The primer is painted onto the prepared teeth, which are kept slightly moist.*

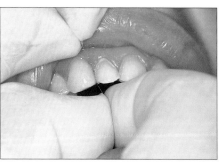

Figure 9.102 *Any surplus resin is removed before light-curing using a plastic strip.*

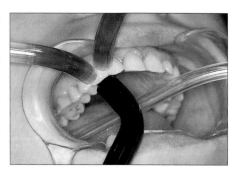

Figure 9.103 *Light-curing is carried out from various angles.*

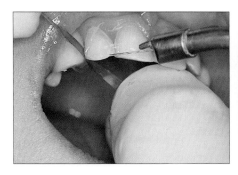

Figure 9.104 *A fine metal strip serves to clean proximal spaces under a water jet.*

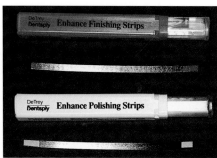

Figure 9.105 *These strips, of two different grain sizes, remain extremely practical for finishing.*

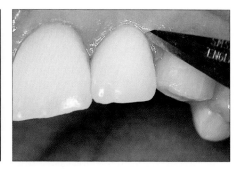

Figure 9.106 *The surplus hardened composite resin is removed using a fine scalpel blade.*

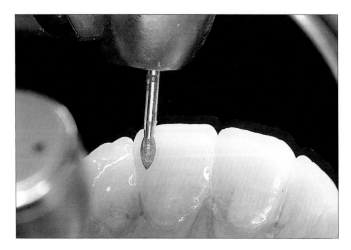

Figure 9.107 *Red- or yellow-banded diamond instruments serve to remove surplus composite resin on lingual surfaces under a water jet.*

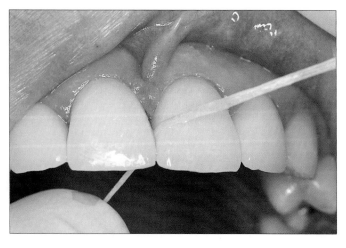

Figure 9.108 *The quality of the finish of each proximal surface can be monitored using silk dental floss.*

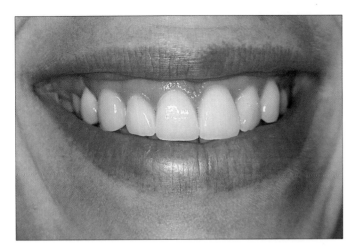

Figure 9.109 Final esthetic effect on the day when seating took place. Note that all stages of cementing and finishing were carried out without any damage to the soft tissue. (Ceramist: Serge Tissier.)

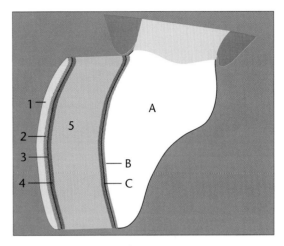

Figure 9.110 Diagrammatic representation of the different stages of treatment to bond a ceramic laminate veneer: (1) ceramic laminate veneer; (2) etching with hydrofluoric acid; (3) silane; (4) adhesive; (5) composite cement. (A) Tooth. (B) Phosphoric acid etching. (C) Dentin–enamel adhesive. (Layers are not to scale.)

- try-in;

- surface treatment;

- bonding and finishing.

The various steps in cementing laminate veneers are summarized in Table 9.3.

Try-in

Before any treatment of the teeth or the laminate veneers, the veneers must be tried-in with the utmost care, and without checking occlusal relationships. The objectives of this stage are to:

- survey the placing of the set of laminate veneers and the relationship between them and with the other (non-prepared) adjacent teeth;

- monitor the color;

- determine the color of the composite cement;

- check the fit of each laminate veneer.

The prepared tooth is first cleaned with a slurry of fine pumice and water. Some authors advocate a mixture of pumice and Mercryl, whch is best applied using a rubber Prophymatic cup. This very practical instrument has an alternating movement which reduces any splashing or spillage, thus avoiding any harm to the gingivae. Contact areas should also be cleaned using very fine metal strips (e.g. Enhance Polishing Strips, Dentsply–DeTrey), moistened with Mercryl.

The tooth is then well rinsed to eliminate any traces of pumice. It is not advisable to use a powder cleaner or brushes, since these two procedures can trigger bleeding, which is detrimental to bonding.

Try-in follows once the laminate veneer has been cleansed. The veneer will normally have been treated in the prosthetic laboratory, but the quality of etching must be checked as a precaution. The surface should be matt. If so, the laminate veneer is soaked in acetone and ultrasonicated for a few minutes to give a perfectly clean surface.

The veneers are tried in one at a time, taking care to moisten them to produce adhesion by surface tension, as with contact lenses.

With a set of several laminate veneers, it is helpful to arrange them in strict order so as to avoid any chance of error. Try-in begins with the most posterior teeth.

No pressure should ever be exerted at this stage. All adjustments will have to be made using either white silicone polishers (Komet) or red-banded diamond instruments combined with a water spray.

Adjustment should be confined to adjusting a contact point or a minor undercut area.

Table 9.3   Steps involved in the cementing of laminate veneers

Bonding procedure	Materials or products	Comments
Cleansing the teeth	Pumice + water or Mercryl: spread by Prophy cups	Eliminates all contamination from the tooth surface
Cleansing the laminate veneer	Stain-removing agent: 1 minute of ultrasonic treatment	Eradicates all contamination caused by manipulation
Try-in	Trying in the moist or Memosil-treated laminate veneer	Allows monitoring of adjustment and esthetic effect, and choice of the bonding composite
Etching the laminate veneer	Hydrofluoric acid: time will depend on the ceramic. Neutralizing: 2 minutes in a sodium bicarbonate gel	Creates micromechanical retention
Silanization of the laminate veneer	Generous moistening of the internal surface of the laminate veneer with silane: left for 2 minutes then dried-off	Sets up chemical bonding between the ceramic and bonding composite
Etching the tooth	37% phosphoric acid for enamel areas (30 seconds); 37% phosphoric acid for dentin sites (15 seconds)	Creates micromechanical retention
Primer on the tooth and the laminate veneer	Spread on 4–5 layers, leave for 30 seconds and dry.	The primer promotes intimate bonding between the tooth, composite and ceramic
Placement	Light-cured composite cement	The laminate veneer is placed in position and the strips pulled off in a lingual direction
Removal of soft surplus matter	Brushes, scalpels (with straight blade), dental floss, plastic strips	One should aim to clear away excess soft composite prior to onset of light-curing
Light-curing	Held in place by wax or Accu-Placer support, light-curing (two lamps): 40–60 seconds	Light-curing must take place from angles to ensure complete cure
Finish	Enhance strips (Dentsply–DeTrey), scalpel, tungsten instruments, yellow-banded diamond instruments, silicone polishers	Wait about 10 minutes before attempting any cleaning procedures
Luster	Diamond polishing pastes (TPS Truluster, Brasseler)	Achieves smooth glossy surfaces

Monitoring the set of laminate veneers

Once the laminate veneers have been checked individually, the whole set is tried-in. If placement is difficult or actually impossible, the contact point must be carefully eased. It is a very delicate operation to make six or eight laminate veneers hold over such unretentive preparations. Water or glycerol can sometimes improve adhesion. At present, the authors prefer to use a transparent silicone (Memosil, Heraeus-Kulzer); this makes the laminate veneer adhere to the tooth once it has polymerized. Moreover, its transparent shade of color does not alter the look of the ceramic.

Occlusion should be neither checked nor adjusted before the laminate veneers have been bonded.

Checking the color and choice of bonding composites

After bonding, the final shade of laminate veneers will depend on

- the color of the ceramic;

- the color of the underlying tooth;

- the color and thickness of the luting composite.

The color of the laminate veneers should therefore be checked during try-in, taking the influence of the tooth color into account. On the basis of this first analysis, either a composite able to correct a minor error in ceramic color will be chosen or one sufficiently opaque to mask the undesirable effect of a stained tooth.

For a tooth not requiring major color transformation, it is estimated that the final color shade depends 80% on ceramic color, 10% on composite color and 10% on tooth color. For a tooth requiring major color transformation, the final color is thought to depend 70% on the ceramic, 10% on the composite and 20% on the tooth. These percentages apply assuming that rules for preparation, spacing and build-up of the ceramic have been observed.

Some authors suggest substantial cement spacing measuring 0.1 or even 0.2 mm (Nixon, 1990), enabling better masking of the color of the tooth. Others prefer to rely on the opacity or translucency of the composite to potentiate or inhibit the color of the underlying tooth. Even with spacing extending to 0.2 mm – and this, too, has its drawbacks – the notion that the color of a laminate veneer can be changed significantly may be illusive.

When composites are placed in fine layers of around 0.1 mm, differences in hue, chroma and translucency are very slight. These observations suggest that the composite cement actually has a relatively slight influence.

By a judicious ceramic build-up, using opaque or translucent dentins, however, tooth color can be successfully altered, fulfilling all the criteria required for good light transmission.

The most translucent composite available should therefore be used to augment light transmission at the interface. This transparent layer will transmit light in all directions, giving a more natural appearance.

If certain color adjustments need to be made through the composite cement, the choice should go to low saturation and opacity. The higher these two factors, the more will this layer act as a barrier to reflect light transmission – and hence affect the final color, with unacceptable results.

It should therefore be remembered that to mask the color of a darkened tooth, it is best to intervene mainly at the stage of ceramic build-up and as little as possible in the area of the bonding composite. Ideally, the most translucent composite available, of a neutral shade, should be employed.

Try-in paste is now available with most veneer bonding kits, to monitor the effect of the composite and the color of the laminate veneer prior to bonding (Dicor, Dentsply–DeTrey; Optec HSP, Jeneric; Variolink, Ivoclar Vivadent and Choice, Bisco, for example). However, it is often found that the color of try-in paste does not exactly match that of the bonding composite, especially after polymerization.

Surface treatment

The laminate veneer

Water-soluble pastes, try-in composites, glycerol, etc., must be completely removed once etching and the different try-in procedures have been completed. After careful rinsing under running water or with alcohol (depending on the product used), the laminate veneers are immersed in a bath of volatile solvent and treated with ultrasound for several minutes.

The internal surface will theoretically have been etched in the laboratory. If this process has been omitted, it should be carried out following the manufacturer's instructions. Each ceramic requires a different substance, concentration and period of time for etching.

Etching is traditionally carried out using commercially available

- 10% ammonium difluoride gel for glass ceramics;

- 2–10% hydrofluoric acid gel for other ceramics.

According to McLean (1980), etching is indispensable, since it eliminates superficial microcracks as well as certain surface flaws on the internal surface by a process of partial dissolution. Impregnation by the bonding resin will provide reinforcement and better distribution of stress; this would explain the improved mechanical properties of ceramics after bonding. Etching also helps to enhance wettability and complete the cleaning process.

Silanization

A fine layer of a silane coupling agent is painted over the internal surface of the laminate veneer once it has been etched and thoroughly cleansed, so as to create a 'chemical link' between the bonding composite and the ceramic.

Silane coupling agents vary considerably in regard to:

- their chemical composition (one or two components);

- degree of hydrolysis;

- how they act during aging.

Some authors postulate a correlation between the degree of silane hydrolysis and adhesion of the composite, which may be summarized as follows:

- with a major level of hydrolysis, cohesive fracture would occur in the ceramic, indicating high efficiency of the coupling agent;

- as silane evaporation occurs with time and hence in aging, fractures would become largely adhesive.

Nicholls (1986, 1988) stressed that:

- when a previously silanized laminate veneer is contaminated by saliva (either accidentally or during try-in for example), 15 seconds etching with 37% phosphoric acid completely restores the qualities of the silane.

- silanization 7 days prior to the bonding session does not diminish the bond.

These observations mean that surface treatment, etching and silanization can be completed in the laboratory, and all that has to be done in the dentist's chair is phosphoric acid etching of the internal surface of the laminate veneer to fully reactivate its coating of coupling agent.

Treating the tooth

The tooth will already have been cleansed prior to try-in. All the same, all residues of composites or any water-soluble paste must be removed, as with the laminate veneer.

The prepared enamel is then etched for 15–30 seconds using a 32–37% phosphoric acid gel. This will be followed by rinsing and drying.

New-generation dental adhesives adhere to the enamel and dentin simultaneously. All products must be applied to a slightly moist surface. Drying without actually drying out is therefore required with these systems.

Bonding and finishing

The composite cement will have already been selected during the preliminary try-in. It is wise to use a sufficiently fluid composite, so as to avoid any undue pressure, which would run the risk of fracturing the laminate veneer.

The etched and cleansed teeth should be insulated interdentally with very fine strips to avoid the composite spilling over onto other preparation sites.

It is useful to pack in a retraction cord if the cervical margin is difficult to access. The cord should be applied before any etching takes place in order to avoid hemorrhage, which would contaminate the prepared tooth surface.

A primer is then spread over the tooth and the laminate veneer and dried off. This may be followed with the bonding resin; the chosen composite is then coated onto the laminate veneer.

The laminate veneer is then eased into place accurately, exerting steady, moderate pressure. It is held in place by a special instrument (Accu-Placer, Hu-Friedy) or a wax ball mounted on a plastic handle. When the laminate veneer is correctly positioned over the teeth, the strips are pulled away in a lingual direction, and any excess composite removed with a brush or probe.

One minute of light curing on all aspects of the tooth (usually using two lamps) is required for complete polymerization.

Any excess material must be completely removed before bonding the next laminate veneer. The use of tungsten or diamond instruments should be minimized; these risk gouging or taking the polish off the ceramic, as well as penetrating into the dental enamel. Scalpel blades are preferable to clean off all margins. Proximal areas, however, should be cleaned off using fine metal strips (e.g. Enhance Polishing Strips, Dentsply–DeTrey; New Metal Strips, GC).

In the case of accessible margins, small white rubber polishers followed by diamond paste (TPS Truluster Brasseler) are used for finishing.

Rotary tungsten or diamond instruments may occasionally be necessary. Multiple-blade tungsten carbide burs included in the Esthetic Trimming (Komet-Brasseler) kit designed by Goldstein, as well as yellow-banded diamond instruments from the TPS Finition (Komet-Brasseler) pack, are very well suited to this procedure.

All the areas touched up (particularly with diamond instruments) should be repolished, first with a rubber polisher and finally with diamond polishing paste.

This entire procedure should be repeated for each laminate veneer.

The following tips may prove helpful in carrying out the cementing procedure:

- Should the etched tooth accidentally become contaminated by blood or saliva, it will need to be etched again for about 10 seconds in order to reactivate the surface prior to bonding.

- All bonding kits offer light-cured composites with the option of adding a catalyst to turn them into dual-cure products. Dual-cure composites do not have to be employed, since laminate veneers are very thin and allow light to be transmitted to the cement. Light-cured materials are generally more color-stable than dual-cure composites.

- With placement of multiple laminate veneers, it is advisable to begin with the most distal, providing a 'test site', thus enabling the bonding composite to be modified for the benefit of the most visible teeth (should this composite appear either too opaque or too saturated).

- Particular attention should be paid to occlusal adjustment, since even slight errors may lead to fracturing.

- Maximum intercuspation as well as lateral contacts

and protrusion must be guided by the occlusal criteria selected.

- Adjustments should be made using red-banded diamond burs for major alterations and yellow-banded diamonds for the remainder.

- A water spray should always be used during this work. Adjustments should be made at least 10–15 minutes after bonding the last laminate veneer in place.

- Once these adjustments have been accomplished, the reworked areas should be carefully polished using small rubber cups followed by diamond polishing paste.

- Patients should be examined 2–4 days after placement to ensure that no excess adhesive remains and to check for correct occlusion. This is also the stage at which one can take postoperative photographs.

- In cases where the occlusal scheme has been changed, or of suspected bruxism, it is wise to arrange for an occlusal splint ('night guard') to be worn at night.

Conclusion

The ceramic laminate veneer remains the prosthetic restoration that best complies with the principles of present-day esthetic dentistry. It is kind to the soft tissue and the adjoining periodontium, avoids the use of any metal structures and posseses excellent esthetic quality. It is also the only prosthetic restoration enabling a significant proportion of the natural enamel to be conserved. This, as emphasized by McLean (personal communication), is the main priority to be respected, natural human enamel being the best restorative material at present.

The ability to replace natural enamel of teeth deficient in structure, shape or color with artificial enamel, intimately bonded to the dental tissue, is an ideal long sought after by researchers, clinicians, ceramic technicians and manufacturers. The first publication on a ceramic jacket crown in 1886 had, even then, a title including the word 'enamelled coating'. Might this ideal have actually been attained one century later? Despite a relatively low failure rate, as confirmed by most authors, longer-term results are needed to answer this question more definitely.

Other progress in surface treatment and materials will undoubtedly contribute further improvements that will make this 'artificial enamelling' simpler and more reliable.

Table 9.4   Mechanical, biological and esthetic failures for 170 patients (1024 laminate veneers) for the period 1984–1994

Mechanical failures		Biological failures		Esthetic failures	
Split (chip fracture)	18	Sensitivity	10	Margins visible	
Cracks	0	Infiltration (microleakage)	15	Proximal	30
Fractures (try-in, bonding)	2	Caries	0	Cervical	18
		Necrosis	0	Influence of underlying tooth	40
Functional fractures				Influence of bonding composite	5
Cervical	1			Influence of ceramic and	
Occlusal	12			build-up technique	28
Debonding	1				
	34 (3.3%)		25 (2.4%)		121 (11.8%)

Analysis of and reasons for failure: a 10-year follow-up

While the use of laminate veneers may now be considered a safe, reliable and completely documented technique (when used by knowledgeable and experienced practitioners), the fact remains that during its 10-year clinical history it has been fraught with incidents, accidents and setbacks. Although minor, these are worth analyzing, since practical lessons may be drawn from them as well as ideas for mechanical, functional and esthetic improvements. The shortcomings may be attributed to many different causes, and may occur at any stage in the process:

- case selection: very dark-colored teeth, bruxism;

- preparation: position and shape of margins, inadequate support, insufficient thickness;

- temporization: ill-adjusted temporary restoration, unsuitable temporary cement;

- laboratory processes: poor choice of ceramic or build-up technique;

- try-in and handling: accidental fracturing;

- choice of cement: opacity, thickness, saturation

- bonding procedure: mishandling, unsuitable products

- communication: poor comprehension of patient's needs, bad communication of data to the prosthetic laboratory.

To obtain a more accurate view of the size and causes of these setbacks, the authors conducted a clinical study over a 10-year period (1984–1994) on 170 patients, wearing a total of 1024 laminate veneers. The mechanical, esthetic and biological failures are presented as percentages in Table 9.4.

Discussion

Mechanical failure
This was very rare, and only reached the rate of 3.3% (Figure 9.111). Failure and fracturing occured most commonly at the incisal edge and mainly affected laminate veneers produced without overlaying the occlusal edge (Figures 9.112 and 9.113). Ceramic veneers hardly ever debond (only once in the authors' experience), and the occurrence can be attributed either to the use of a product after its expiry date or to a serious error during the bonding procedure (Figures 9.114 and 9.115).

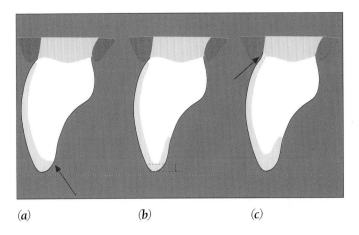

(a) (b) (c)

Figure 9.111 *Three causes of fracturing of ceramic laminate veneers:* (***a***) *poor positioning of incisal finishing margin;* (***b***) *insufficient thickness of incisal ceramic;* (***c***) *margin extends too far sub-gingivally.*

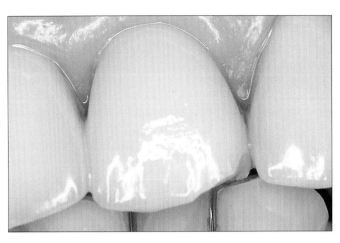

Figure 9.112 *Fracture of the veneer edge due to insufficient coverage of the incisal edge.*

Figure 9.113 *In mandibular teeth, it is essential to produce an incisal overlay so that the veneer can work under compression. The fracture is very noticeable in this instance.*

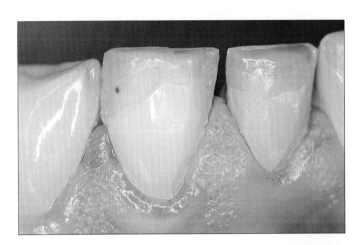

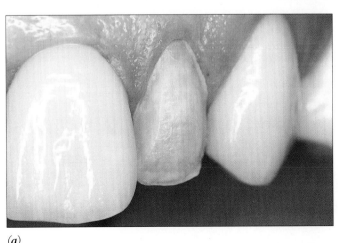

(a)

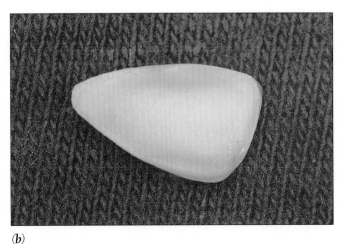

(b)

Figure 9.114 (***a, b***) *A debonded ceramic laminate veneer. All the composite stayed on the tooth surface; faulty etching of the veneer was responsible in this case.*

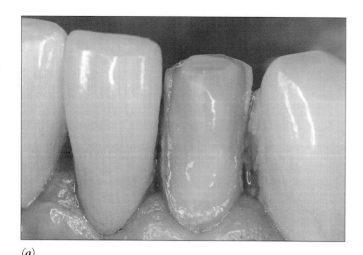

(a)

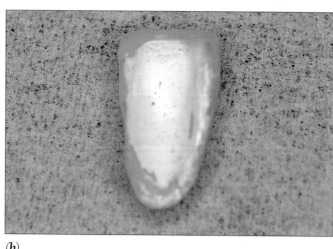

(b)

Figure 9.115 (*a, b*) *In this case of debonding, most of the composite cement has remained on the laminate veneer; faulty tooth surface treatment was the causative factor.*

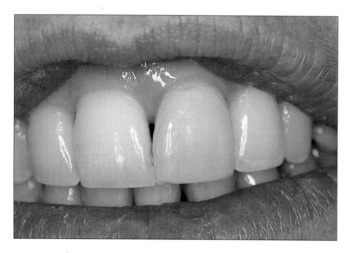

Figure 9.116 *Eight years post veneer placement, slight leakage is noted at the cervical margin.*

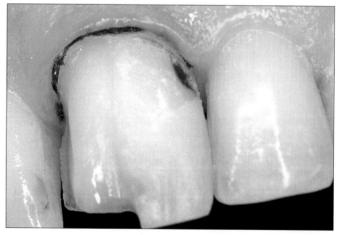

Figure 9.117 *Once the veneer has been removed, the leakage is seen to have been very limited.*

Biological failure

This, too, occurred extremely rarely, in only 2.4% of cases.

Most instances of postoperative sensitivity affected laminate veneers made between 1984 and 1990. This has now become very rare with the use of modern adhesives, and usually fades within a few days. The percentage of cases with marginal microleakage (Figures 9.116 and 9.117) also shows a downward trend at present due to the improved precision of ceramic laminate veneers, as well as to the use of more resistant adhesive cements and, finally, to better adhesion.

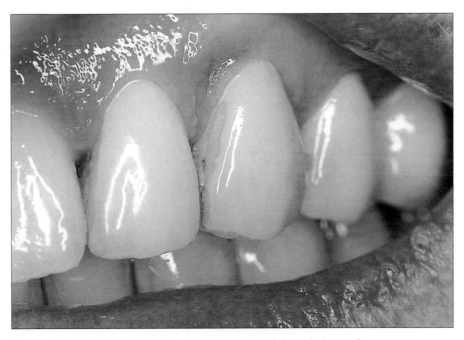

Figure 9.118 *Esthetic failure due to the recession of the soft tissue after seven years.*

Esthetic failure

This is not structural failure, but is the result of non-pleasing esthetic effects.

In cases of tooth discoloration, any visible margin constitutes a major source of esthetic problems, often jeopardizing the end result.

The proportion of visible margins increases some years after the placement of laminated veneers, and depends on the degree of recession of the marginal gingiva and the interproximal papillae (Figure 9.118). This recession is difficult to predict, and it is therefore wise, in the case of a major change, to draw the proximal margins back as far as possible in a lingual direction.

Very dark colors (Figures 9.119 and 9.120) or greatly varying supporting teeth (Figure 9.121) also complicate the esthetic result; it is perhaps in this area that most difficulties have been encountered in obtaining correct light transmission. Although the patient may often be happy with the overall color change, the esthetic effect does not appear natural (Figure 9.122).

Progress now being made in ceramics and ceramic build-up techniques, as well as wiser selection of cases suitable for treatment (Figure 9.123), has reduced esthetic failures significantly.

Mechanical and biological failures together in the authors' study amount to a total of 59 instances, or about 6%, which is equal to the failure rate of metal ceramics. At present, the percentage of esthetic failures does not exceed that found with any other type of ceramic restoration.

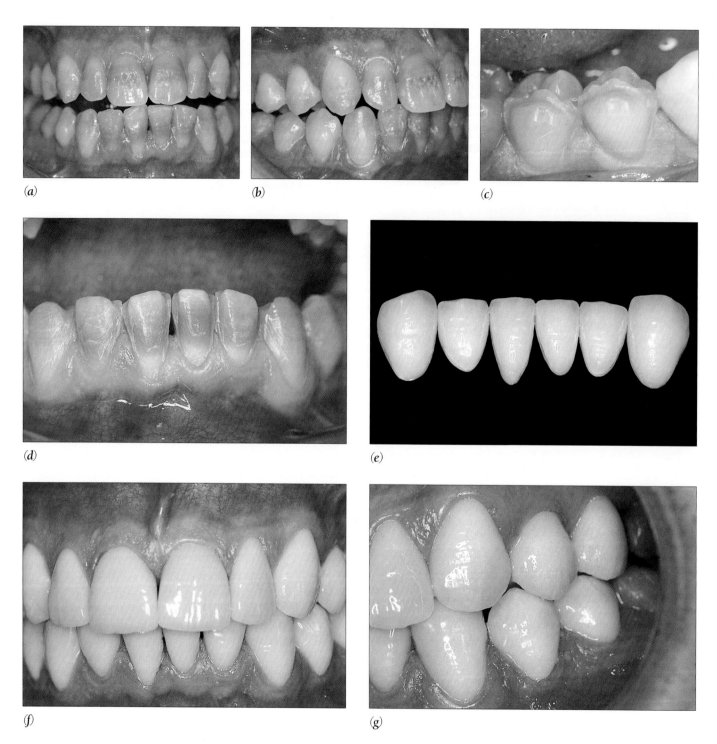

Figure 9.119 *A natural light-transmission effect cannot always be achieved in cases of severe discoloration, since it requires the use of opaque ceramic 'dentins' and composite cements of low translucency.* (**a**) *Severe tetracycline staining associated with major dysplasia.* (**b**) *Note the difference in staining between the inciso-canine and premolar groups.* (**c**) *Preparation for laminate veneers; note the even color of the teeth.* (**d**) *Teeth are severely stained in this case.* (**e**) *Laminated Empress veneers.* (**f, g**) *To suppress any encroachment of the underlying tooth, it was necessary to opaque these laminate veneers heavily and to use a fairly opaque film of thick composite resin; this eliminates any natural translucency. (Ceramist: Laboratory GH, Paris.)*

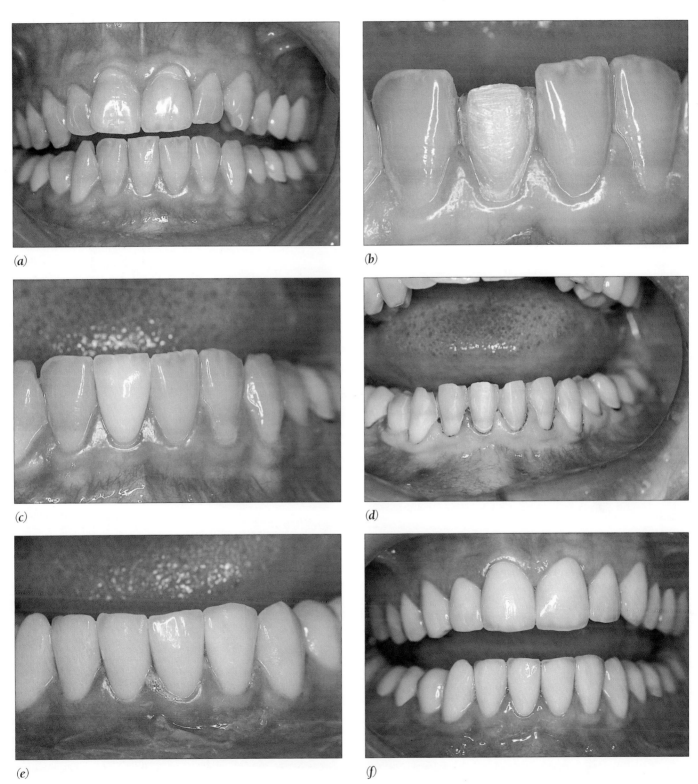

(a)

(b)

(c)

(d)

(e)

(f)

Figure 9.120 *In cases of severe discoloration, the viability of the lamination and the composite cement can usefully be tested prior to completion on an individual laminate veneer. (**a**) Severe tetracycline staining. (**b**) Preparation of a single laminate veneer. (**c**) The laminate veneer is tried in then seated without any surface preparation in order to test the final effect. (**d**) Preparations are then carried out. (**e**) This technique enables stratification, choice of composite cement and final color to be tested; this is essential to achieve the right effect. (**f**) Veneers in place: an acceptable esthetic effect can be achieved despite very heavy discoloration. (Ceramist: Jacques Diligeart.)*

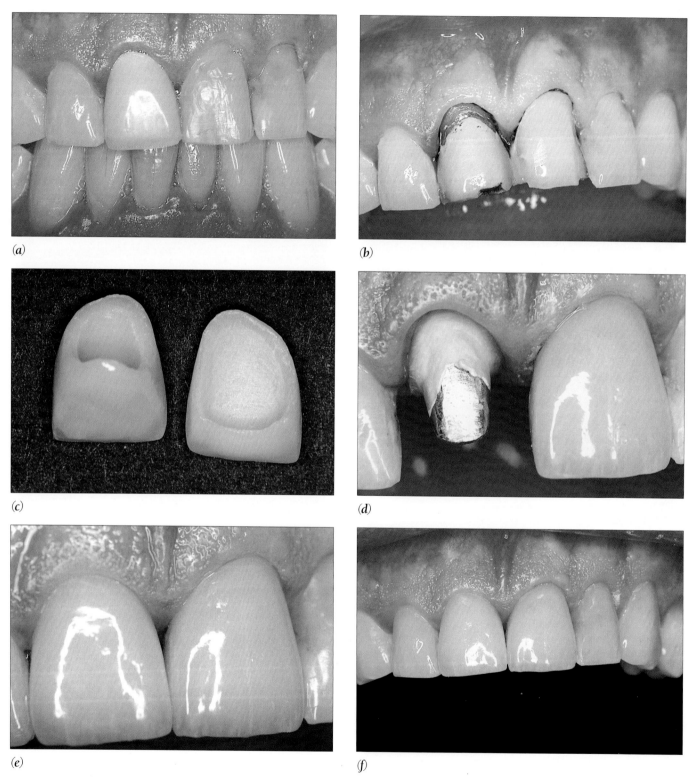

(a)

(b)

(c)

(d)

(e)

(f)

Figure 9.121 *The same light-transmission properties can be achieved by a judicious choice of ceramic material using stratification techniques, despite widely varying thicknesses and tooth structure.* (**a**) *This patient wishes to change the look of the two central incisors only.* (**b**) *A ceramic laminate veneer overlay will be carried out for the left central; an all-ceramic crown is more appropriate for the right central because of the presence of an endodontic post and core.* (**c**) *The jacket crown and the veneer have been fabricated in Empress by stratification.* (**d**) *The veneer is bonded.* (**e**) *Good esthetics, despite widely differing underlying tooth structure.* (**f**) *This result could only be achieved because of the high chroma of this color.* (Ceramist: Jacques Diligeart.)

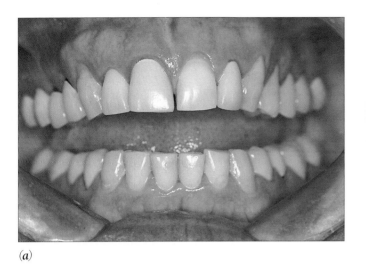

(a)

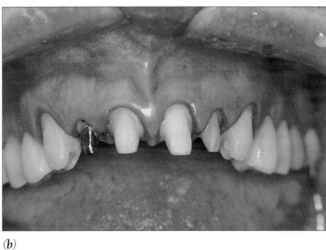

(b)

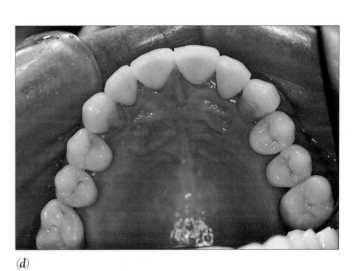

(c)

(d)

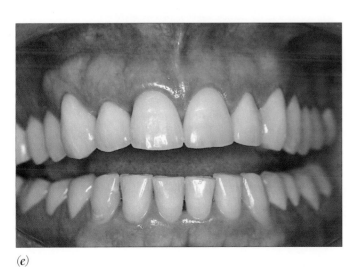

(e)

Figure 9.122 *This patient wishes to improve the color and esthetic properties of his teeth; despite widely differing tooth structure, all-ceramic restorations will be used. (***a***) In this case eight Empress jacket crowns and two laminate veneers over the maxillary canines are produced. In the lower arch, bleaching only will be performed. (***b***) Illustration of the wide disparity between underlying tooth structure. (***c***) A model with crowns. (***d***, ***e***) Final esthetic effect. (Ceramist: Jacques Diligeart.)*

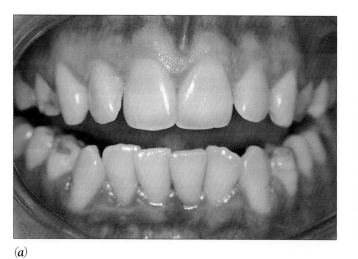

(a)

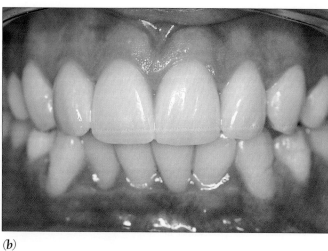

(b)

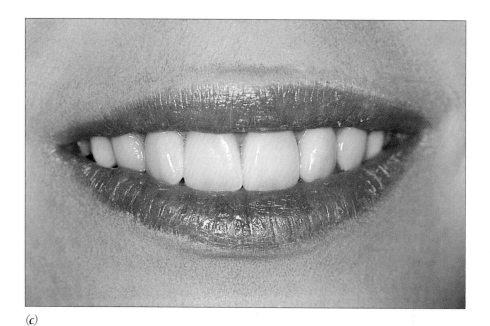

(c)

Figure 9.123 (a–c) *When the teeth are only slightly stained, the final esthetic effect is more natural. In this case, six maxillary laminate veneers were placed (bleaching was previously performed on both upper and lower arches). (Ceramist: Serge Tissier.)*

References

Buonocore MGA, Simple method of increasing the adhesion of acrylic filling materials to enamel surfaces. *J Dent Res* 1955; **34**: 849–53.

Calamia JR, Simonsen RJ, Effect of coupling agents on bond strength of etched porcelain. *J Dent Res* 1984; **63**: 162–362.

Crispin BJ, Esthetic moieties: enamel thickness. *J Esthet Dent* 1993; **5**: 37.

Garber DA, Rational tooth preparation for porcelain laminate veneers. *Compend Contin Educ Dent* 1991; **12**: 316–22.

Goldstein RE, *Change Your Smile.* Chicago: Quintessence, 1984.

Greggs TS, *Method for Cosmetic Restoration of Anterior Teeth.* United States Patent No. 4,473,353. Filed 15 April 1983; Date of Patent 25 September 1984.

Highton RM, Caputo AA, Matyas J, Effectiveness of porcelain repair systems. *J Prosthet Dent* 1979; **42**: 292.

Horn HR, Porcelain laminate veneers bonded to etched enamel. *Dent Clin North Am* 1983; **27**: 671–84.

Lustig PL, A rational concept of crown preparation revised and expanded. *Quintessence Int* 1976; **11**: 41.

McLean JW, *The Science and Art of Dental Ceramics.* London: Quintessence, 1980.

Nicholls JI, Esthetic veneer cementation. *J Prosthet Dent* 1986; **56**: 9–12.

Nicholls JI, Tensile bond of resin cements to porcelain veneers. *J Prosthet Dent* 1988; **60**: 443–47.

Nixon RL, Porcelain veneers: An esthetic therapeutic alternative. In: Rufenacht CR. *Fundamentals of Esthetics.* Chicago, IL: Quintessence, 1990: 329–50.

Nixon RL, IPS Empress: the ceramic system of the future. *Signature* 1994; **1**: 10–15.

Pincus CR, Building mouth personality. *J Calif S Dent Assoc* 1938; **14**: 125–29.

Rochette A, Attachment of a splint to enamel of lower anterior teeth. *J Prosthet Dent* 1973; **30**: 418–23.

CHAPTER 10

Ceramic and Modified Metal–Ceramic Crowns

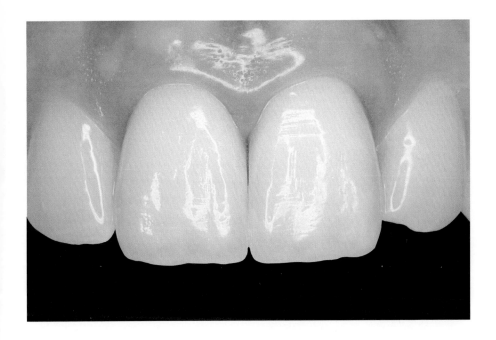

The ceramic jacket crown is certainly one of the most esthetically successful restorations available; it was also the first crown ever invented. Jacket crowns were first produced in 1886 by Land, who designed a technique for firing ceramics on a platinum matrix in a furnace that he had patented. This innovation marked the onset of a period devoted to the development of ceramic inlays and onlays, which relied on the same technology. Unfortunately, these prostheses were simply cemented on, often by means of zinc phosphate cement, and resulted in a very high failure rate. A high fracturing incidence of ceramic jacket crowns caused these prostheses to lapse into temporary obscurity. During the 1960s, these intrinsically fragile crowns were improved upon by McLean, who increased their mechanical resistance by reinforcing them with an alumina base. The aluminous porcelain jacket crown served as an esthetic point of reference for almost 20 years. The improvement in ceramics, refractory investments, and bonding techniques led to the development of all-ceramic restorations directly bonded to tooth structure for crowns. The bonding reinforces the mechanical resistance of jacket crowns and reduces

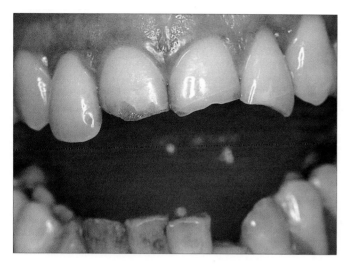

Figure 10.1 *A female patient, in her 30s, following a severe car accident. The mandibular incisors have been reimplanted, and three maxillary incisors are fractured, without pulp exposures. Figures 10.2–10.6 detail aspects of the treatment.*

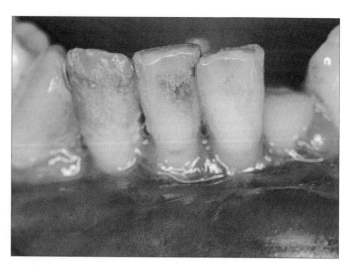

Figure 10.2 *The mandibular anterior teeth, after removal of the splint.*

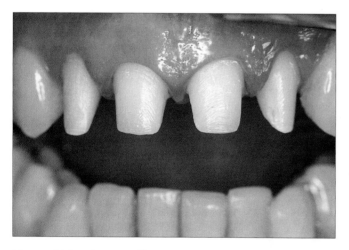

Figure 10.3 *Four maxillary anteriors prepared for all-ceramic jacket crowns.*

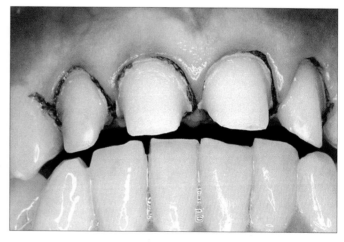

Figure 10.4 *Gingival displacement is achieved by the use of two cords : a surgical suture silk thread and a threaded cotton cord, the diameter of which will vary according to the volume of the gingival sulcus.*

the risk of fracture. The bonding also significantly improves esthetic properties, since the composite resin cement has the advantages of adjustable color and opacity, as well as light transmission properties resembling those of natural teeth (Figures 10.1–10.6).

It was the growth in the development of ceramic laminate veneers during the mid-1980s that heightened awareness of this technique.

A bonded ceramic jacket crown is now the treatment of choice for restoration of single anterior teeth that are

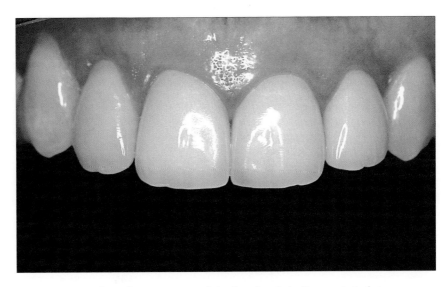

Figure 10.5 *The esthetic outcome of the four-bonded all-ceramic jacket crowns: note the balance between the central and the lateral incisors, and the subtle texture.*

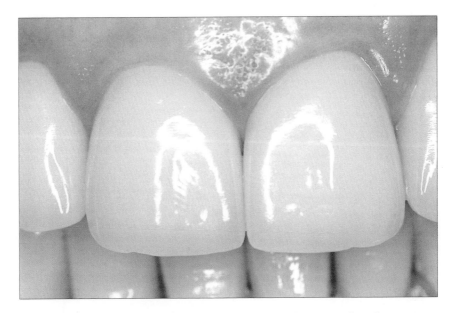

Figure 10.6 *Close-up of the central incisors. The jacket crowns have been adhesively luted. (Ceramist: Gérald Ubassy.)*

unsuitable for treatment with laminate veneers, for the following reasons:

- the absence of a metal substructure confers optical qualities resembling those of natural teeth;

- they can be successfully blended in with bonded laminate veneers;
- their gingival margins and diffuse light reflection to the gingivae ensure that the surrounding periodontal tissues appear healthy.

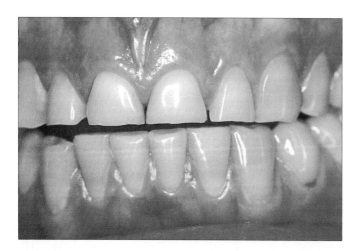

Figure 10.7 *This female patient, in her mid-20s, suffered from bulimia and bruxism when she was a teenager. Her maxillary anterior teeth show severe attrition and a yellowish color (A3.5 Vita).*

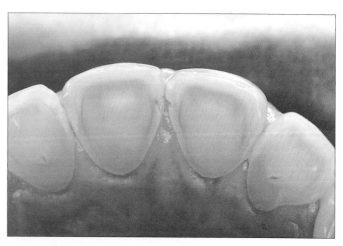

Figure 10.8 *Lingual view of the maxillary incisors showing the loss of hard tissue due to hyperacidity (same patient as shown in Figure 10.7).*

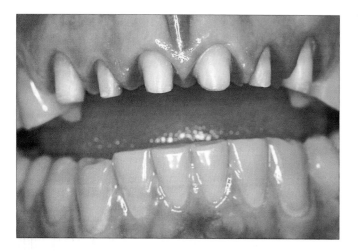

Figure 10.9 *The preparations for the all-ceramic jacket crowns: all teeth are vital and protected by a hybrid layer (dentin infiltrated by a hydrophilic dentin primer).*

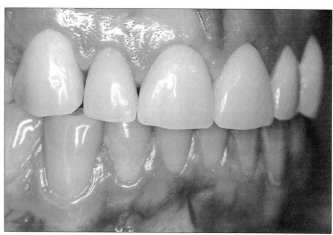

Figure 10.10 *Immediate temporization according to the preliminary diagnostic wax-up. Since only minor alterations are desired by the patient, a second set of temporary crowns and a treatment wax-up are not necessary.*

However, this technique is not yet widely used because preparation of these ceramic jacket crowns requires strict, delicate precision. In addition, the bonding techniques employed, mainly to the dentin, are somewhat complex, and adverse effects to the pulp are of concern.

This chapter describes techniques designed to minimize the risk of mechanical failure (fracturing of the ceramic) and biological failure (pulpal inflammation or necrosis) (Figures 10.7–10.15).

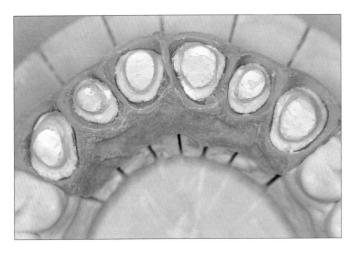

Figure 10.11 *The 'soft-tissue' master model.*

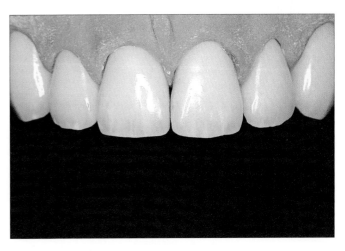

Figure 10.12 *All-ceramic jacket crowns (IPS Empress, Ivoclar) on the 'soft-tissue' model. Note the harmonious shape of the teeth. (Ceramist: Gérald Ubassy.)*

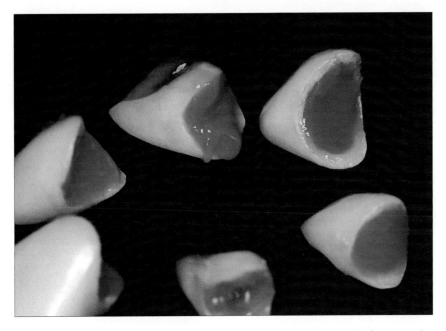

Figure 10.13 *The crowns are etched in the laboratory using a hydrofluoric acid gel. After try-in, and before positioning, they are conditioned at chairside with 37% phosphoric acid.*

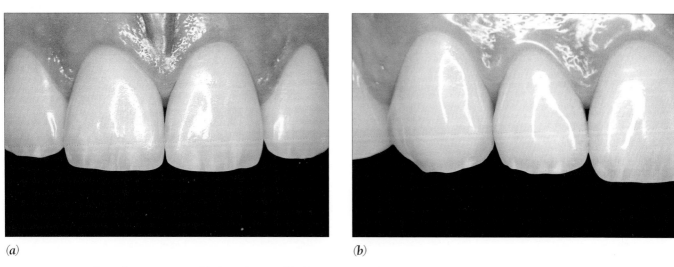

(a)

(b)

Figure 10.14 *The esthetic outcome: (**a**) frontal view; (**b**) close-up view of right side. The soft tissue is healthy and the incisal thirds of the ceramic jacket crowns are natural and opalescent.*

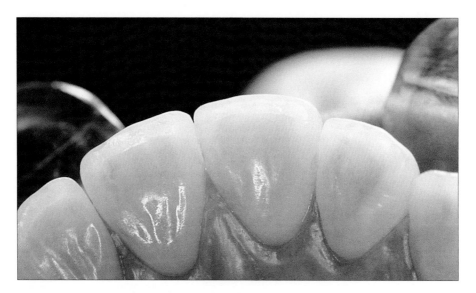

Figure 10.15 *Lingual view showing the light transmission and the cervical aspect – an example of some of the esthetic advantages of all-ceramic crowns.*

Clinical considerations

Different types of jacket crowns

The introduction of new ceramics in recent years has led to various applications for these materials and has given rise to several types of jacket crowns:

- the feldspathic ceramic jacket crown fired over refractory investment (Fortune, Williams; G Cera, GC; IPS Classic, Ivoclar; Lamina, Shofu; etc.)

- the heat-pressed leucite-reinforced ceramic jacket (IPS Empress, Ivoclar) crown;

- the glass–ceramic castable jacket crown (Dicor/Dicor Plus, Dentsply-Caulk);

- the jacket crown produced by slip casting (In-Ceram, Vita);

- the jacket crown produced by mixed techniques: a core cast in glass–ceramic is later veneered with a ceramic such as Vitadur N (Willi's glass);

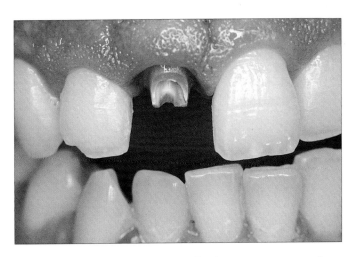

Figure 10.16 *An example of a difficult case to restore, with a dark root, bright dentin and strongly opalescent incisal edge with mamelons, halo and white spots.*

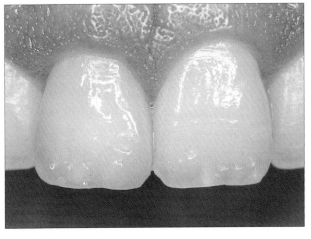

Figure 10.17 *After etching and silanating the ceramic margins, the modified metal–ceramic crown (low-fusing ceramic Duceram-LFC, Ducera) is bonded on to the tooth, which has been previously restored by a metallic dowel and core. (Ceramist: Marc Cristou.)*

- the 'low-fusion' jacket crown – a feldspathic ceramic core veneered by a low-fusing (660°C) ceramic (Duceram LFC, Ducera) (Figures 10.16 and 10.17).

Indications

Establishing indications for the jacket crown requires special attention beyond the customary clinical examination that precedes all prosthetic restorations. Many failures could be avoided by examination of the support teeth, occlusal relationship and other less obvious parameters.

Ceramics are brittle materials, basically of high compressive and low flexural strength, and they should therefore be applied only when appropriate. Jacket crowns are generally indicated on slightly damaged anterior teeth with good clinical crown height, in the absence of bruxism or parafunctional activity.

Posterior teeth

Modified metal–ceramic crowns Esthetics and light transmission are less important in the posterior region, where reliability remains the chief clinical parameter; a metal–ceramic crown would therefore be the restoration of choice.

Winter (1990, 1992), Geller and Kwiatkowski (1987) and Geller (1991) have recently described a metal framework vertically shortened at the cervical level,

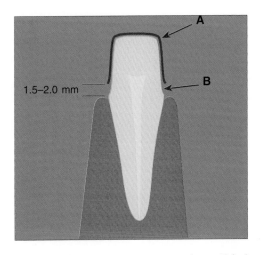

Figure 10.18 *Schematic representation of a modified coping for a metal–ceramic crown: A, metal substructure; B, natural tooth. The reduced metal coping ends 1.5–2.0 mm short of the chamfer, allowing a more translucent porcelain margin, which increases the diffusion of light to the soft tissue.*

where the metal substructure finishes at about 2 mm from the shoulder. This arrangement allows the use of semitranslucent margins, giving the cervical zone a more natural color and allowing light to pass through at gingival level (Figure 10.18). These reduced-frame-

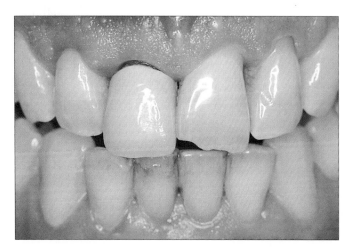

Figure 10.19 *A defective crown, with poor margins, on a male patient in his mid-50s. Note the level of the gingiva around the upper right central incisor.*

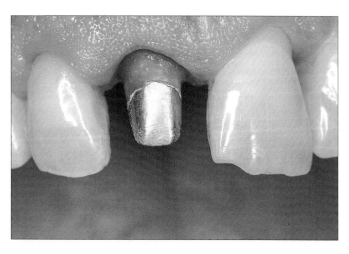

Figure 10.20 *Gingivoplasty has been carried out, and a dowel-core cemented in.*

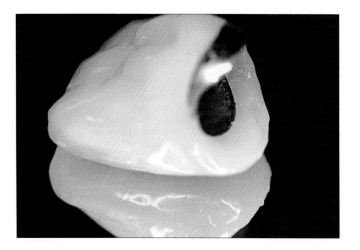

Figure 10.21 *The crown has a ceramic margin butt-joint on the mesial, distal and buccal aspects. The metal coping is vertically shortened at the cervical level, and ends at about 2 mm from the deep chamfer.*

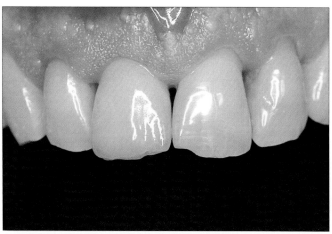

Figure 10.22 *The esthetic result, although not ideal, is harmonious and pleasing. The authors chose not to restore the broken angle of the left incisor, but to emulate it for improved personalization of the patient's smile.*

work metal–ceramic crowns are presently proving to be an excellent compromise between esthetic properties and mechanical resistance (Figures 10.19–10.22). They also allow the fabrication of bridges, and are compatible with cast metal cores, which cannot be used with jacket crowns because of their negative esthetic effect. Statistics recently reported by Peter Schärer (personal communication) show that the reduced framework does not lower the mechanical resistance of these prostheses.

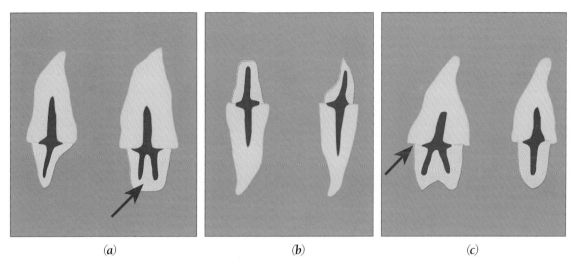

(a)   (b)   (c)

Figure 10.23 *Examples of a metal–ceramic dowel-core. (a) For maxillary incisors, a framework with two extensions is recommended because of the width of the tooth (arrow). (b) In mandibular incisors, a single extension is used. (c) In this bicuspid framework, one extension is buccal while the other is lingual. The core leaves space for a shoulder margin (arrow).*

Anterior teeth

The following factors should be considered during clinical examination.

Caries and restorations   The presence of caries or old restorations requires that a prognosis be established regarding the pulp; if damage has become too extensive, peripheral preparation will leave behind a fragile core, and such additional invasive procedures could bring about devitalization of the pulp. Prior treatment of the canal therefore becomes a necessity under these circumstances. Fortunately, pulp vitality can often be preserved when lesions are small to moderate. If in doubt, restorations should be replaced, producing as good a seal as possible. Very small lesions are often eliminated during preparation.

Pulpless teeth   In the case of pulpless teeth, all-metal core restorations (cast post and core or amalgams) should be avoided. In view of the translucency of jacket crowns and the effects of light transmission, these metal restorations will inevitably make the ceramic appear gray after bonding, resulting in esthetic failure.

The choice is therefore between restoration using composite resins or a metal–ceramic post and core. The latter is made up of one or two cast metal posts, extended inside the core by ceramic retaining pins,

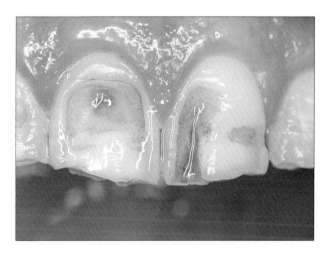

Figure 10.24 *A severe case of occlusal attrition and facial abfraction in a female patient in her 50s with bruxism.*

opaqued and colored to blend with the abutment dentin. This metal–ceramic post and core can be cemented with traditional cement or, better still, bonded, especially in cases where the root is short (Super-Bond, Morita) (Figure 10.23).

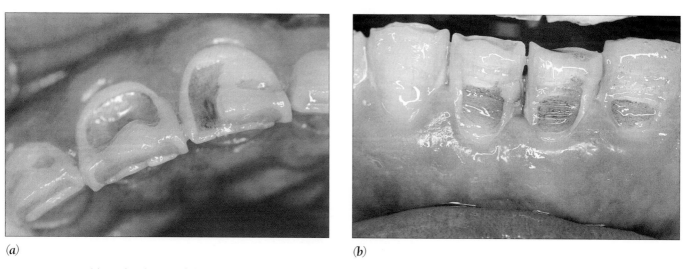

(a)   (b)

Figure 10.25 *(a) Occlusal view of the maxillary incisors and (b) facial view of mandibular incisors showing further damage.*

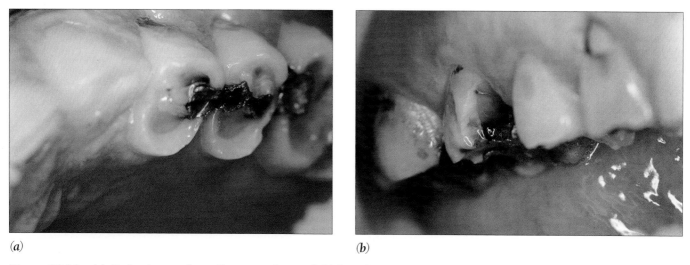

(a)   (b)

Figure 10.26 *(a) Occlusal view of maxillary premolars and (b) buccal view of molars. This case is an indication for metal–ceramic single crowns, with vertically reduced copings and circumferential ceramic butt-joint margins.*

If examination of the radiographs shows that removal of an existing cast post and core is likely to damage the root, this must be considered to be a contraindication for an all-ceramic jacket crown.

Occasionally, use of an opaque ceramic such as In-Ceram (Vita) or Optec (Jeneric) combined with more extensive (over 1.5 mm) preparation will be sufficient to conceal a metal core, but this option is always a risk, the

consequences of which can be assessed only after bonding.

Occlusal factors

Occlusal factors are decisive as to whether or not a jacket crown is indicated (Figures 10.24–10.31). Bruxism, of medium or pronounced severity, is a frequent contraindi-

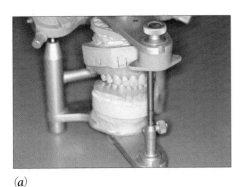
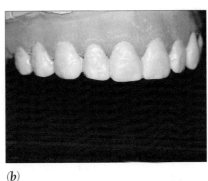
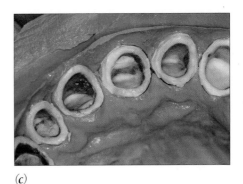

(a)   (b)   (c)

Figure 10.27 (a) *The models are mounted on a semi-adjustable articulator.* (b) *The preliminary diagnostic wax-up is recorded on the dies prior to the waxing of the metal substructures.* (c) *At the biscuit bake stage every crown is carefully tried in the mouth, and the ceramic margins are checked for fit, with adjustments made as necessary using a special silicone material as an indicator. A full impression is then made to fabricate a model, and the cervical contour and emergence profile will be finalized.*

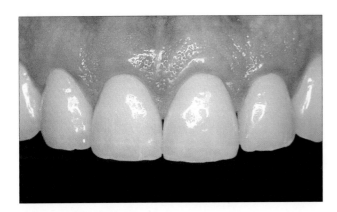

Figure 10.28 *The modified metal–ceramic crowns one week after cementation. The soft tissues are still maturing. (Ceramist: Gilbert Moricet.)*

cation, since this will increase the risk of fracture. These repetitive occlusal contacts in eccentric movement produce fissuring of the ceramic by enlarging structural microdefects and connecting existing porous sites. Bruxism, in the absence of gold occlusal surfaces, requires a metal substructure that will serve as a barrier against the propagation of microcracks. The use of uncast metal substructures obtained by electrical deposition or capil-

larity (Captek) have reawakened interest in this type of metal–ceramic crown. The reinforcing property of bonding using composite resins is now fairly well established, although it is not known if bonded jacket crowns can withstand anything more than slight bruxism. If there is any doubt, the wearing of a night-guard is advisable, as in the case of ceramic laminate veneers.

Too short a tooth is a further contraindication: after 1.5 mm (minimum) occlusal preparation, a tooth height commensurate with the requirements of retention and stabilization must still remain. This arrangement can be circumvented by resorting to coronal lengthening by periodontal surgery.

'Edge-to-edge' occlusion is also a contraindication for jacket crowns.

Periodontal condition

The periodontal condition is also a decisive factor in the choice of jacket crowns, and in this respect their use does not differ from that of any other type of fixed prosthesis. Good periodontal health either has to exist or has to be re-established before any impression procedure. In addition, the degree of gingival recession is also significant. A full discussion of this is given at the end of the chapter.

When the anterior teeth show a high degree of bone recession, preparation of a 1.2 mm shoulder could prove detrimental to the pulp. If a supragingival margin

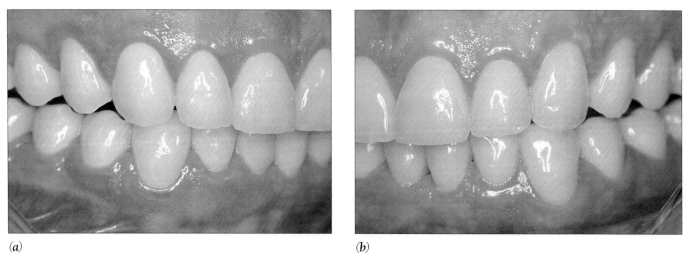

(a)   (b)

Figure 10.29 *(a,b) Lateral views of the completed maxillary and mandibular restoration.*

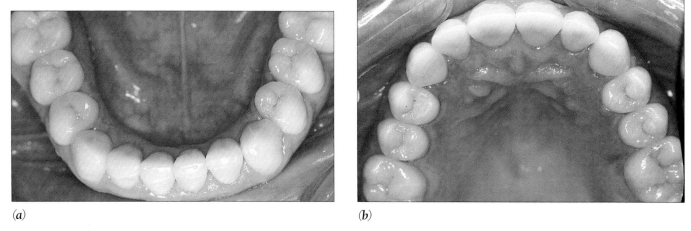

(a)   (b)

Figure 10.30 *Occlusal views of completed restorations: (a) mandibular; (b) maxillary. Metal–ceramic crowns provide a high level of reliability.*

cannot be set at the cemento-enamel junction for esthetic reasons, such as embrasures and visibility of the root, it is often preferable to prepare metal–ceramic crowns, the cervical margins of which can vary from one surface of the tooth to another.

The same can also be said of a partial coronal fracture well within the subgingival zone: every time a shoulder is contraindicated, because of insufficient space for

example, metal–ceramic crowns will be indicated. They have the basic clinical advantage of being compatible with all shapes of cervical margin.

Color of the underlying tooth

As previously mentioned, the color of the underlying tooth, whether a tooth stump or a metal core, should

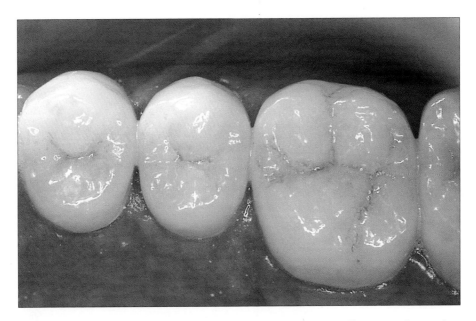

Figure 10.31 *Close-up view of the occlusal surfaces of the maxillary premolars and molars.*

be carefully considered before provision of any bonded ceramic prosthesis. Heavy discoloration of the teeth, as may result from tetracycline treatment, will have a detrimental influence on final tooth color if the following steps are not taken (Touati and Miara 1993):

- selection of a less translucent ceramic and use of slightly opaqued dentins;

- dental preparation involving a minimum of 1.5 mm enamel reduction;

- use of slightly opaqued composite cement;

- emphasizing depth characterizations and incisal area effects so that jacket crowns do not have a dull appearance after bonding.

It is essential to enter the color of the underlying tooth on the shade prescription form passed to the laboratory so that the ceramicist can gauge the factors mentioned above. Ivoclar has recently developed colored stumps for the laboratory model, which the authors consider to be an excellent initiative. Similarly, all models should ideally be fabricated with artificial soft tissue, the coloring of which should be chosen from a shade card to match the patient's gingival color.

The most difficult type of clinical situation is the existence of a discolored tooth between healthy teeth. When the latter are to be given laminate veneers, it is often preferable to bond them initially, and subsequently finalize the shade of the jacket crown. Final adjustment depends on the composite cement chosen, although this can only provide fine tuning, not a major change in color.

In cases of very darkly colored stumps, a metal–ceramic core may often be preferred for the sake of simplicity. This restoration combines both functional and esthetic advantages, due to the presence of a reduced-metal substructure overlaid in ceramic. The cores are made in dentin ceramic over a miniature metal–ceramic substructure. The dentin ceramic can be saturated and opaqued, depending on the individual case.

A merely opaqued stump is esthetically inadequate since no light transmission can take place – a drawback experienced with metal–ceramic crowns.

Planning and execution of crown preparations

Tooth preparation is a key element in the provision of any prosthesis, particularly in esthetic dentistry.

Before preparing the tooth, care should be taken to ensure that all information useful to the laboratory technician, dentist and patient has been recorded, since many errors can be avoided by so doing. The following concerns will repeatedly arise:

- Should tooth shape and/or color be reproduced?

- Should new esthetic conditions be created?

- Should existing features be partially reproduced?

In any event, it is important to make an accurate record of all data obtained prior to treatment, and, before the start of any preparation, the following information must be carefully recorded:

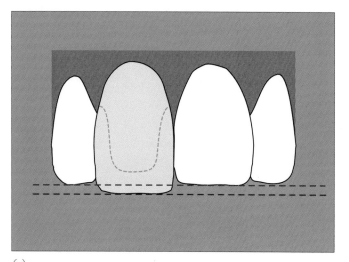

(a)

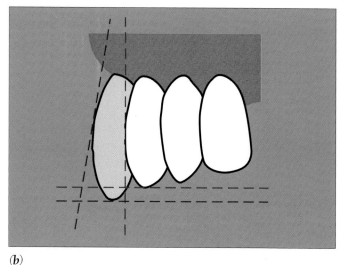

(b)

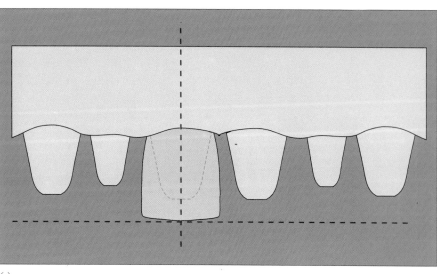

(c)

*Figure 10.32 A 'provisional reference restoration' is made for the technician's use only, before the preparation of the adjacent teeth. The patient approves the length and width of this temporary crown before the final restoration is carried out. (**a**) In this example, the crown is lengthened in contrast to the adjacent teeth; (**b**) the protrusion is also increased. (**c**) This temporary reference crown is then used in the laboratory to provide information concerning the axis, length, width, protrusion, occlusion and even shape of the final restoration.*

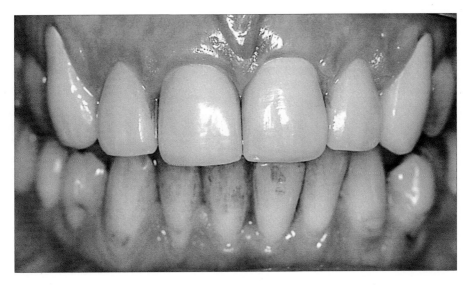

Figure 10.33 *Defective metal–ceramic crowns exhibiting poor cervical margins, an opaque appearance, unesthetic smile line, short teeth and grayish gingivae. The patient, a female in her mid-50s, is a heavy smoker.*

- impressions of arches and study casts;

- occlusal relationship;

- tooth color;

- photographs with shade guide;

- silicone index of buccal and lingual surfaces;

- radiographs.

With esthetic prostheses, the operator is faced with the need for reference points throughout the whole procedure. These will optimize the clinician's sense of security as well as his or her relationship with patients and the laboratory. Objective reference points serve as a guarantee of success, whether existing presentations need to be copied or modified.

The esthetic questionnaire is a basic element in dentist–patient communication, and should be completed at this stage (see Chapter 7, 'Transfer of Esthetic Information').

Patients will often wish to preserve their individual smile, and may only expect improved tooth color from any anterior prosthesis. Whether for provisional or permanent prostheses, study casts are indispensable for copying and conveying this information to the laboratory. Some patients may, for instance, wish to have the incisors lengthened or have a more pronounced labial–buccal axis – in all cases, a reference for use on the laboratory model is required.

The authors have therefore designed a provisional reference restoration as follows (Figure 10.32): before proceeding to preparation of the teeth, one or two units, to suit the circumstances, are prepared at some distance from each other. The temporary restoration is made to blend in with the esthetic design: it is very carefully adjusted with regard to occlusal relationships, and is relined at the cervical margins (Figures 10.33–10.37).

This provisional reference restoration can have an incisal edge identical to that of the original tooth, or may be lengthened, developed in a labial–buccal or lingual direction, or shortened, according to the clinical presentation and/or the patient's requirements.

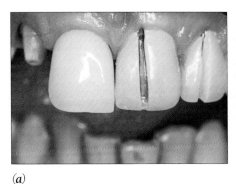

(a)

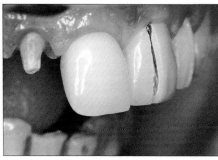

(b)

Figure 10.34 (a) Before removing the left central incisor crown, one reference tooth is fabricated in acrylic resin at chairside for the technician's use, following the patient's expectations in terms of new length and protrusion. (b) Lateral view showing the new protrusion and lip support. The reference tooth can also register the occlusal relationship and the incisal guidance after removal of the previous crowns.

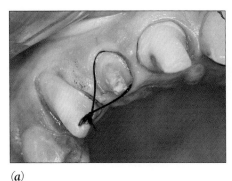

(a)

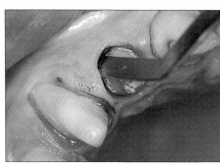

(b)

Figure 10.35 (a,b) A black silk suture thread is inserted in the sulcus and will be left there, after removal of the retraction cord, during the impression procedure.

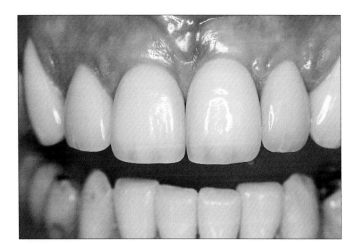

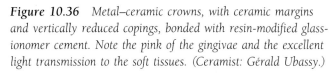

Figure 10.36 Metal–ceramic crowns, with ceramic margins and vertically reduced copings, bonded with resin-modified glass-ionomer cement. Note the pink of the gingivae and the excellent light transmission to the soft tissues. (Ceramist: Gérald Ubassy.)

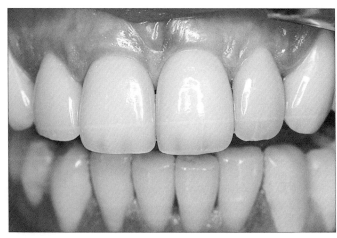

Figure 10.37 The mandibular anterior teeth have been veneered, and the maxillary central incisors dominate the adjoining teeth well and produce a pleasing smile line.

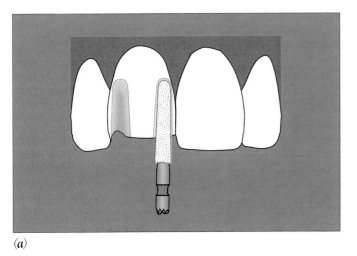 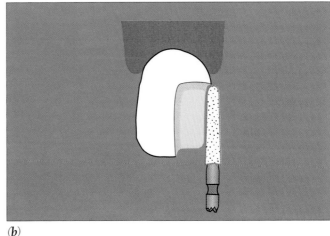

Figure 10.38 (*a*) *In order to gauge the depth of preparation, penetration grooves are prepared using a rotary instrument according to the Stein technique.* (*b*) *Alternatively, a half-tooth may be prepared.*

With this provisional reference restoration repositioned on the laboratory model, the technician will possess a spatial reference point and anterior guidance. Ceramic for adjoining teeth can then be produced with confidence.

Tooth preparation

A labial silicone index can serve as a guide for coronal reduction, but it cannot always be accurately repositioned in the mouth; on a trimmed and sectioned model, this often becomes impossible. The authors have therefore adopted the habit of preparing a half-tooth to monitor and quantify reduction (Figure 10.38).

In fixed prosthetics, the choice of instrument combinations is important. An instrument is an extension of the clinician's hands and puts his or her concepts into practice, forming shapes and margins on the abutment appropriate to individual clinical situations.

As the underlying concepts governing tooth preparation evolve with time, and particularly with advances made in biomaterials, so instrumentation evolves. Goldstein and Lustig greatly contributed to the concept of logical ordering of instrumentation from the middle of the 1970s; more recently Touati has progressively assembled the entire armamentarium required in esthetic dental practice, and has arranged them in kits, according to their purpose:

- TPS for fixed prosthetics and rotary curettage (Komet-Brasseler 4040);

- TPS finishers (Komet-Brasseler 4055);

- TPS bonded laminate veneers (Komet-Brasseler 4182);

- TPS2 (Komet-Brasseler 4180).

Few instruments are required for jacket crown preparations – two or three at the most. The shouldering instrument is the most important of these, since it is the cervical margin that distinguishes jacket crown preparation.

The following configuration is required for a bonded all-ceramic jacket crown (Figure 10.39):

- approximately 1.2 mm shoulder (or deep chamfer);

- rounded internal edges and angles;

- occlusal clearance of at least 1.5 mm.

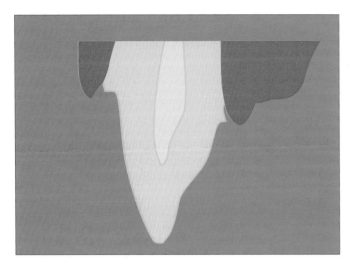

Figure 10.39 *The classical form of preparation for an all-ceramic crown.*

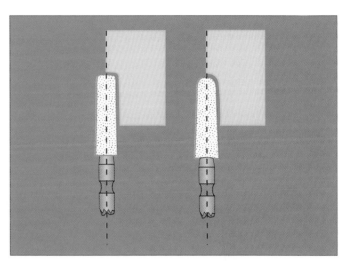

Figure 10.40 *The difference between a shoulder (left) and a deep chamfer (right) is not always obvious, and depends on the instrument used.*

The shoulder requires a rounded shouldering or a deep chamfer instrument (Figure 10.40). A pear-shaped instrument will be needed for lingual reduction; the coarseness of these instruments averages between 70 and 140 µm.

It is unwise to choose too narrow an instrument (of less than 1 mm) to create the shoulder, since this could risk leaving a raised enamel edge at the periphery of the cervical margin. However, were this to occur, the area could be flattened again with an identical instrument of larger diameter, to even off the shoulder.

General principles for preparation

The general principles for jacket crown preparation are governed by the mechanical properties of the ceramic material: high compressive but low flexural strength, and lack of elasticity. Preparation must include a 1.2 mm (average) unbevelled peripheral shoulder, a 1.5–2 mm reduction of the incisal edge, and 1.5–2 mm occlusal reduction with rounded, gentle angles (Figure 10.41).

The general contour of the preparation must match the natural tooth as closely as possible, which will give the jacket crown a uniform thickness, and hence a

certain homogeneity, and will enable the incisal edge to return to its initial position if necessary (this is very important for the final esthetic result) (Figure 10.42).

Matching the contour of the natural tooth implies reduction of the labial surface with double convergence, that is, double orientation of the instrument (Figure 10.43). The prepared surfaces must remain unpolished so as to maximize bonding (Figure 10.44).

Preparation techniques

Gingival tissue

In general, for all-ceramic jacket crowns intended for non-discolored teeth, the preparation should not extend deep into the gingival sulcus: cervical margins will end at or slightly below the gingival crest on the four tooth surfaces. This arrangement significantly facilitates the stages of making impressions, checking the temporary restoration, try-in, bonding and finishing. The only use for a gingival retraction cord would then be to enhance the recording of subgingival areas during the impression, and facilitating the quest for the ideal emergence profile in the laboratory. In many cases, 0 or 00 black silk suturing thread can act as a protective measure during preparation procedures.

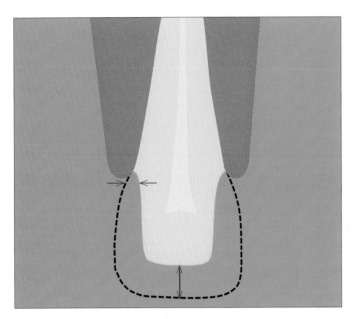

Figure 10.41 *The contour of the preparation must be consistent with the natural tooth, with a deep chamfer or shoulder of approximately 1.2 mm, and an occlusal reduction of between 1.5 and 2.0 mm.*

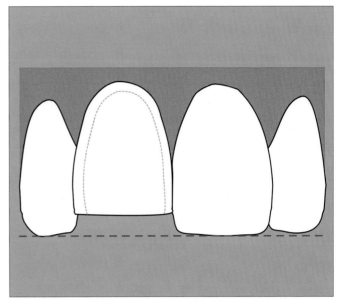

Figure 10.42 *When several preparations are necessary, and the purpose of crowning is only to correct a color problem (not form or position), it is essential to reduce one incisal edge only, and to assess the result before preparing the adjacent teeth.*

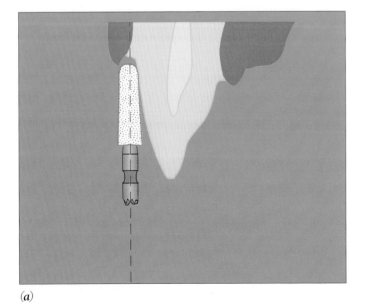

(a)

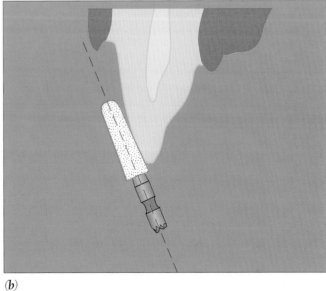

(b)

Figure 10.43 *When reducing the labial surface of the tooth, its exact contour must be emulated in order to avoid the removal of too much tissue and to allow for a crown of regular thickness. The instruments must be applied in two directions: (a) the first orientation involves the cervical two-thirds of the tooth; (b) the second involves the incisal third of the tooth.*

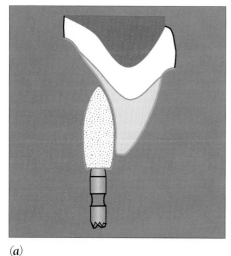

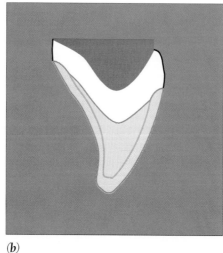

(a)   (b)

Figure 10.44 *(a,b) The same rules apply to the lingual surface of the tooth as to the labial surface: the tooth must be reduced to allow sufficient space for the crown and for the re-establishment of normal occlusal and protrusional relationships.*

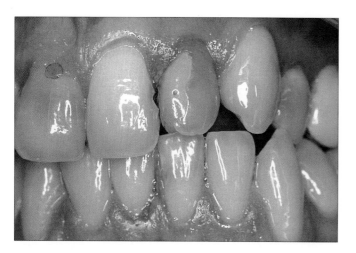

Figure 10.45 *A difficult case for prosthetic restoration, involving severely decayed, devitalized and discolored teeth. The maxillary left central incisor and canine are vital teeth.*

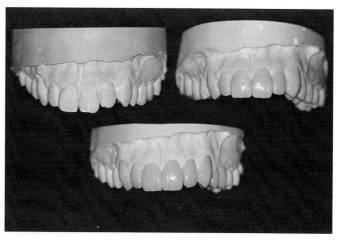

Figure 10.46 *The incisal midline has to be moved slightly to the left. As usual, the temporary crowns replicate the shape and position of the teeth in the diagnostic wax-up.*

With any discoloration of the underlying teeth, devitalized teeth or tetracycline staining, it becomes essential to position the cervical margin slightly into the gingival sulcus for esthetic reasons (Figures 10.45–10.48).

Dental tissue

After color determination, preliminary photographs and collection of all essential data, the teeth will be prepared under local anesthesia. Occasionally one or two units will be prepared first to provide a reference guide, as previously described. The authors always create the outline of a half-tooth (see Figure 10.38b), using the following procedure:

- 1.5-2 mm reduction of incisal edge;

- preparation of the deep chamfer (1.2 mm on average) (Figure 10.49);

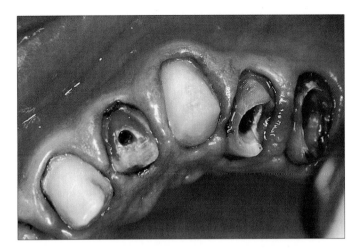

Figure 10.47 *Most of the teeth will be restored by cast dowels and cores. The margins are located 0.5 mm into the gingival sulcus.*

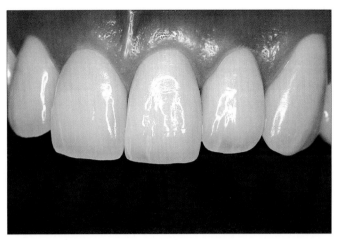

Figure 10.48 *The metal–ceramic crowns (IPS Classic, Ivoclar) with ceramic margin butt-joints are bonded with a resin cement. The cervical light transmission is optimal, and the color of the gingivae is dramatically improved. Note the characterizations of the incisal edges, the texture and the opalescence effect. (Ceramist: Gérald Ubassy.)*

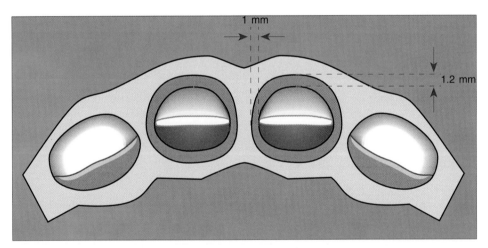

Figure 10.49 *Occlusal view of modified metal–ceramic preparations, showing that the shoulder and deep chamfer are consistently 1 mm in the mesial and distal aspects, and 1.2 mm in the lingual and buccal aspects.*

- 'double orientation' of the labial surface;

- 'channel' section of the proximal contact area so as not to touch the adjoining unaffected tooth;

- preparation within the axis (with a taper of 6°–8°) of the subcingulum area to increase retention and stabilization;

- scooped reduction of the supracingulum area appropriate to the occlusal relationship.

The degree of preparation can be visually monitored using this half-tooth preparation technique, which has proved useful for avoiding over- or under-preparation.

This rough outline is then completed, and the margins finished and checked for their relationship with the free gingival crest, and the taper (averaging 6°–8°) is monitored.

For finishing, red-banded diamond instruments are used without resorting to polishing, which could detract from bonding, while care should be taken to round-off

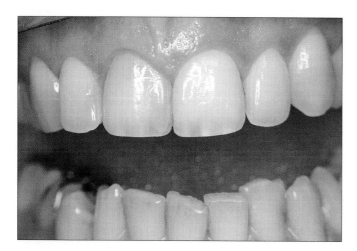

Figure 10.50 *The maxillary right central incisor has undergone root canal therapy and is severely compromised.*

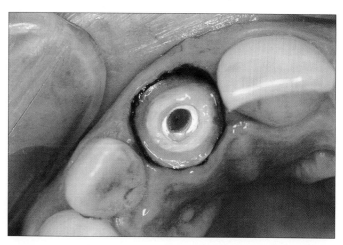

Figure 10.51 *The preparation just before the impression is made. A cotton retraction cord (00) is placed in the gingival sulcus over a silk suturing thread, which will be left in situ during the impression.*

all angles and corners to reduce the number of weak points in the ceramic.

Gingival retraction

The prerequisite for any gingival retraction procedure is the presence of healthy periodontal tissue, enabling reversible gingival deflection to take place, causing little or no damage to the gingival margin. Both horizontal and vertical gingival retraction allow access of sufficient thickness of the impression material at the cervical margin to avoid tearing or deformation when removed. In the event of injury to or bleeding from the gingivae following preparation, it is wise to wait a few days until the healing process has completed; this will facilitate gingival retraction considerably.

Of the numerous methods of gingival retraction now in existence, such as electrosurgery, rotary gingival curettage and retraction cords, the use of retraction cords is the most suitable for jacket crowns because of the minimal degree of permanent gingival recession they cause (0.1 mm in general). Retraction cords can be coarse or fine, impregnated or non-impregnated, woven or knitted. The use of impregnated cords is recommended, and knitted types are easier to lodge in place, thus preserving the junctional epithelium and supracrestal

connective fiber attachments. This compaction must be gentle and can employ one or two cords, according to the depth of the sulcus and the tone of the gingival margin. Retraction of free gingiva on proximal surfaces often requires two cords (Ultrapak 0 or 00, Ultradent), impregnated with Hemodent (buffered aluminum chloride solution, Premier Dental Products) (Figures 10.50–10.54).

Any bleeding must be staunched before taking an impression. It can sometimes be useful to replace the provisional crown over cords in place within the gingival sulcus for about 5 minutes, to add compression.

Retraction cords are generally withdrawn prior to impression taking, but it is not unusual to leave an extra-thin cord (Ultrapak 000) at the bottom of the sulcus to check for and prevent any bleeding. Some clinicians routinely leave suturing thread (American silk 0 or 00) at the bottom of the gingival sulcus throughout preparation and impression-taking.

Jacket crown impressions

The choice of impression tray should preferably tend toward Rimlok or perforated metal stock trays, previously coated with a suitable adhesive. These are rigid enough to avoid accidental deformation. Partial impres-

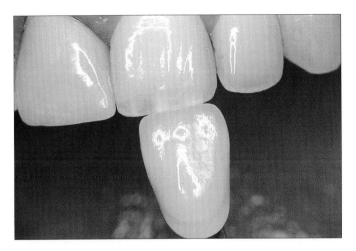

Figure 10.52 *An example of the type of photograph that is sent to the to ceramist to assist in his or her work. Note the highly characterized incisal aspect of the tooth. (Ceramist: Jean-Marc Etienne.)*

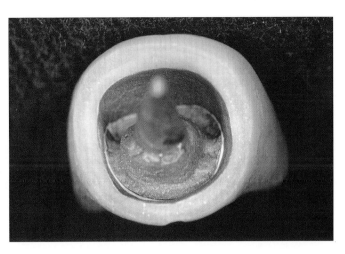

Figure 10.53 *The ceramic margin (Creation) is etched and silanated, and the crown bonded onto the conditioned dentin and sandblasted post and core.*

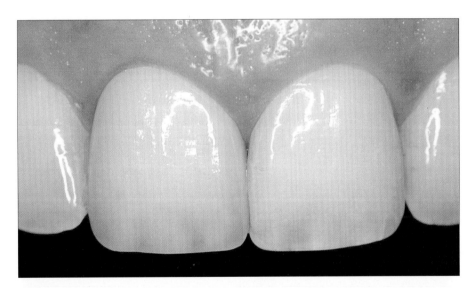

Figure 10.54 *The completed metal–ceramic crown. (Ceramist: Jean-Marc Etienne.)*

sion trays such as Kwik Tray (Kerr) can be used for single jacket impressions.

Impressions can be taken in a double-mix (one-stage dual-viscosity), or using the 'wash technique' (two-stage dual-viscosity). Reversible hydrocolloids or addition silicones can be used with the former technique, but silicones (conventional) only with the latter.

Double-mix technique

The double-mix technique is fast and simple, but requires some experience. In view of recent advances, this type of impression can be taken by an unassisted clinician.

The low-viscosity material, stored in cartridges, is loaded into an injection syringe. It is mixed automatically during the course of injection. The nozzle should always be kept in contact with the preparation during injection. The impression tray is loaded up with malleable, high-viscosity silicone putty. The latest nitrile gloves are particularly practical, since they do not stick or interfere with silicone polymerization.

'Wash' technique

With multiple preparations, and when cervical margins are subgingival, the 'double-impression' or 'wash' technique can be adopted. An initial impression is taken with no spacing, using a high-viscosity silicone (hard putty). After curing, rinsing, and drying, undercut areas and impressions of intradental spaces are eliminated. An 'over-impression' is then taken, using low-viscosity injectable silicone, taking care to replace the impression tray accurately in the same position as before, without extensive finger pressure.

Provisional restorations

This is an important stage for biological and esthetic reasons. The seal of cervical margins, the extent of areas in contact with the periodontium and the accuracy of occlusal contact are all decisive for esthetic reasons, and these factors will inspire the patient with confidence in the treatment. For these reasons, the authors generally prefer to use jacket crowns produced in the laboratory, even for as little as a two-week period.

Tooth preparation, resembling that performed in the mouth, is carried out on a duplicate provisional study cast. The temporary crowns are then fabricated in heat-cured resin, with flasking, in consultation with the ceramist who will produce the final prosthesis.

Experience has shown that time devoted to provisional crowns is not wasted. As well as demonstrating the ability to conduct the treatment according to the patient's wishes, the final esthetic effect can be tested 'live', including also phonation and, above all, periodontal response to the contours of the prosthesis. This technique may be considered essential in the case of implant-supported prostheses.

The provisional crowns are carefully polished with cotton thread wheels and suitable polishing pastes, and then cemented using a eugenol-free cement, such as Nogenol (Dentsply-Caulk), Freegenol (GC) or Temp-Bond ND (Kerr). The external resin surfaces are coated with Xynon, a microfilm separator that prevents adhesion of the cement and helps in cleaning cement from the provisional restorations. Orange solvent can be used successfully to dissolve any excess cement.

Try-in

The try-in procedure is intended to monitor the successful completion of the prosthesis in the laboratory, as well as esthetic and functional integration.

Jacket crowns are often unretentive, so temporary stabilization may be useful during try-in. The same transparent silicone (Memosil, Heraeus-Kulzer) used for bite registration or try-in of laminate veneers can be used for this purpose. The patient is asked to smile and talk so that the esthetic effect and phonation can be observed.

Occlusal relationships can then be checked without any risk of fracturing the ceramic, and fine adjustment is possible at this stage, generally with aluminous silicone polishers and tips.

The transparent silicone, while providing optical continuity, also makes it possible to appraise the final shade of color independently of the composite cement, and will guide one's choice of cement color. Chroma is easier to raise than to reduce, and the cement cannot be relied upon to bring about a significant transformation, but even if its influence only accounts for 10–20% (depending on the degree of opacity of the ceramic in question), this can be the difference between success and failure.

Water-soluble try-in pastes will assist the clinician's choice, even though total accuracy cannot be achieved since pastes do not always show exactly the same shade as the definitive cured composite. It could be claimed that the 'try-in/bonding' stages are frequently at the root of failure, and should therefore be handled with care. Again, failure can only be avoided by experience; it is rare when the abutment is of a normal color, but frequent when teeth are not all of the same shade. The latter situation may be considered a contraindication for ceramic jacket crowns.

Bonding of ceramic jacket crowns

Bonding of ceramic jacket crowns can be achieved using three different techniques.

Traditional luting techniques

Traditional luting cements (i.e. zinc phosphate, glass ionomers) were used routinely with porcelain jacket crowns up until the late 1980s, and were simple to use. However, in light of evidence that resin cements and bonding can enhance the strength of etched ceramic restorations (Nathanson, 1994; Burke, 1995), the conventional cements are no longer indicated for routine use with these crowns. The newer resin-modified glass-ionomer luting cements are contraindicated since they expand in wet environments and can cause fracturing of all-ceramic crowns (*CRA Reports*, November, 1996).

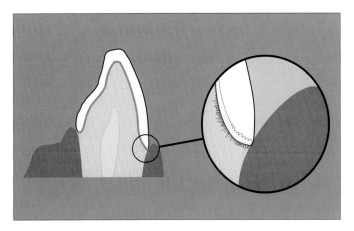

Figure 10.55 *The bonding process reinforces the strength of the all-ceramic jacket crown due to the resin cement film which penetrates the microretentions of both the conditioned dentin and enamel on one side, and the etched ceramic on the other. This film helps to diffuse the stresses across the tooth.*

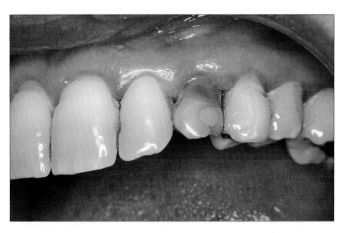

Figure 10.56 *After extraction of the deciduous canine, a bridge will be placed from the lateral incisor to the first bicuspid.*

Bonding using one material only

Bonding, using a chemically cured 4-meta-MMA+TBB resin is described fully in Chapter 11 'Ceramic Inlays and Onlays'. In this technique, resin cement acts both as a dentin–enamel adhesive and as a filler between the preparation and the jacket crown (Figure 10.55). It enables a hybrid layer, as described by Nakabayashi (1992), to be formed with conditioned dentin, and bonds to the etched cervical enamel collar.

Etching solutions from Sun Medical, as well as the dual-component adhesives consisting of silane and 4 meta monomer, should be used. Although this cement does not come in a wide variety of shades (fortunately it is supplied as a fairly translucent 'clear' powder) and is not easy to clear at the cervical margin, it has excellent rheological properties, and has proved successful over 10 years of experience in Europe.

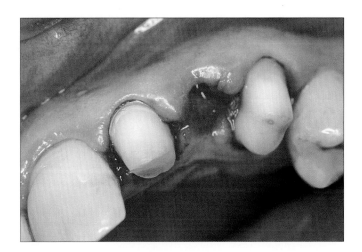

Figure 10.57 *The canine is extracted on the day that the preparations are performed, and the impressions made (a silk suture thread is in place in the gingival sulcus).*

Bonding using modern dentin–enamel adhesives

This procedure involves the use of a resin cement in combination with a modern dentin–enamel adhesive.

The tooth (Figures 10.56–10.60)

• Careful cleaning of the prepared tooth to eliminate any trace of the temporary cement.

• Etching of the prepared tooth (cervical enamel and dentin) for 15 seconds using 10% phosphoric acid, followed by thorough rinsing and dabbing dry using absorbent paper.

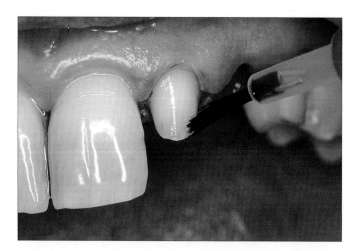

Figure 10.58 *Hybridization: the conditioned and disinfected preparation is coated with a fifth-generation single-component primer-adhesive (One-Step, Bisco) in order to create a protective hybrid layer.*

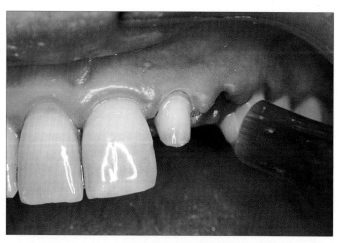

Figure 10.59 *Light polymerization of the primer-adhesive prior to the impression being made.*

- Application of 2–3 layers of primer onto the slightly moist tooth surface; after 10 seconds the primer is gently dried with air. With single-component adhesive systems, this is the only step required.

- If a dual-component adhesive is used, a fine layer of adhesive resin is applied to the tooth (not light-cured).

- Etching of the jacket crown with hydrofluoric acid (concentration and application time will depend on the type of ceramic), followed by rinsing, immersion in an ultrasonic bath and neutralizing with sodium bicarbonate. If the internal surface of the jacket crown has been merely sandblasted rather than etched, the ceramic surface should be treated with phosphoric acid and then rinsed to optimize silanization.

- Coating the inner crown surface with a primer or silane solution, which is allowed to dry.

- Coating the jacket crown internally with adhesive resin and the resin cement (e.g. Variolink, Ivoclar Vivadent; Choice, Bisco or Enforce, Dentsply-Caulk).

- Placement of the jacket crown and cleaning of excess resin cement. A glycerol gel can be coated onto the

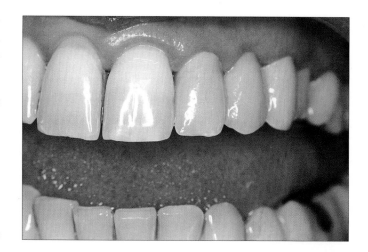

Figure 10.60 *The finished result: the ovate pontic allows for the conservation of the interdental papillae. (Ceramist: Gilbert Moricet.)*

margins. Light-curing is conducted for about two minutes, on every aspect of the tooth.

More recently, fifth-generation adhesives have appeared on the market that simplify the bonding procedures, since the primer and bonding material can

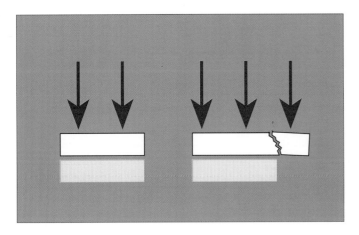

Figure 10.61 *The key to success with ceramic restorations is the understanding that the ceramic is brittle, and must always be supported to produce a compressive stress. Creating excessive flexural stresses will dramatically increase the risk of fracture.*

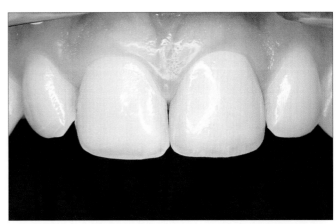

Figure 10.62 *The left incisor shown here is a metal–ceramic crown of the 1980s, whose framework goes down to the chamfer. Note the resulting shadowing in the cervical area, and the increased opacity.*

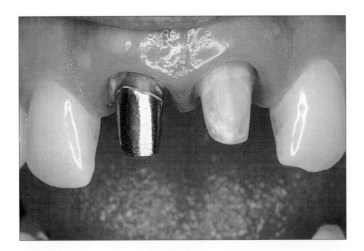

Figure 10.63 *In this case, because the underlying cores are of different colors, one being metal, all-ceramic crowns are contraindicated.*

now be mixed in one bottle (One-Step, Bisco; Prime & Bond, Dentsply–Caulk; Syntac SC, Ivoclar Vivadent). Two steps are still required: etching and priming/bonding. Some adhesives are radio-opaque, filled and release fluoride (e.g. Optibond FL, Kerr; Clearfil Liner Bond, Cavex).

Finishing

For ceramic jacket crowns, finishing involves only the cervical areas where the cement has oozed out during placement.

Before light curing, all surplus cement is brushed off or removed with dental floss or polyethylene foam pads. One should not be too zealous over the margin, however, because a fine layer of resin inhibited by oxygen from the air will inevitably be produced during polymerization. A layer of glycerol can be painted over the cervical margins prior to polymerization in order to limit the formation of this inhibited layer.

Final finishing should take place only after the hardening process has been completed. Rotary multiple-bladed instruments (Goldstein's ET Brasseler-Komet) should be used, followed by yellow-banded diamond rotary instruments (Touati's Brasseler-Komet TPS finishing instruments), scalpels, polishing wheels, aluminous silicone caps, diamond polishing paste, and strips (Enhance Polishing Strips, Dentsply–DeTrey). Occlusal relationships are again checked and adjusted as required.

While enabling us to achieve the highest esthetic standards in the anterior area, ceramic jacket crowns require much skill (Figure 10.61). The final stage of bonding is cardinal in achieving optimal results. The elimination of metal substructures optimizes the 'natural' appearance of these restorations (Figure 10.62).

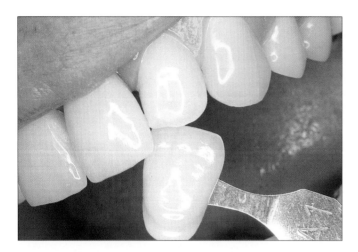

Figure 10.64 *The shade guide in place for the ceramist's use: the appropriate color in this case is A1 Vita.*

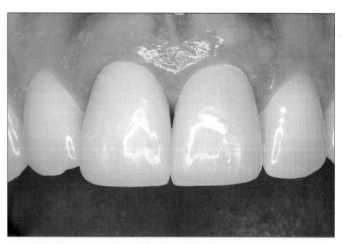

Figure 10.65 *The provisional restorations.*

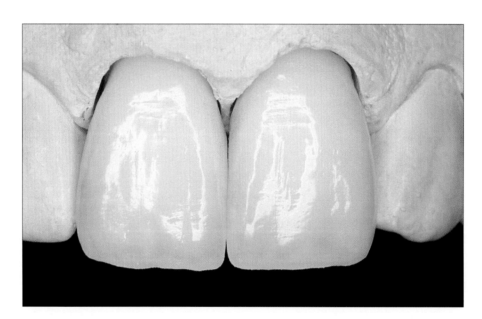

Figure 10.66 *The final metal–ceramic crowns (Creation), with vertically reduced copings. (Ceramist: Willi Geller.)*

The presence of underlying tooth structure varying greatly in color is a constraint on this technique, and the same applies to cast metal cores. Crowns with a metal framework vertically reduced at the cervical area are a better alternative. The same applies to posterior teeth, where jacket crowns do not offer sufficient esthetic advantages to justify taking risks at the mechanical level (Figures 10.63–10.68).

At our present state of knowledge and length of clinical experience, it still appears logical to use metal–ceramic crowns in molar and premolar teeth. However, where patients demand a natural appearance on both the lingual and labial surfaces, jacket crowns may occasionally be used. But, as elsewhere in adhesive dentistry, they require experience and meticulous attention to detail.

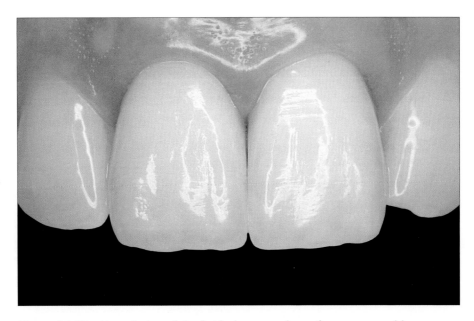

Figure 10.67   *Frontal view of the finished crowns: the surface texture and luster are very pleasing. Note that the broken angle of the left lateral incisor has not been restored, since creating a harmonious look does not necessarily require complete symmetry. (Ceramist: Willi Geller.)*

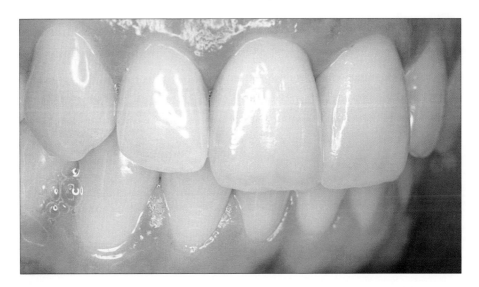

Figure 10.68   *Lateral view: the chroma gradually increases from central incisor to canine.*

CASE PRESENTATION: 1

A case presentation follows (Figures 10.69–10.74) showing that excellent clinical results can be achieved, even when supporting teeth are very short (Touati, 1997; reproduced with permission from *PPAD*, Montage Media).

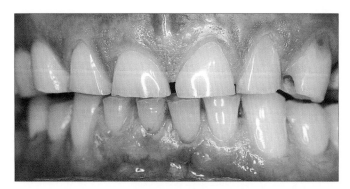

Figure 10.69 *Preoperatrive view of worn-out dentition with reduced vertical dimension of a 60-year-old male patient, requiring complete oral rehabilitation.*

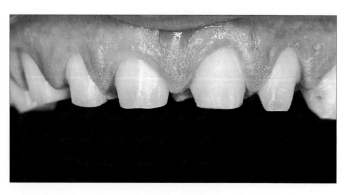

Figure 10.70 *Preparations are performed on vital teeth, despite the reduced height of the teeth.*

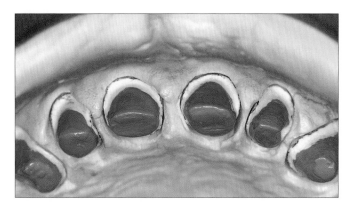

Figure 10.71 *Once the metal–ceramic crowns with vertically reduced frameworks are tried in at the biscuit stage, a silicone impression is taken and a second plaster model is poured. The emergence profile achieves an accurate intimate contact with the soft tissues during the last bakes.*

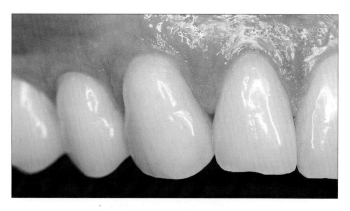

Figure 10.72 *A pleasing emergence profile has been created, reducing the black triangular spaces by bringing the proximal contact towards the soft tissues.*

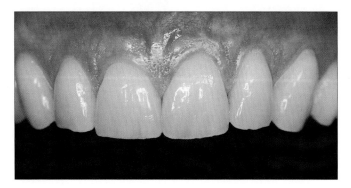

Figure 10.73 *Due to the second model technique, the transmucosal aspect of the ceramic restorations is biologic and naturally esthetic.*

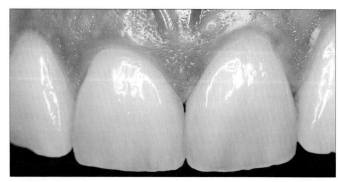

Figure 10.74 *The final result displays harmonious intimacy between the crown restorations and the soft tissues. (Ceramist: Willi Geller.)*

CASE PRESENTATION: 2*

Presentation and diagnostic evaluation

A 30-year-old male patient presented requesting esthetic and functional restoration. His primary complaint was the dark-gray color of his teeth and a severe overbite (Figures 10.75 and 10.76). Otherwise, he was content with the shape of the individual teeth, except for the maxillary left lateral incisor, which was pulpless and had been temporarily restored by direct application of composite resin on the buccal aspect. The patient's concern was that, because of the pronounced overbite, the mandibular incisors were touching the anterior aspect of the palate and causing pain. In addition, the mandibular incisors and canines were abraded by bruxism resulting from the malocclusion. The patient declined orthodontic treatment and requested prosthetic rehabilitation with ceramic restorations.

The maxillary premolars and molars displayed extensive coronal restorations, gold inlays, several onlays, and large direct composite resin fillings (Figure 10.77). A treatment plan was formulated that required the maxillary arch to be restored with single ceramic crowns in order to open the vertical dimension and return the palate to its natural state. All teeth were to remain vital. Mandibular incisors and canines were to be treated with ceramic laminate veneers. Silicone impressions were taken to pour two sets of articulated plaster models: one set was to be retained as a reference model, particularly for the shape of the teeth; the second set was to be prepared for the fabrication of the provisional restorations. Occlusion was registered and transferred to the articulator. Intraoral photographs were taken of the initial clinical conditions.

In cases like this, the aim of treatment is to reproduce the shape, emergence profile, and spatial arrangement of the natural dentition, with minor alterations being allowed in order to improve the alignment or to correct any chip fractures. Here the patient requested that the appearance of the restored teeth be similar to the natural dentition, except for color and length. Therefore the pretreatment diagnostic model was duplicated in order to retain a reference of the shape.

To fabricate the provisional crowns, the second model was utilized in the following manner. The vertical dimension was slightly augmented on the articulator. Silicone indices were taken of the buccal aspects and incisal edges of the teeth. The acrylic resin crowns were fabricated by the laboratory technician. One side of the dental arch was prepared first, and rough preparations were made of the abutments using the silicone indices to provide a 1.2–1.3 mm reduction. Teeth were joined two-by-two for improved retention, and great care was taken to restore the natural protrusion. This procedure is generally easier when one side is completed first, using the other side as a reference for alignment. For comfort (phonation, lip support, occlusion and proprioception), it is of critical importance to restore the natural vertical axis of the teeth.

All preparations were performed in one session (Figure 10.78). The vertical dimension was to be opened, side by side, to retain a reference of the position of the incisors and of the occlusion. Provisional restorations were seated and adjusted, side by side. The teeth were prepared with a peripheral chamfer of average depth 1.3 mm, retaining their vitality. The maxillary left lateral incisor was prepared for a cast post and core. Gingival displacement was made using the two-cord technique (one silk suture thread and a second knitted one). Several impressions were taken with additional silicones (Reprosil, Dentsply–Caulk) for each group of teeth. To allow complete healing of the soft tissues, the impressions are generally taken one or two weeks following the preparations.

Cementation and evaluation of provisional restorations

Figure 10.79 shows a one-week postcementation view of the provisional crown restorations, joined in two-by-two manner to reduce the risk of debonding. The crown surface was varnished (Palaseal, Jelenko). All internal effects and characterizations were created with intensive colors (Artglass, Jelenko) in a special light oven.

The form and occlusion of the provisional restorations were carefully evaluated, and an impression was taken to serve as a reference during the fabrication of all frameworks using silicone templates. All provisional restorations were cemented with a eugenol-free provisional cement (Temp-Bond ND, Kerr) (Figure 10.80). All vital teeth were disinfected with a chlorhexidine gel and hybridized (One-Step, Bisco) *following* the completion of provisional restorations to prevent adherence of the acrylic resin (Provipont, Ivoclar Vivadent) to the dental adhesive during the rebasing process (Figures 10.81 and 10.82).

At the next appointment, occlusion was registered. Using a face-bow, the maxillary laboratory model was accurately repositioned on the semi-adjustable articulator

*From Touati and Etienne, 1998; reproduced with permission from *PPAD*, Montage Media.

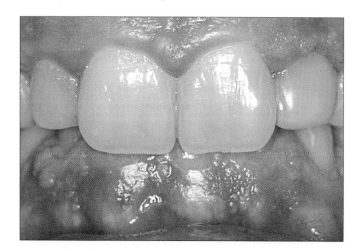

Figure 10.75 *Discolored dentition*

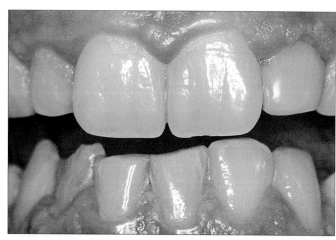

Figure 10.76 *Severe overbite*

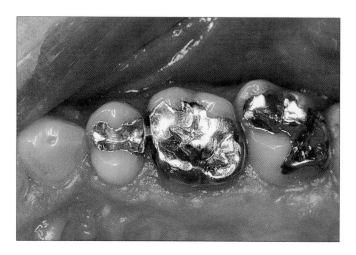

Figure 10.77 *Previous restorations, including gold inlays*

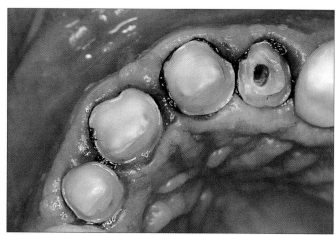

Figure 10.78 *Gingival displacement*

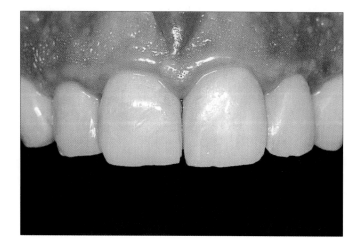

Figure 10.79 *Provisional restorations, one week postcementation*

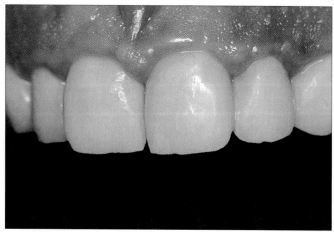

Figure 10.80 *One week postcementation, left side*

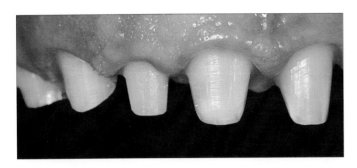

Figure 10.81   Vital teeth are disinfected and hybridized (right side)

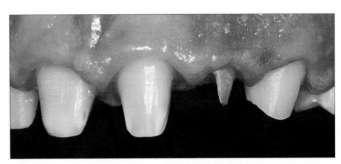

Figure 10.82   Vital teeth are disinfected and hybridized (left side)

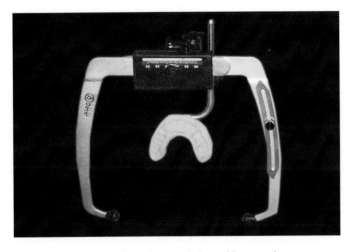

Figure 10.83   Face-bow for semi-adjustable articulator

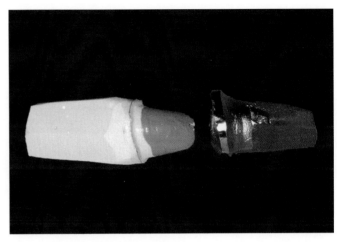

Figure 10.84   A tranfer coping

(Figure 10.83). All occlusal relationships, which had been established and checked in the provisional restorations (centric occlusion, vertical dimension, anterior guidance, lateral excursions, etc.), were transferred to the articulator. Several recordings were made with Moyco beauty wax and silicones, with the provisional crowns being removed, region by region, in order to utilize the anatomy of the remaining crowns.

In a complex case, particularly in a full-arch rehabilitation, it is difficult to register every detail of the preparations accurately in one global impression. Therefore, in this case, several impressions were prepared, region by region. These impressions were used to fabricate transfer copings (Figure 10.84). Dies were made of epoxy resin and coated with a die spacer that did not extend to the cervical margins. The transfer copings were perforated in the occlusal surface to allow access

for evaluation. All transfer copings were placed on the prepared teeth and checked carefully; special attention was paid to ensure accurate seating.

Model and framework fabrication

A silicone impression was taken utilizing the double-mix technique to allow the fabrication of the first working model in epoxy resin. All epoxy dies were prepared and repositioned accurately in their respective transfer copings by the ceramist. Wax was used to secure the position of the dies and the copings (Figure 10.85). The anterior preparations display a peripheral deep chamfer intended for a 360° ceramic butt joint every time the occlusion is favorable (Figure 10.86).

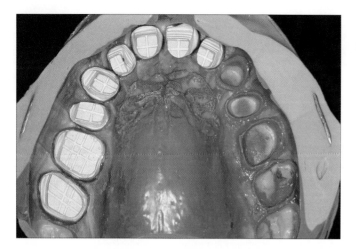

Figure 10.85 Securing position of copings and dies

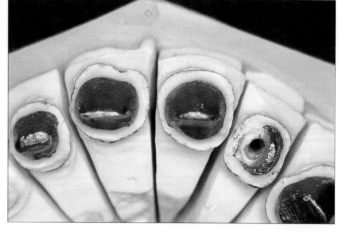

Figure 10.86 Anterior preparations on the model

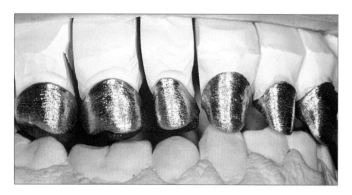

Figure 10.87 Castings in precious alloy

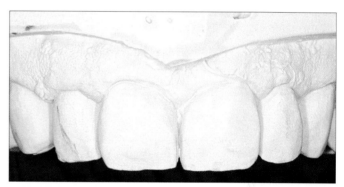

Figure 10.88 Model fabricated from the impression of the provisional restorations

At this stage, dies were separated for improved access to all cervical margins during waxing. It was not necessary for the first model to provide information regarding the free gingiva and interdental papillae.

The frameworks were fabricated by the laboratory technician. For mechanical and esthetic reasons, these frameworks had to be homeotypic reductions of the definitive shape of the dentition. Therefore it was essential that the technicians worked with silicone indexes obtained from the model displaying the provisional restorations, after these had been tested and accepted by the patient.

Frameworks were waxed according to silicone indexes originated from the model of the temporary restorations. Each individual framework was cast in a precious alloy (Figure 10.87). Once its accuracy had been carefully evaluated, the cervical aspect was cut back. The casting was thereby vertically reduced (1.5 mm on average) to allow a complete ceramic butt-joint margin, with no shadowing effect on the marginal gingiva, as a result of the opacity of the metal framework (Geller technique). The ceramic material used in the butt-joint was 'margin ceramic': it is a high-fusing ceramic with improved fluorescence properties.

Intraoral try-in and adjustment

A model was fabricated from the impression of the provisional crowns to guide the shape of the frameworks and the layered buildup of the ceramic bisque (Figure 10.88).

At this stage, the dentist evaluated the occlusal relationships, marginal accuracy and esthetic properties of the bisque restorations, and subsequently provided the ceramist with the anatomy of the soft tissues and

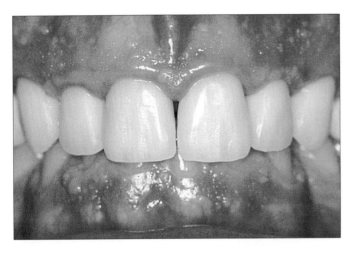

Figure 10.89   *Bisque restorations for assessing emergence profiles*

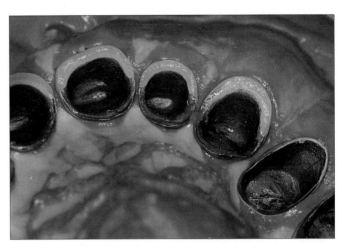

Figure 10.90   *Second impression: fine-tuning emergence profiles*

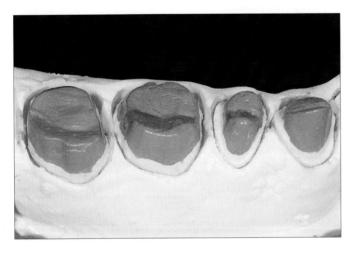

Figure 10.91   *Second model: establishing cervical contours*

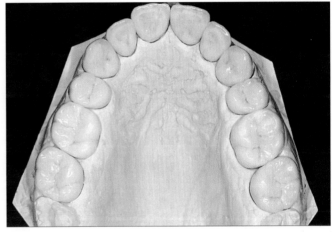

Figure 10.92   *Modified metal–ceramic crowns on the model*

interdental papillae to allow fine tuning of the cervical aspect of the teeth, i.e. the crucially important emergence profile (Figure 10.89).

Every bisque crown was tried-in at chairside, with the dentist controlling the complete seating of the crown and the accuracy of the ceramic margins. If the cervical fit was not optimal, the internal aspect of the modified porcelain-fused-to-metal crown restoration was relined with a white silicone (Fit Checker, GC). When a new die was poured in the investment material, the ceramic margins were adjusted. All corrections for form were performed at this stage with the patient's cooperation.

Once the margins and the proximal contacts had been evaluated, the dentist proceeded to the occlusal adjustment, and again registered the centric occlusion on a special silicone material (formulated for bite registration). An impression was taken using the double-mix technique. This second impression provided the anatomy of the soft tissues and interdental papillae (Figure 10.90). The second model was not separated in dies (Figure 10.91). It served to establish cervical contours, particularly those of the emergence profile. This step is essential in order to achieve a natural and harmonious soft tissue integration of the crown restorations.

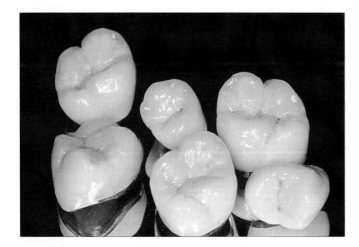

Figure 10.93   Modified metal–ceramic crown restorations

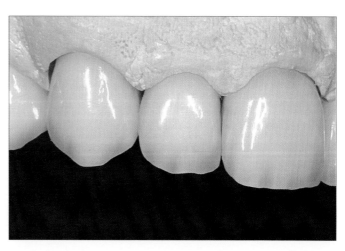

Figure 10.94   Simulation of optical characteristics: texture

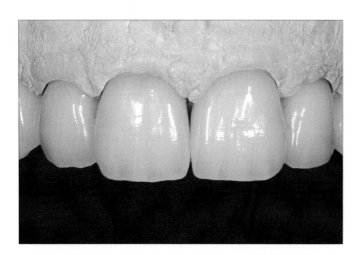

Figure 10.95   Mamelons resulting from the stratification

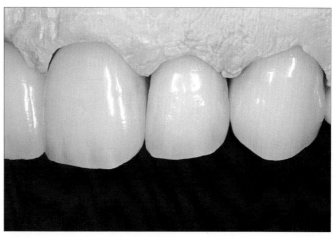

Figure 10.96   'Halo' and opalescence

Simulation of innate optical characteristics

The ceramist concentrated on utilizing dentins of appropriate opacity for the depth and to give the right value (Figure 10.92), employing several 'incisal' and 'transparent' dentins with a range of opalescent effects, depending on the expected result. The occlusal anatomy had been meticulously tried and adjusted intraorally at the bisque stage to provide natural results and patient comfort (Figure 10.93). Internal effects and characteristics are clearly visible – lobes, mamelons, and halo

('make-in' ceramic) – in order to provide a vital and youthful appearance (Figures 10.94–10.96). The restoration of the surface texture is particularly important and must be accomplished in accordance with the age of the patient and the position of the teeth in the arch.

The proximal surfaces were evaluated individually (Figure 10.97). On the anterior teeth, these surfaces are vertical, which is essential for recapturing the pyramidal form of the interdental papillae. Figure 10.98 shows a facial view of the preparations for laminate veneer restorations on the mandibular incisors. The ceramic laminate veneers were carefully sandblasted to remove the refractory investment (Figure 10.99). They were then

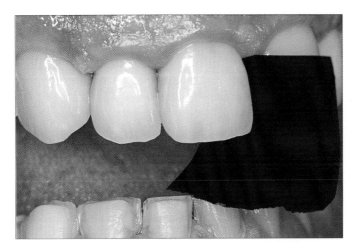

Figure 10.97 *Evaluation of proximal surfaces*

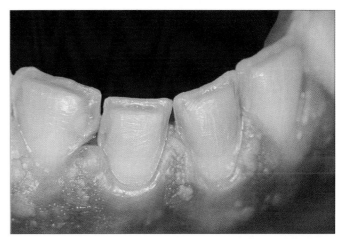

Figure 10.98 *Preparations for laminate veneer restorations*

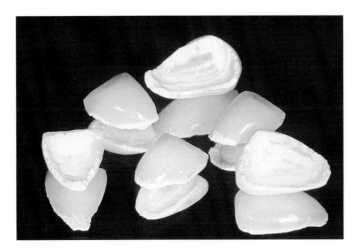

Figure 10.99 *Ceramic laminate veneers*

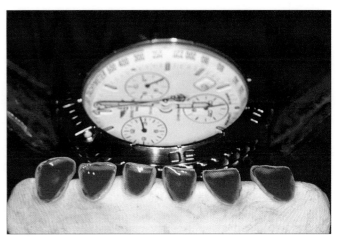

Figure 10.100 *60-second etching of veneers*

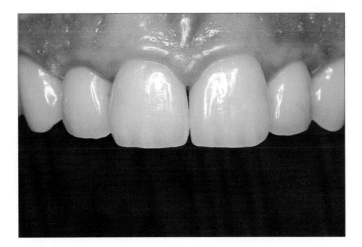

Figure 10.101 *Metal–ceramic crowns following cementation*

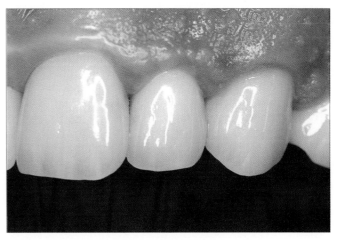

Figure 10.102 *Ceramic margins: etched and salinated*

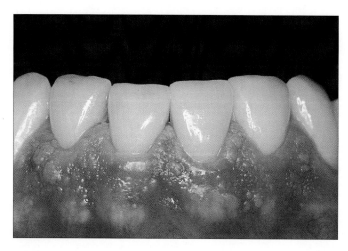

Figure 10.103 *Luting of veneers*

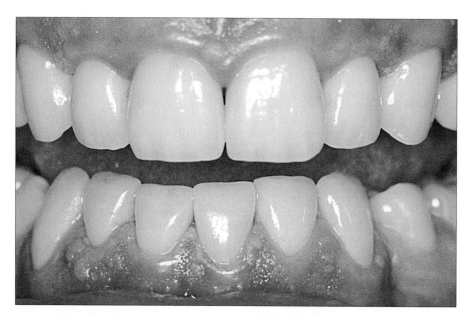

Figure 10.104 *The completed restorations, several months postoperatively*

Seating and cementation of definitive restorations

Figures 10.101 and 10.102 show the modified metal–ceramic crowns immediately following cementation with a resin-modified glass-ionomer cement (Fuji Plus, GC America). All ceramic margins were etched and silanated. Prior to cementation, every vital tooth was hybridized again with a dentin primer. The ceramic laminate veneers were individually luted with a composite resin cement (Variolink II, Ivoclar Vivadent) (Figure 10.103).

The postoperative views shown in Figures 10.104–10.108 demonstrate the definitive result several months following completion of the restoration. The result is pleasing: gingival integration is present, and, owing to meticulous oral hygiene, the soft tissues are

etched for 60 seconds with a hydrofluoric acid gel, and then rinsed and neutralized with baking soda (Figure 10.100).

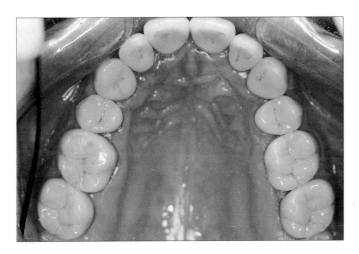

Figure 10.105   *Completed restoration: upper arch*

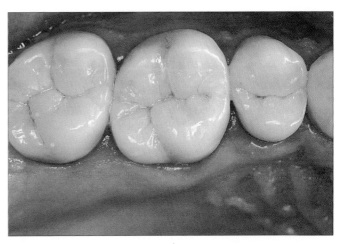

Figure 10.106   *Gingival integration is achieved*

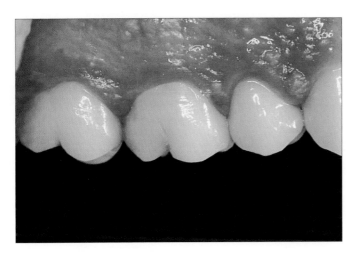

Figure 10.107   *Postoperative hygiene aids recovery of soft tissues*

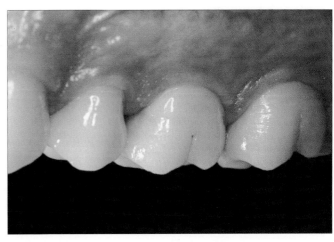

Figure 10.108   *Esthetic and pleasing natural appearance*

considerably less inflamed compared with the immediate preoperative status.

Conclusions

Such an extensive prosthetic treatment as that described here requires excellent understanding of the requirements and expectations of the patient, along with a good team approach. Use of numerous references is mandatory throughout the procedure in order to avoid errors, particularly in the position and occlusion of the teeth. Provisionalization is a crucial step for the assessment of the esthetic parameters. The authors agree with Amsterdam (personal communication, Israel, 1997) when he states that all prosthetic goals should be reached during temporization. Modified metal–ceramic crown restorations (with a vertically reduced framework) provide strength and cervical translucency, and can compete with all-ceramic restorations in terms of the esthetic results achieved. Like all-ceramic restorations, modified ceramic crowns can be bonded with composite cements, which further enhances the effects of marginal sealing and biocompatibility. Emergence profile and interdental embrasures are factors of critical importance in the esthetic result and the natural appearance of the restorations.

Esthetic aspects of periodontal tissues

The aim of this section is to briefly discuss the factors influencing the well-being of the marginal periodontium. Healthy gingival tissues are an essential condition for the esthetic success of any fixed or bonded prosthesis. Relatively simple procedures can help to restore morphological conditions that are conducive to healthy periodontal tissues. Periodontal surgery prior to crown preparations may be an important treatment option to consider.

Periodontal disease has been defined as a disorder marked by inflammation affecting the periodontium, manifesting as loss of connective tissue attachment. This pathological process leads to the formation of a periodontal pocket accompanied by the destruction of dental support tissues.

Biological width is a vital concept in prosthetics, and must be respected where any subgingival restorations such as ceramic jacket crowns are concerned. Any disturbance will induce pathological and unesthetic alteration of the gingival margin, and impressions should never be made before recovery of a healthy biological width. This anatomical feature has been defined as the dimension existing between the most coronal portion of the epithelial attachment and the alveolar crest (Figures 10.109–10.111).

In corono-apical order, it includes:

- junctional epithelium averaging 0.97 mm;
- supracrestal connective tissue fibers averaging 0.107 mm;
- depth of the gingival sulcus averaging 0.69 mm.

Any violation of this space will induce inflammatory effects, resulting in it being re-established at a more apical level following bone resorption. Bearing in mind that 1–2 mm of healthy dental structure must be added on top of the junctional epithelium for placing the prosthetic cervical margin, it would appear essential to have 3–4 mm between the osseous (alveolar) crest and the most coronal portion of the tooth fragment intended for restoration.

The place of initial therapy

This simple treatment of the causes of periodontal disease precedes the provisional phase of the prosthesis, and does not necessitate intervention by a periodontal specialist.

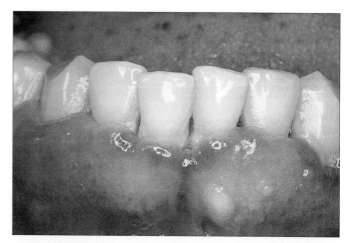

Figure 10.109   *Periodontitis with severe gingival inflammation.*

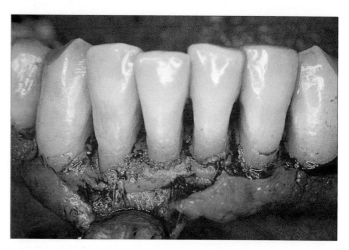

Figure 10.110   *The flap helps to show the extent of the osseous defects.*

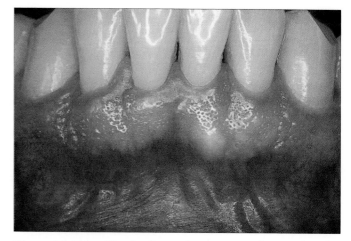

Figure 10.111   *After healing and maturation, the periodontal condition is adequate for potential prosthetic treatment. (Courtesy of Dr Sylvain Altglas.)*

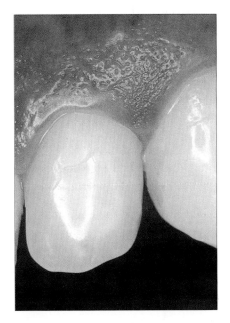 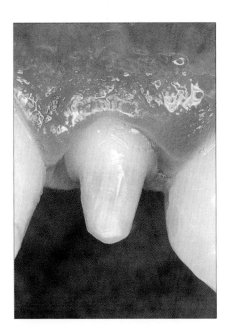 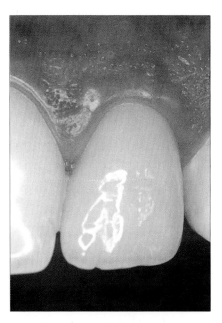

Figure 10.112   Unesthetic gingival morphology due to a poorly adapted and contoured temporary crown.

Figure 10.113   The papillae are compressed and are starting to collapse.

Figure 10.114   After a new temporary crown has been fabricated, with a harmonious cervical contour and well-situated proximal surfaces, the soft tissues regain their original anatomy, showing sharp interdental papillae. (Courtesy of Dr Sylvain Altglas.)

This stage of eradicating supra- and subgingival microbial plaque resolves gingival inflammation within a few days and reverses the tendency to bleed. It also restores the normal morphological characteristics of the tissue. It arouses the patient's motivation to initiate a strict oral hygiene technique, which can ensure elimination of calculus and bacterial deposits by scaling of the supra- and subgingival root surfaces.

Healing 'marginal' gingivitis restores a harmonious gingival outline of a pale pink shade with healthy papillae. Permanent eradication of gingival inflammation can often require elimination of plaque-retaining factors such as restorations with overhanging margins, poorly fitting crowns, etc. The use of well-fitting and properly polished temporary prostheses is also cardinal.

The periodontal role of provisional restorations

The diagnostic and therapeutic role played by provisional prostheses is considerable; they serve as models for the final prosthesis and to measure the suitability of tooth shape, emergence profile, function, phonation, etc. (Figures 10.112–10.114).

The response of the gingivae guides progressive modification of the temporary prosthesis by either addition or subtraction through realignment or polishing respectively. The goal is to obtain prosthetic biointegration, and sometimes this will require two sets of temporary crowns.

It is evidently unsafe to embark on the definitive prosthesis before the periodontium has returned to normal and the patient feels satisfied with the esthetic appearance of the teeth and gingivae.

Impressions of the temporary crowns adapting gradually to the periodontium will be a helpful guide to the ceramist as to the shape and bulk required for the cervical third of final prostheses – a crucial factor for biological esthetic success.

Surgical steps prior to prosthetics

Crown-lengthening procedure

The crown-lengthening procedure enables healthy dental structure to be exposed. Indications for this technique

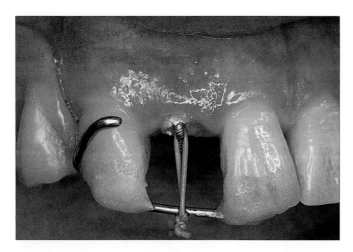

Figure 10.115 *Orthodontic appliance for controlled extrusion of a fractured tooth.*

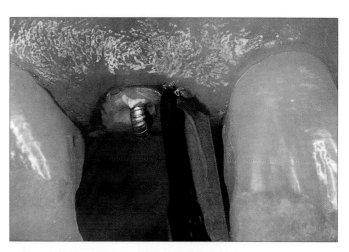

Figure 10.116 *Circumferential sulcular fibrectomy is performed.*

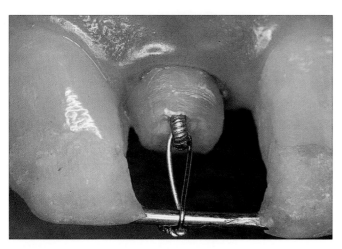

Figure 10.117 *The root has been successfully extruded.*

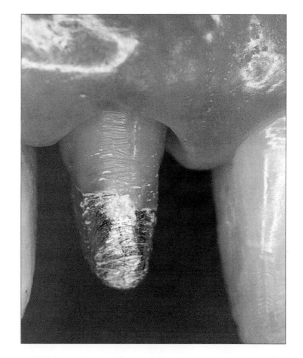

Figure 10.118 *The tooth can now receive a cast dowel and core, and can be prepared for a ceramic crown.*

include partial or complete subgingival fracture, and the need to regain biological width. Generally, a full-thickness flap is raised to allow for ostectomy and osteoplasty. Particular care should be taken when festooning the osseous alveolar contour, which will promote a good periodontal margin outline and hence the harmonious and natural appearance of the prosthesis.

Forced eruption (Figures 10.115–10.119)

Recovery of teeth or roots with deep subgingival fractures may require the use of orthodontics. Should a single tooth in the anterior area be affected, the forced eruption technique can produce sufficient extrusion of the tooth to allow cervical margins to be prepared in the usual way.

This technique requires the fitting of a segmented orthodontic appliance made up of a supporting bar,

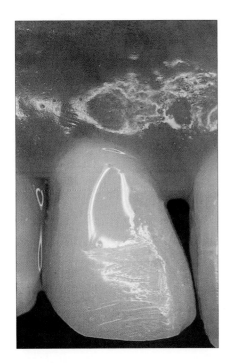

Figure 10.119 *The acrylic provisional restoration. (Courtesy of Dr Sylvain Altglas.)*

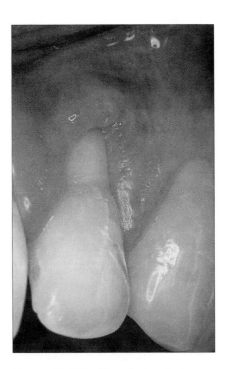

Figure 10.120 *Unesthetic soft-tissue recession in the anterior region.*

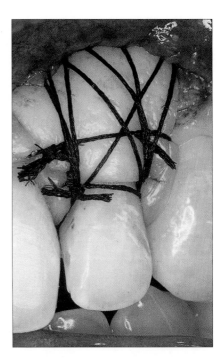

Figure 10.121 *The epithelial connective tissue graft sutured in place.*

bonded by composite resin. An elastic traction cord is stretched between the root post and the bar, which will induce extrusion. Circumferential sulcal fiberectomy is carried out every 6 days so as to surgically section Sharpey's supracrestal fibers. After a 3–4-week stabilization period, the tooth can be prepared to receive a temporary crown.

Eruption, as described, can also help to increase the amount of alveolar bone for implants. Under these circumstances any traction would use an intraosseous implant as support after completion of the osseointegration.

Root coverage procedure (Figures 10.120–10.122)

When unesthetic recession takes place in the anterior area, especially if the recession affects an isolated tooth, mucogingival surgery can considerably improve the appearance.

Impacted graft technique A constant thickness corresponding to that of the periosteal base must be observed

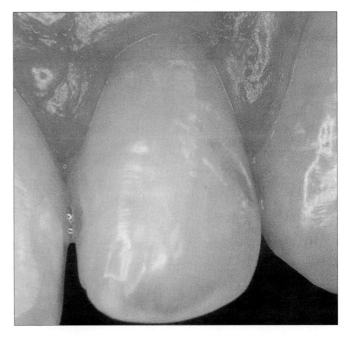

Figure 10.122 *The esthetic result, 6 months postoperatively. (Courtesy of Dr Sylvain Altglas.)*

when taking a graft. The recipient site is prepared with a peripheral shoulder so as to contain the carefully sutured epithelial connective tissue graft. Several months will be required before the final result can be appreciated.

Connective-tissue grafting technique The graft, consisting solely of connective tissue, is placed between the root and the external flap. The epithelial cells of the outer flap recolonize the connective-tissue graft, enabling the ambient shade of color to be recovered.

Microabrasion can sometimes help to improve the results of these grafts.

References

Burke FJT, The effect of variations in bonding procedure on fracture resistance of dentin-bonded all-ceramic crowns. *Quintessence Int* 1995; **26**: 293–300.

Geller W, Dental ceramics and esthetics. Presented at Chicago Midwinter Meeting, February 15, 1991.

Geller W, Kwiatkowski SJ, The Willi's glass crown: A new solution in the dark and shadowed zones of esthetic porcelain restorations. *Quintessence Dent Technol* 1987; **11**:233–42.

Goldstein RE, Esthetic principles for ceramo-metal restorations. *Dent Clin North Am* 1977; **21**:803.

Lustig PL, A rational concept of crown preparation revised and expanded. *Quintessence Int* 1976; **11**: 41.

McLean JW, *The Science and Art of Dental Ceramics.* London: Quintessence, 1980.

McLean JW, Hughes TH, The reinforcement of dental porcelain with ceramic oxides. *Br Dent J* 1965; **119**:251.

Nakabayashi N, The hybrid layer: resin–dentin composite. *Proc Finn Dent Soc* 1992; **88(Suppl 1)**: 321–9.

Nathanson D, Principles of porcelain use as an inlay/onlay material. In: *Procelain and Composite Inlays and Onlays: Esthetic Posterior Restorations* (ed DA Garber, RE Goldstein). London: Quintessence, 1994.

Touati B, Miara P, Light transmission in bonded ceramic restorations. *J Esthet Dent* 1993, **5**: 11–17.

Touati B, Etienne JM, Improved shape and emergence profile in an extensive ceramic rehabilitation. *Pract Periodont Aesthet Dent* 1998, **10**: 129–35.

Winter R, Achieving esthetic ceramic restorations. *J Calif Dent Assoc* 1990; September 21.

Winter R, Creation porcelain: negating the need for an all-ceramic restoration. Lecture given at the 17th Annual Session of the American Academy of Esthetic Dentistry, Sante Fe, NM, USA, 1992.

CHAPTER 11

Ceramic Inlays and Onlays

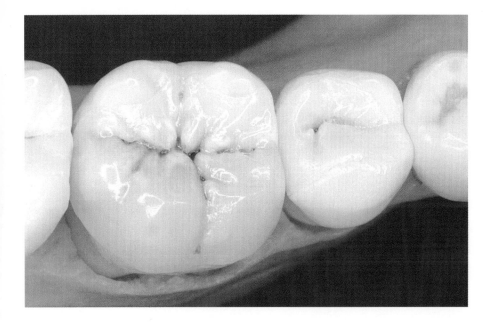

Interestingly, ceramic inlays go further back in modern dental history than gold inlays. They came into use in the late nineteenth century as an esthetic means of restoring carious lesions. It was only natural to aim for a substance of the same color as human teeth (Figure 11.1). Unfortunately, the use of porcelain inlays was halted by too high a failure rate; these inlays were made on a metal matrix and then simply luted using a conventional (e.g. zinc phosphate) cement. Early porcelain inlays had poor marginal fit, and the conventional cement could easily wash out. The advantages of the lost wax casting technique combined with the accuracy and reliability of gold alloys put a stop to the use of ceramic inlays for about 50 years (Figure 11.2).

Having been tentatively reintroduced in the 1960s for certain cervical cavities (and luted with silicate cements), ceramic inlays made further advances during the l980s as a result of several technological developments:

- advances made in refractory investments;
- the use of silane coupling agents;
- the use of composite resin cements;
- improved bonding techniques.

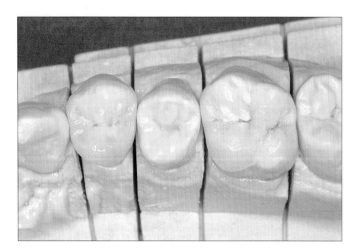

Figure 11.1 *It has always been the goal of dentistry to find an ideal esthetic and functional material for posterior restorations. An example of esthetic restorations fabricated by ceramist Gérald Ubassy.*

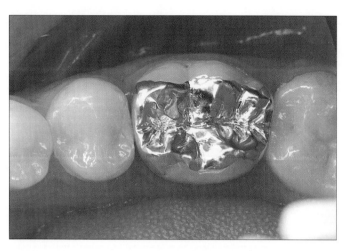

Figure 11.2 *Cast gold restorations have set the standard for decades, but unfortunately cemented gold inlays do not reinforce the tooth structure, and while cemented gold onlays do reinforce tooth structure, they are unesthetic in appearance.*

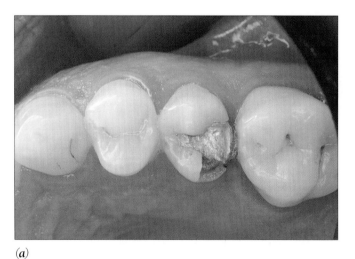

(*a*)

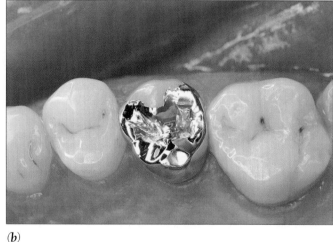

(*b*)

Figure 11.3 (*a*) *An amalgam restoration does not reinforce the tooth structure. Here the lingual cusp has fractured.* (*b*) *The same tooth restored with a gold onlay provides more resistance to occlusal stresses.*

The current state of the art of ceramic inlays and onlays, based on a 10-year experience with modern materials, is much more positive than in earlier generations (Figures 11.3 and 11.4) (Dietschi and Spreafico, 1997). Providing there is good case selection, accurately defined cavity design, and strict bonding procedures (relying on the latest dentin–enamel adhesives), ceramic inlays and onlays can produce very satisfying results. However, the technique remains delicate and laborious, requiring collaboration with a good ceramist and a good understanding of the ceramic material. While giving an esthetically pleasing result, ceramic is subject to critical clinical constraints due to its lack of elasticity. (Figures 11.5 and 11.6).

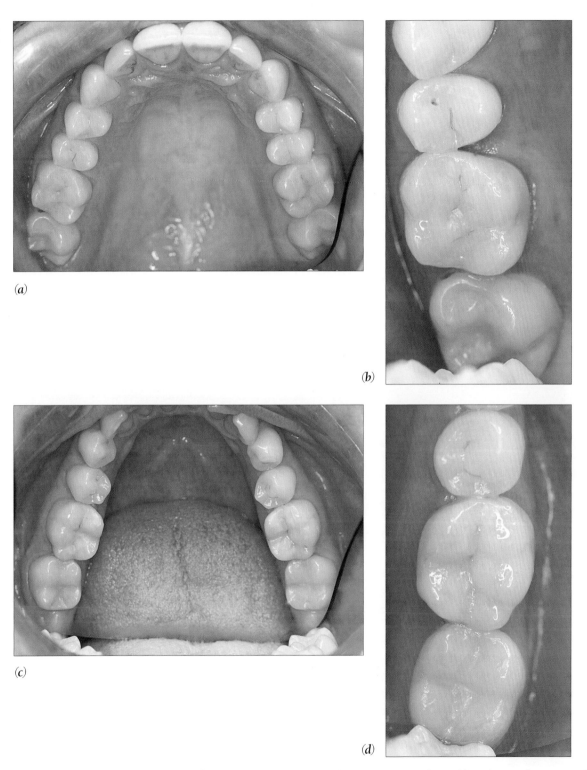

(a)

(b)

(c)

(d)

Figure 11.4 (**a**) *Maxillary arch esthetically restored with two all-ceramic crowns (centrals) and several ceramic inlays and composite restorations.* (**b**) *Close-up at 5-year follow-up.* (**c**) *Ceramic inlays in the first molars; direct adhesive composite restorations in the second molars.* (**d**) *Close-up at 5-year follow-up.*

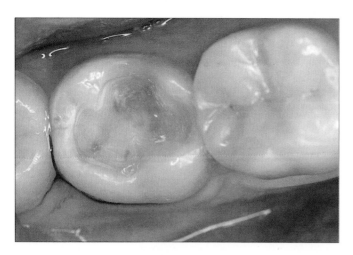

Figure 11.5 A large cavity in the second molar: the first molar has had a feldspathic ceramic inlay (MOD) for six years. Only a little cement erosion is noticeable.

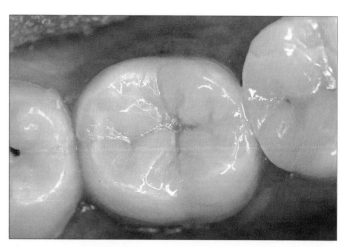

Figure 11.6 Ceramic inlay in the second molar; there is good color integration with a translucent resin cement (Choice, Bisco). (Ceramist: Serge Tissier.)

Case selection

It is first and foremost the selection of cases suitable for treatment that determines the ultimate medium- and long-term success rate of ceramic inlays, and the clinician must concentrate effort on the selection process. This process will evolve as the clinician gains experience, but a few basic rules can be usefully singled out:

- ceramic inlays/onlays are indicated for medium-level damage to vital molars or premolars (Figures 11.7–11.10);
- ceramic inlays/onlays must be prepared so as to leave an outer enamel margin, which is needed to provide a reliable seal;
- the margins of inlays/onlays must never coincide with occlusal contacts. This is a root cause of medium-term failures. The avoidance of these contacts may sometimes require a change in cavity design, and even transforming to an onlay preparation (Figures 11.11 and 11.12);
- extensive unsupported overhangs must be avoided; these inevitably lead to fractures due to the poor flexural strength of the ceramic material (Figures 11.13 and 11.14);
- parafunction activity in general and bruxism in particular must be considered as strict contraindications; the same is true of poor oral hygiene;

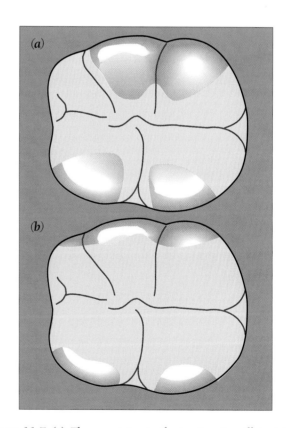

Figure 11.7 (a) The remaining tooth structure is sufficient to withstand the stresses that result from normal dental function. (b) Here the remaining tooth is too thin to withstand normal function, and an onlay will provide more strength.

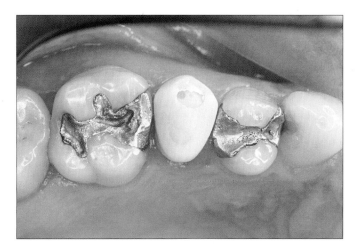

Figure 11.8 *A worn-out acrylic provisional crown between two teeth with failing amalgam restorations.*

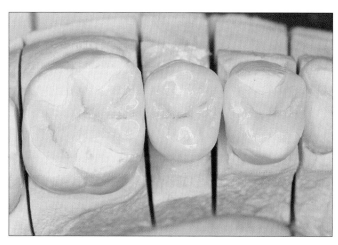

Figure 11.9 *Ceramic inlays and a metal–ceramic crown shown on the model. (Ceramist: Gérald Ubassy.)*

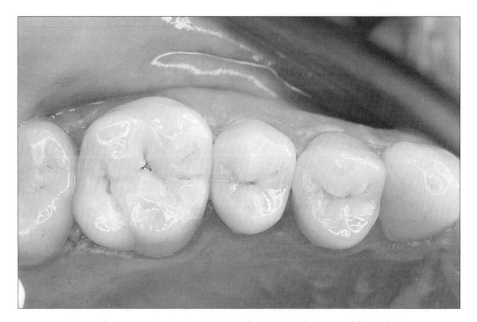

Figure 11.10 *The restorations cemented in the mouth: the same feldspathic ceramic has been used for the metal-ceramic crown and the inlays.*

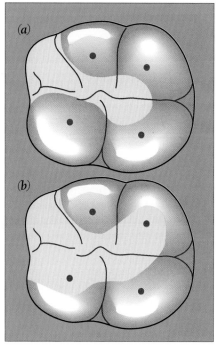

Figure 11.11 *Occlusal contacts should be situated away from the margins of the cavity: (**a**) correctly placed occlusal contacts; (**b**) two contacts incorrectly placed within the cavity.*

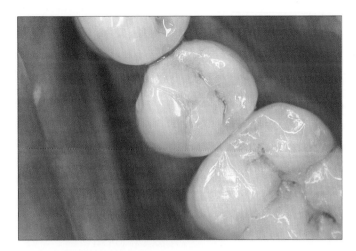

Figure 11.12 The buccal occlusal contact coincides with the margin, leading to the formation of a fracture.

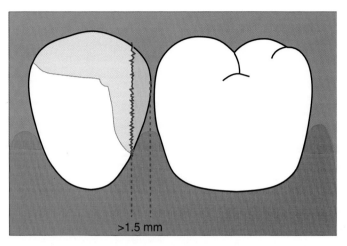

>1.5 mm

Figure 11.13 An unsupported proximal section that extends over 1.0–1.5 mm from the tooth support, especially in high stress-bearing areas where the floor of the cavity is not wide enough, can result in fracture because of the lack of elasticity of the ceramic material.

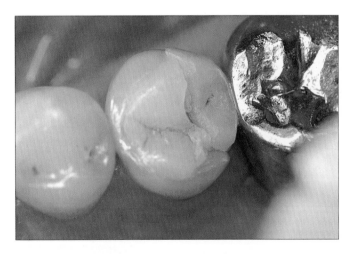

Figure 11.14 Bruxism (see wear facets on the gold crown), and excess unsupported ceramic in the distal aspect lead to inevitable failure of the restoration.

- ease of access to the cavity is essential to the success of careful preparation, making impressions, and bonding under a rubber dam;
- if teeth are too short, this can often be considered a contraindication, since insufficient depth would then be allowed for the ceramic material (1.5 mm is the

minimum thickness allowable). This concept of coronal height also relates to the level of cervical margins: it is extremely difficult to place inlays/onlays with subgingival margins in view of the special conditions required for bonding and the requirement to finish on enamel margins.

Modifiable adverse clinical conditions

Certain adjustments can often improve the clinical presentation considerably, thus making ceramic inlays/onlays a viable option (Figures 11.15–11.19).

Very deep (especially undercut) cavities can be dealt with using protective bases. If the remaining dentin appears to be insufficiently thick (less than 0.5 mm), the clinician may choose to use a calcium hydroxide lining as a pulp dressing. This should then be covered with a resin-modified glass-ionomer cement, which will fill the undercuts at the preparation stage, thus minimizing further coronal destruction. If the remaining dentin is thicker, and not transparent enough for the pulp to show through, the glass-ionomer base can be applied directly. There is no particular need to resort to these bases for moderate-sized cavities, especially in view of advances in modern dentin adhesives. Use of glass ionomer was advocated at a time when we were clinically poorly equipped to deal with frequently occurring

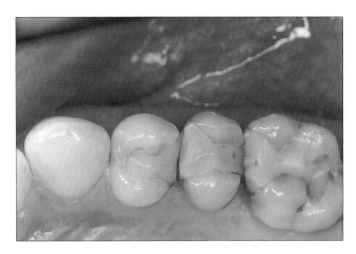

Figure 11.15 *Defective composite restorations exhibiting microleakage.*

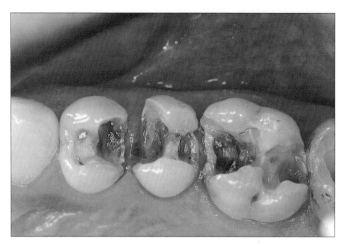

Figure 11.16 *Removal of the composite reveals underlying caries.*

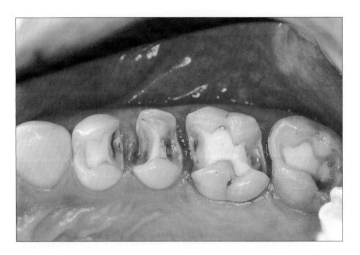

Figure 11.17 *As the cavities are deep, and feature undercuts, a glass-ionomer base is used (Fuji II, GC).*

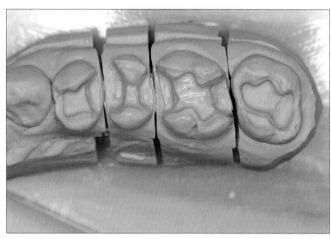

Figure 11.18 *The master model showing the prepared teeth.*

postoperative sensitivity associated with inadequate seal. In the past, postoperative sensitivity and pulpal inflammation were said to be consequences of the contact between vital dentin and acid etchants. It has now been proved that bacterial infiltration is the main cause of pulpal inflammation and postoperative sensi-

tivity. Since the introduction of more reliable dentin adhesives that, after dentin etching and suppression of the smear layer, create a half-resin half-dentin hybrid layer, we have confined the use of bases to deep cavities where undercuts are often present close to the pulp.

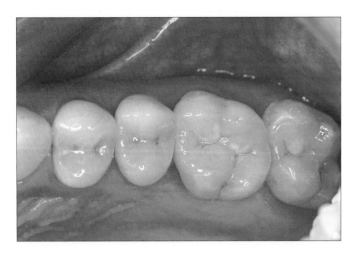

Figure 11.19 The final result after the four ceramic restorations have been bonded.

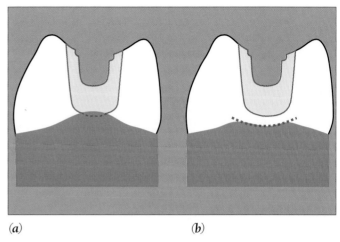

(a)   *(b)*

Figure 11.20 (a,b) Occasionally, when cavities are deep, it is necessary to carry out a partial gingivectomy so that the margins are rendered supragingival.

Subgingival margins may be dealt with by partial gingivectomy, thus rendering them supragingival, so as to fulfil the conditions required for bonding (Figure 11.20).

Ceramic inlays or onlays?

The choice of whether to prepare for an inlay or an onlay will depend on the presentation. When remaining walls of the tooth become fragile, opinions may differ over the course to take:

* some prefer to prepare an inlay cavity wherever possible, in view of the cuspal reinforcement effect achieved by bonding (Figure 11.21);
* some opt for cuspal overlay (Figures 11.22–11.24).

While the former must be the first choice, the authors have opted for the latter view at times, for the following reasons:

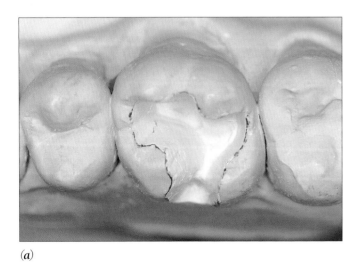

(a)

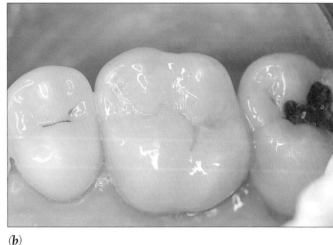

(b)

Figure 11.21 (a) A large cavity in a first molar. (b) Thanks to adhesion, this inlay has esthetically restored and reinforced the tooth.

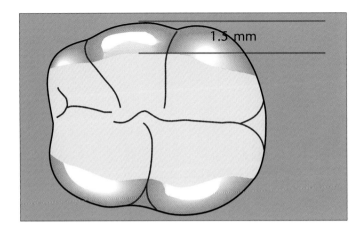

Figure 11.22 *When the thickness of the remaining tooth structure in a molar is less than 1.5 mm, the risk of fracture increases, especially if the patient has some parafunction. In such a case, it is safer to cover the cusps with an onlay.*

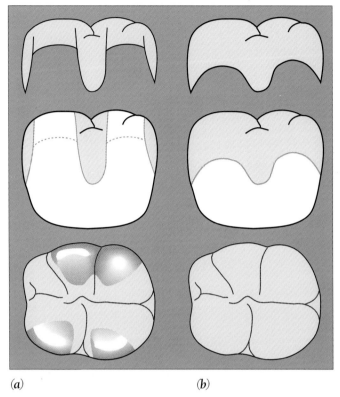

(a)   (b)

Figure 11.23 (**a**) *In some cases where there is an inlay preparation with extensions that are creating a complex and tortuous contour, it can be difficult to form an accurate marginal fit, and thus it is best to use an onlay – not to strengthen the tooth, but to avoid unnecessarily extensive margins (**b**).*

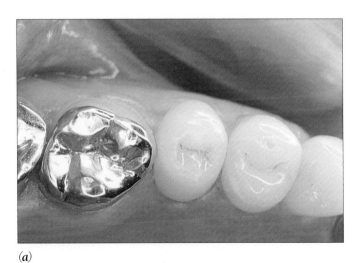

(a)

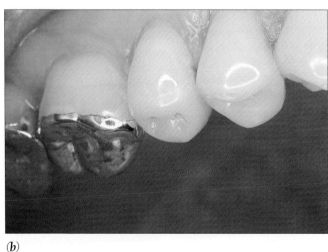

(b)

Figure 11.24 (**a**) *An onlay was indicated, for occlusal reasons, on the 2nd bicuspid. Unlike the molars, and thanks to the progress of adhesion, a ceramic onlay can be bonded on the tooth with a translucent cement (Variolink translucent, Ivoclar Vivadent). (**b**) Compared with the molars, the result is esthetic and conservative, and only a chamfer has been prepared on the buccal aspect of the tooth.*

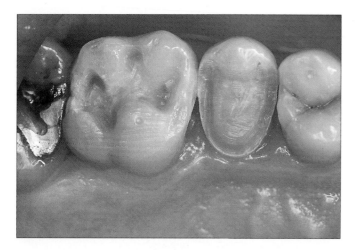

Figure 11.25 *Extensive onlay preparation on the 2nd bicuspid, and an inlay preparation on the first molar.*

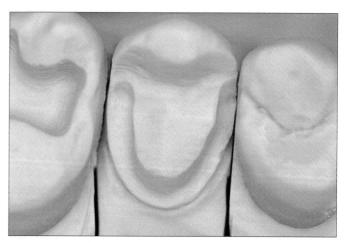

Figure 11.26 *This type of preparation is indicated when a lingual cusp is broken. The deep chamfer will provide a compression effect inside the ceramic material.*

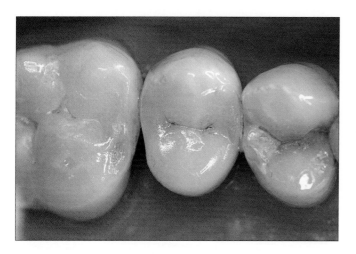

Figure 11.27 *The Empress (Ivoclar) onlay and inlay, after luting.*

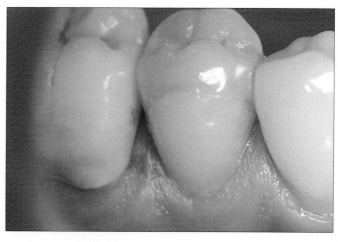

Figure 11.28 *Follow-up of a ceramic onlay at 5 years. Even though not subjected to direct occlusal forces, the buccal margin has slightly deteriorated. The causes are the micromovements of the restoration during function and the lack of elasticity of the ceramic material.*

- When the margins are located away from occlusal contacts, on the labial and lingual surfaces, the tooth–ceramic interface is less fragile, being less subject to functional wear and tear, and the composite resin cement is longer-lasting (Figures 11.25–11.27). However, despite being protected from occlusal loading, onlay margins may still deteriorate (Figure 11.28).

- Esthetically, onlays are superior, and in addition, since onlay margins have less tortuous contours, they may be clinically more reliable. The option is more invasive, however, and can only be justified in the case of fragile walls – certainly not as a routine choice.

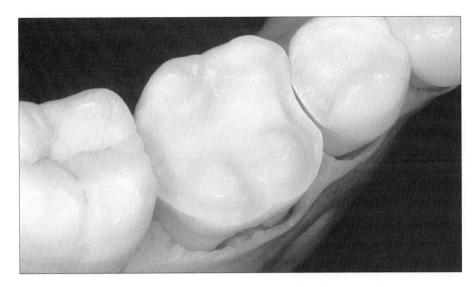

Figure 11.29 Typical onlay and inlay cavity design: note the rounded angles and cusps, the soft contours, and the enamel chamfer. One aim of these preparations is to reduce tensile and flexural stresses, and to increase compression within the ceramic restoration.

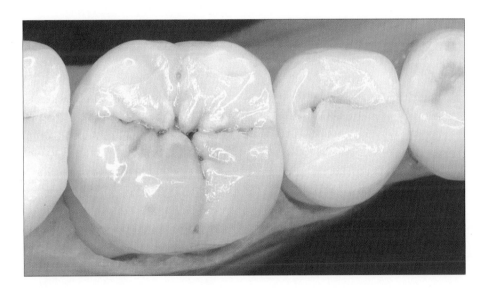

Figure 11.30 Ceramic is an outstanding material in the dentist's armamentarium, and allows for natural effects and characterization. (Ceramist: Gérald Ubassy.)

Tooth preparation

Tooth preparation for ceramic inlays and onlays differs markedly from that for cast metal inlays (Figures 11.29 and 11.30) (Magne et al, 1996). This is due to the properties of the ceramic biomaterial, and is especially designed to compensate for the shortcomings of the material, particularly its fragility, when used in a thin layer.

Inlays

The following modifications to a conventional inlay cavity preparation are required for ceramic inlays:

• a proximal cavity with no slice cut or bevel edge;
• axial walls with a roughly 10° angle of taper;
• an enlarged isthmus (not less than 2 mm wide);

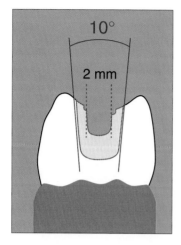

Figure 11.31 *A typical cavity design leaves a wall divergence of around 10°, and an isthmus not less than 2 mm.*

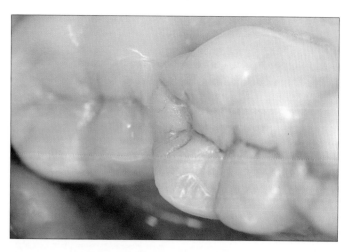

Figure 11.32 *A proximal fracture has occurred resulting from the proximal overhang and the lack of elasticity of the ceramic material.*

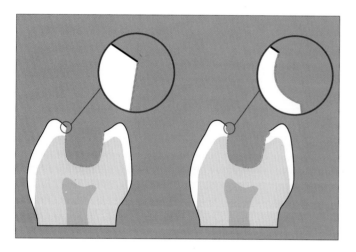

Figure 11.33 (**a**) *The standard cavo-surface design has a 90° butt margin.* (**b**) *A hollow-ground chamfer is sometimes indicated in low-stress-bearing areas and where the occlusion is favorable.*

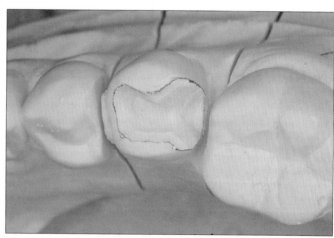

Figure 11.34 *Example of a preparation with a hollow-ground chamfer clearly visible on the stone die.*

- rounded internal angles (Figure 11.31).
- the base of the main cavity should be flat to enhance compression of the material lying above (Figure 11.32);
- occlusal margins may not coincide with occlusal contact sites;

- margins should be prepared to a 90° cavosurface line angle; alternatively, they should present a hollow-ground chamfer (occlusion permitting), in an attempt to create an 'invisible' margin (Figures 11.33 and 11.34).

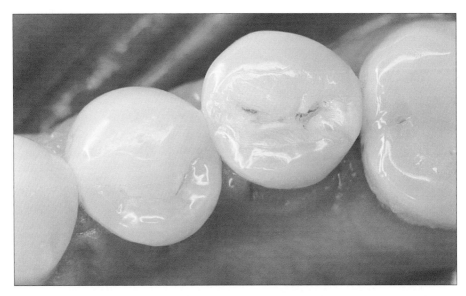

Figure 11.35 *The cemented restoration: note that this is a feldspathic ceramic inlay. The margins are hardly visible due to the translucent enamel used, and a truly camouflaged effect is achieved by using several chromas and values inside the inlay. (Ceramist: Gérald Ubassy.)*

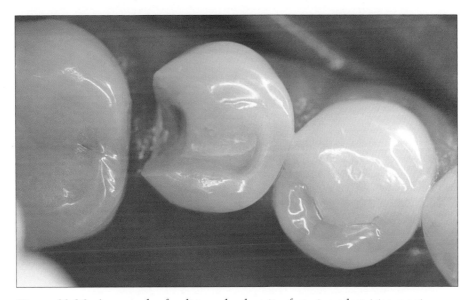

Figure 11.36 *An example of a disto-occlusal cavity, featuring a butt-joint margin.*

Butt-joint cavosurface line angle

An edge-to-edge relationship at an angle of 90° between the margin of the inlay and that of the preparation is simpler to create and less fragile during fabrication of the inlay (Figures 11.35 and 11.36). It is suitable for short teeth and unretentive preparations and for cast or heat-pressed ceramic techniques such as Dicor and Empress, and produces an acceptable esthetic effect.

Visually there appears to be an abrupt transition between the ceramic and the enamel, often resulting in difficulties with color integration if the cement film at the interface is not sufficiently translucent. However, with the steady improvement in the accuracy of refractory investments and ceramic inlays, far better esthetic effects can be achieved now than were possible in the early 1980s (Figure 11.37).

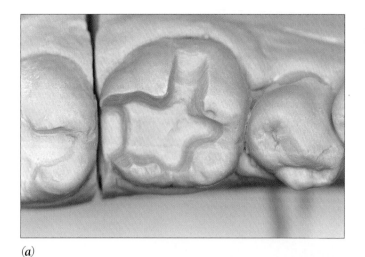

(a)

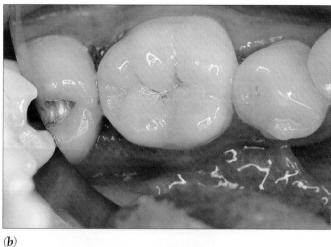

(b)

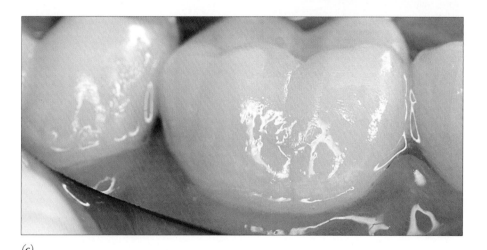

(c)

Figure 11.37 (a) *Inlay preparation with a buccal extension and a 90° cavo-surface margin.* (b) *The cemented ceramic inlay exhibits good esthetic color integration.* (c) *Due to the accuracy of modern investments, a good marginal fit can be achieved even with a highly complex contour.*

Hollow-ground chamfer

In a number of publications on composite inlays (Touati, 1984; Touati and Pissis, 1984; 1986), the authors first described a rounded-hollow-ground chamfer (Figures 11.38–11.41). This has been used where possible with ceramic inlays and, more than a decade later, the results are satisfactory given the following requirements: adequate cavity height, non-obtrusive occlusal contact sites, and a skilful laboratory technician. Nonetheless, this type of margin is definitely more fragile and restricted to cases with suitable occlusion (Figure 11.42). The esthetic effects are superior to those of the butt margin due to the color gradation between tooth and inlay, which are further optimized by placing semitranslucent ceramic near the margins, allowing the color of the underlying tooth to show through and to enhance light transmission (Figures 11.43–11.44, and see also Figure 11.35). Fairly translucent resin luting cements should be used to enhance this effect.

With current material technology, it is possible to achieve better esthetic results even with 90° cavo-surface margins (butt-joints) on occlusal surfaces. On the other hand, on buccal surfaces where color integration is crucial and difficult, it is advisable to use deep chamfer margins for increased color blending and larger enamel surfaces.

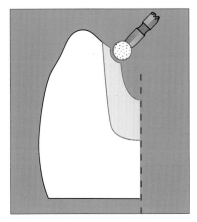

Figure 11.38 *The hollow-ground chamfer should be deep enough so that it is not fragile. It is usually formed using a round diamond instrument.*

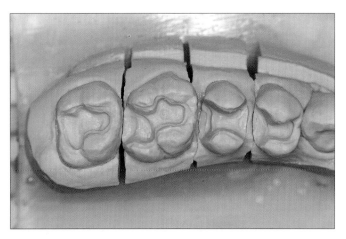

Figure 11.39 *A quadrant of inlay preparations on the master model. Note the hollow-ground chamfer finishing margin.*

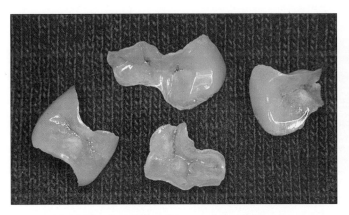

Figure 11.40 *The four feldspathic porcelain inlays.*

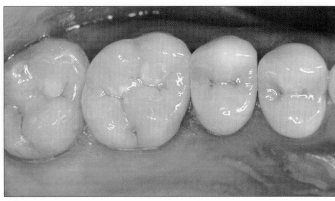

Figure 11.41 *The four porcelain inlays cemented in the mouth.*

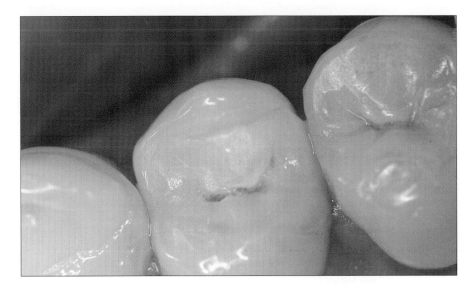

Figure 11.42 *Fracturing of the ceramic margin on the buccal aspect of the inlay, at the location of the hollow-ground chamfer.*

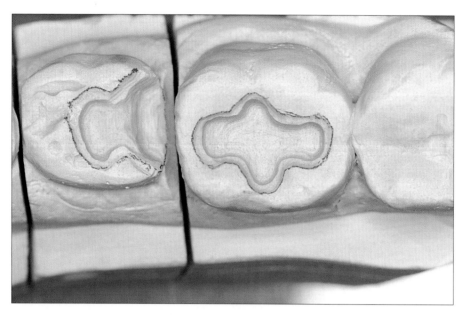

Figure 11.43 *Preparations with a hollow-ground chamfer seen on a stone model.*

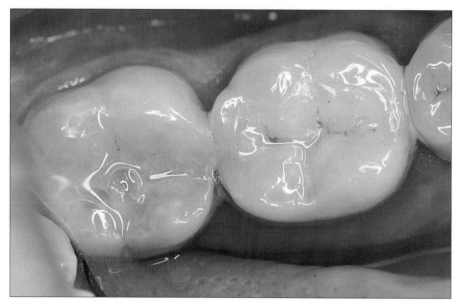

Figure 11.44 *An excellent color blending of the inlay on the first molar. (Ceramist: Serge Tissier.)*

Proximal finish

As previously mentioned, a proximal slice, as used with gold inlays, is not indicated for ceramic inlays. This is in order to minimize ceramic extensions, which may induce fracture due to brittleness. The proximal cavity, however, is sufficiently open to allow access for brushing. It should be noted that the cervical margin of this proximal cavity is not bevelled but merely flat, like a shoulder, and located within the enamel; at the present stage of development it is preferred not to rely on joints bonded to dentin or cementum.

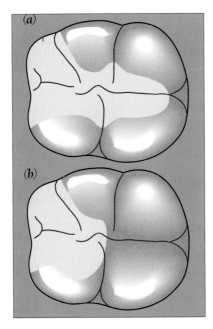

Figure 11.45 (**a**) *Conventional cemented metal inlays must incorporate most of the occlusal grooves, to provide adequate retention.* (**b**) *In contrast, the contour of a cavity for a bonded ceramic inlay does not need such stabilization, and is therefore more conservative.*

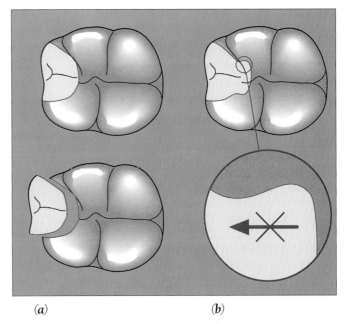

(**a**)   (**b**)

Figure 11.46 (**a**) *However, no stabilization at all would increase the risk of premature displacement of the inlay, even if it were properly bonded.* (**b**) *The design must therefore incorporate vertical grooves ('dovetail') for greater stability.*

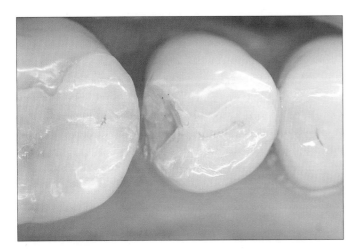

Figure 11.47 *A narrow isthmus may have contributed to the fracture of this restoration.*

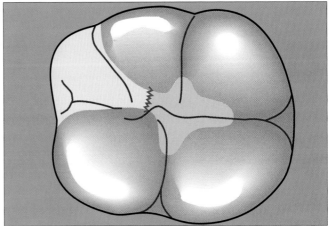

Figure 11.48 *If the isthmus is too narrow, it can create a tension zone, which will cause the brittle ceramic to fracture.*

Isthmus

These should not be too narrow, to avoid fracture sites within the inlay. An ideal inlay cavity has few tortuous contours and a bulky shape. 'Extension for prevention' to healthy grooves is no longer the norm (Figures 11.45 and 11.46). An isthmus should not measure less than 2 mm (preferably 2.5 mm for molars) bucco-lingually. A balance should exist between the volume of the ceramic and the width of the isthmus (Figures 11.47 and 11.48).

Onlays

Cuspal overlaying should allow a clearance (thus thickness of ceramic) of at least 1.5 mm, preferably 2 mm (Figure 11.49). All cuspal angles should be rounded, and margins should consist of a shoulder with a rounded internal angle or a deep chamfer. Rotary tools for this purpose consist mainly of tapered round-end diamond instruments and an olive-shaped or spherical instrument designed for the hollow-ground chamfer (Figure 11.50).

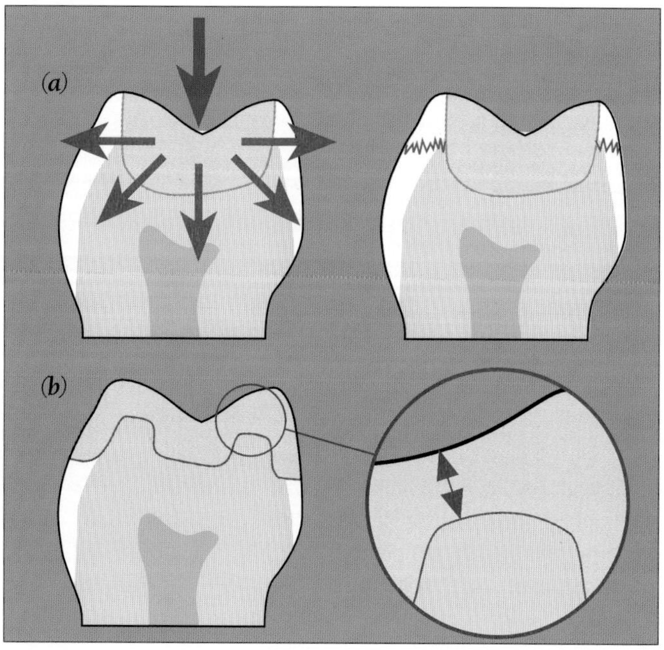

Fabrication of inlays/onlays

Impression taking and duplicates

Impressions of supragingival cavity preparations are simple to take, and lend themselves to techniques familiar to the operator, such as the use of hydrocolloids and silicones. Addition silicones are the impression materials of choice.

The fabrication of ceramic inlays/onlays often requires preparation of duplicate dies of refractory material. These may be obtained by duplicating the laboratory model if the impression material is too unstable for repeated pouring (such as hydrocolloids). Hence there is a preference for addition silicones, with which the technician can make two casts: one of extra hard plaster and the other of refractory investment. This technique is simpler as well as more accurate than those involving duplicates.

Temporization

Temporization is an indispensable stage in the creation of inlays and onlays, since any oversight here can affect the well-being of the pulp and/or the final adhesion of the ceramic restoration. The best solution consists of direct, chairside creation of light-cured resin inlays/onlays after lubrication of the teeth. This enables the thickness of the cosmetic material and the width of the isthmus to be checked directly using a micrometer. The temporization stage must therefore precede that of impression taking, so that any correction of cavity depth can be made subsequently.

After trimming and adjusting the margins and occlusal contact sites, this resin inlay is cemented using a eugenol-free temporary cement. Eugenol has the disadvantage of inhibiting the setting of composites.

It is sometimes tempting to fill a small inlay cavity using a eugenol-free temporary cement, but experience has shown that the limited mechanical properties of

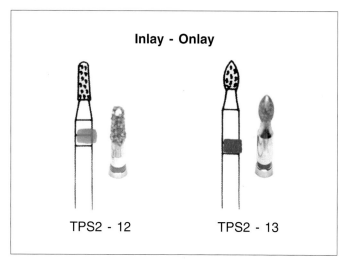

Figure 11.49 *Ceramic does not absorb much of the stress applied to it, and will instead transmit it to the surrounding tooth structure. (**a**) If the tooth structure is too thin, it will fracture. (**b**) If the onlay overlays the cusp, it will protect the tooth, providing that it is strong enough to withstand everyday wear and tear. There should be a minimum occlusal clearance of around 1.5–2.0 mm.*

Inlay - Onlay

TPS2 - 12   TPS2 - 13

Figure 11.50 *The two diamond instruments most commonly used for inlay and onlay preparations, from the TPS2 Kit (Brasseler-Komet).*

such cements lead at least to disappearance of the edges, if not fracturing of a portion of the temporary filling. Failure of the seal at this stage will inevitably bring about dentin–pulp sensitivity, subsequently vulnerable to infiltration by bacteria. It is the pump-like effect on the odontoblasts and differences in intrapulpal osmotic pressure that heighten sensitivity, with the bacterial infiltration being the cause of the pulpal necrosis that is occasionally observed.

It is possible to seal and reinforce the trimmed dentin at this stage using a dental adhesive. After removal of the smear layer, the surface dentin can be hybridized by the adhesive. The solvent should be allowed to evaporate, and the adhesive polymerized either chemically or by light; it will then serve as an effective protection, and will be left in place at the final bonding stage. This hybridization must be thin so as not to hinder placement of the inlay or, better still, be produced prior to making impressions.

A few years ago new provisional composite materials (Fermit and Fermit N, Ivoclar Vivadent) were formulated. These new materials must be inserted, carved and light-cured directly in the mouth on the preparation. When using these materials, it is important to avoid hybridization at this stage as they might bond to this protective layer.

Try-in

Try-in allows the fit of the inlay or onlay to be tested. This stage requires care and accuracy owing to the fragility of the ceramic restorations prior to bonding. The inlays/onlays are inserted using a small globule of wax of low melting point attached to a plastic instrument handle, or using a placing instrument such as the Accu-Placer, Hu-Friedy. (All instruments used up to the point of bonding, such as spatulas or pluggers, are made of plastic, since they are flexible and less likely to cause fracturing of the ceramic.) Both try-in and bonding are facilitated if a vertical stabilization groove has been incorporated in the preparation (Figure 11.51).

During try-in it may be necessary to adjust interproximal contact areas, and any areas of friction on the internal surface (Figures 11.52 and 11.53).

Interproximal contact areas

A sheet of carbon paper may be used for detecting the contact area, or, better still, the proximal surface can be stained with pillar-box red dissolved in chloroform,

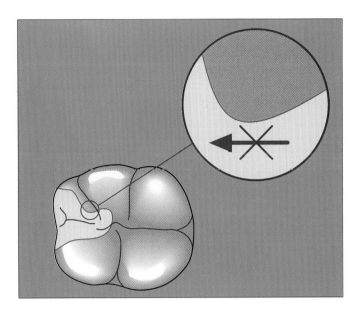

Figure 11.51 One advantage of a vertical stabilization groove is that it facilitates try-in and bonding by keeping the restoration in position.

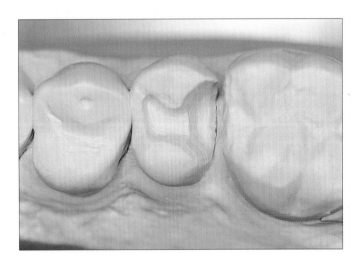

Figure 11.52 DO inlay preparation, shown on a model.

for example. Correction should be carried out slowly, using aluminous silicone wheels or cups (Figures 11.54 and 11.55).

Friction on the internal surface

A white silicone fluid (Fit Checker, GC) is used for detection of discrepancies, and any adjustments are made by

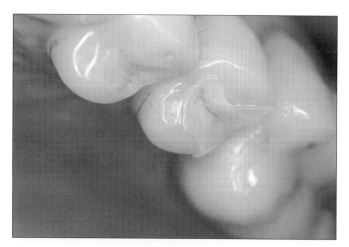

Figure 11.53 A difficult and risky stage is the try-in, especially the detection of tight proximal contacts.

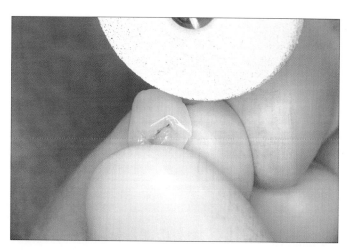

Figure 11.54 Adjustment of the contact with a silicone wheel (TPS Finition Kit, Brasseler-Komet).

red-banded medium-speed diamond instruments under a water spray. It is not recommended to check occlusal contact prior to bonding of the inlay/onlay, because of the risk of fracturing the ceramic. However, if this procedure appears to be vital, a silicone fluid film (Memosil, Bayer) should be used to soften occlusal impact.

Not all ceramics have the same mechanical resistance to stresses. Feldspathic ceramics are less resistant than leucite-reinforced or glass ceramics. The two latter groups should always be selected when mechanical requirements appear to be a major factor.

Cementing

Attaching the ceramic restoration to the prepared tooth by means of bonding with a resin cement will provide not only retention but also added resistance to the inlay/onlay

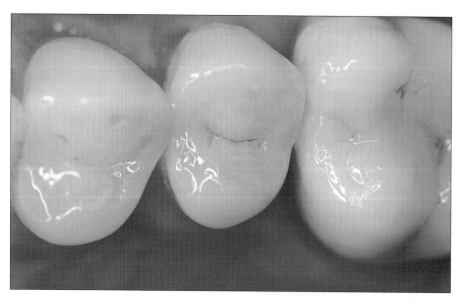

Figure 11.55 The esthetic outcome: due to the transparent resin cement, the margins of the ceramic inlay in the second premolar are virtually invisible. (Ceramist: Laboratory GH, Paris.)

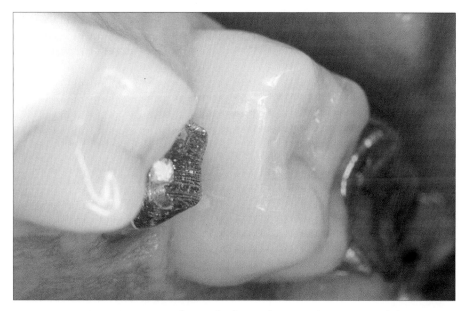

Figure 11.56 An MO ceramic inlay in the first molar: note the precision of the proximal margins.

(Degrange et al, 1994a,b; Dietschi and Spreafico, 1998). At this stage the tooth is also being sealed and its shade finally determined. Bonding can thus be considered a multipurpose stage.

Choice of Cement

Providing the recommended preparation technique has been followed, the inlay/onlay will seldom be more than 2 mm thick, and the cement of choice will be a dual-cure (i.e. autocuring and light-activated) resin cement.

With thicker restorations, such as ceramic inlays and onlays that extend 3 mm or more from the surface, an autopolymerizing cement may be the material of choice. At these thicknesses ceramic restorations may limit the transfer of light energy, and 'dual' resin cements may not reach a high enough monomer-conversion rate to guarantee bonding quality and the well-being of the pulp. The thicker the ceramic layer the higher the light absorption rate.

Resin cements should be used in conjunction with appropriate dentin–enamel adhesives. The operator should be familiar with the properties and instructions for use of these materials.

Choice of color

The choice of resin cement color is an important consideration in view of the favorable or unfavorable effects it can produce (Figures 11.56 and 11.57). Considering the thickness of inlays/onlays, the authors prefer the luting cement to be only faintly colored and translucent enough to bring out the natural color of the remaining dentin and enamel. This takes into account the fact that the color of try-in pastes seldom matches exactly that of the fully cured resin cement. If the cement is opaque or of high chroma, its esthetic properties decline and the margin becomes visible. It may be beneficial to subtly correct the inlay color, especially toward the edges, although the choice is less important with inlays/onlays than with laminate veneers, which are only a quarter as thick. Should any opaquing be required in the ceramic material, the authors recommend that it is confined to the deeper-lying layers of the inlay/onlay.

Viscosity

The authors have previously used microfilled composite cements because of the fluidness and fineness of the cement layer. However, it became apparent that the weak-point of inlays/onlays bonded with a microfilled cement lies in the composite resin lute, this being liable to medium-term breakdown, wear and hydrolysis. The manufacturers have responded by supplying highly filled and viscous micro-hybrid composite cements. These are certainly less fluid, and some require ultrasonic placement (Sono-Cem, ESPE and Variolink Ultra,

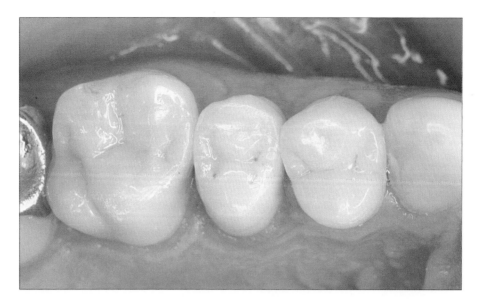

Figure 11.57 The occlusal view, also showing a metal–ceramic crown on the second premolar and a DO ceramic inlay on the first premolar. (Ceramist: Gérald Ubassy.)

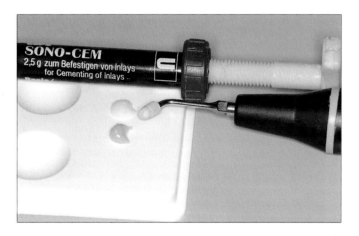

Figure 11.58 The Sono-Cem cement (ESPE) and the sonic insert.

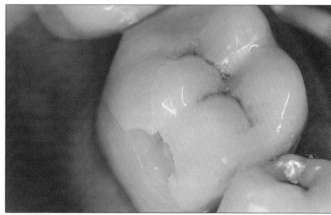

Figure 11.59 This occlusal crack was started by a marginal fracture, which was probably due to a defect at the tooth–ceramic interface.

Ivoclar) (Figure 11.58). Better mechanical properties would appear to result from their structure, but this cannot be fully evaluated at this early stage of clinical development. Their anticipated superior longevity, especially in the marginal area, might be confirmed in the future.

Marginal fit

The more accurate the margins, the smaller the thickness devoted to the composite cement and the more limited marginal defects will be (Figure 11.59). A relationship has been shown to exist between the width of the ceramic–tooth interface and horizontal erosion of the

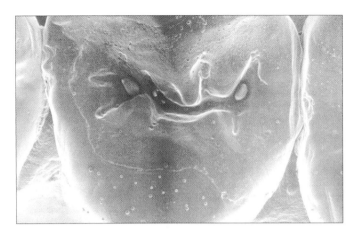

Figure 11.60 SEM (×20) of a replica after 5 years – the ceramic inlay exhibits good marginal integrity.

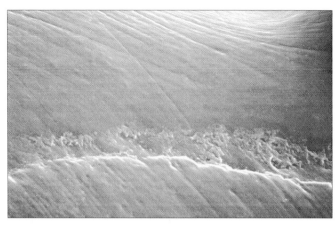

Figure 11.61 SEM (×100) of the margin: when occlusal conditions are good, there is little wash-out of the resin cement after 5 years.

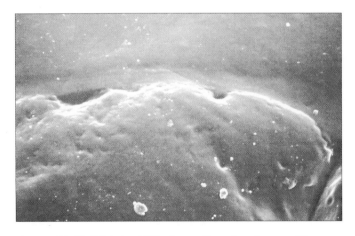

Figure 11.62 SEM (× 100) of a replica after 5 years. The tooth–ceramic interface exhibits small defects.

composite; the latter appears to stabilize at a level equal to 50% of the former (K Leinfelder, personal communication, 1994). The accuracy of investments and refinement of ceramics and composite cements permit mean lute thickness values of 50 μm, conducive to extending the life of these margins (Figures 11.60–11.62).

Margin failure results from:

• wear and loss of the composite;
• insufficient thickness of the ceramic;
• microscopic cracks in the ceramic;
• microscopic distortion of the margins due to concentration of stress;
• coincidence of margins with functional occlusal contact sites.

Marginal gap size must be kept to a minimum (Mormann et al, 1982). It has a noticeable influence on loss of the composite lute, which is not only a result of mechanical abrasion but also arises from hydrolysis, thermocycling and the polishing techniques used after polymerization. These problems also affect non-functional sites (the cervical margins) and extend to the margins of onlays located on the buccal–labial or lingual surfaces (see Figure 11.28).

Quality of adhesion and seal

Adhesion and seal are certainly associated, but can evolve completely independently of each other. Both can have an effect on the success of ceramic inlays/onlays.

Debonding can obviously be considered a failure, especially in the event of the inlay chipping or breaking in the process. This occurs only rarely, however, stealthy infiltration being more common; this could originate from a defect of the margin, such as splitting, wear at the interface, a poor fit, etc., or from a cervical margin bonded onto the dentin or cementum.

By potentiating hydrolysis of the composite, destruction of the base, recurring caries, etc., an unsatisfactory seal can mediate fracture of the ceramic, which will thereby have lost its essential support.

Clinical bonding procedures

The rubber dam is mandatory at this stage of the procedure. After removal of the provisional inlays, the cavities are cleaned with hand instruments, with ultrasonic instruments, and finally with an air–powder abrasive device, which has proved to be the most effective clinical method for removing contaminants and residues of eugenol-free temporary cement.

Inlays and onlays are tried and contact points are adjusted. Occlusion will be checked after the luting procedures.

For luting, it is most convenient to use a single-component enamel–dentin adhesive such as Prime & Bond (Dentsply–Caulk), One-Step (Bisco) or Scotchbond 1 (3M), and a dual-cure luting composite such as Variolink Two (Ivoclar Vivadent), Choice (Bisco) or Nexus (Kerr).

The inlay, or onlay, which has been sandblasted in the laboratory, is protected externally by a layer of wax, extending right up to the margins.

The internal aspect is then etched for 90 seconds with a 10% gel of hydrofluoric acid, thoroughly rinsed in running tap water, and neutralized in a sodium bicarbonate solution. All of the operations require gloves, since hydrofluoric acid is a very dangerous substance. The internal aspect is dried and silanated. After evaporation of the silane, it is brushed with a primer/adhesive solution (One-Step, Bisco), carefully air-dried, and then light-cured.

The tooth surfaces are treated as follows. First, they are disinfected with a chlorexidine gel, Plak Out gel (Hawe Neos) is commonly used, but one can also use other disinfectants. After this, the surfaces are etched with an 'all-etch' technique. The cavity is then prepared to receive the inlay. Dental floss and a clear matrix stabilized with a translucent reflecting wedge are put in place. It is important always to leave the dentin slightly wet. Onto the moist dentin, two very thin coats of One-Step are successively brushed and light-cured, after evaporation of the solvent.

The composite cement (base + catalyst) is mixed and applied onto the preparation.

The inlay is inserted, and the excess composite is removed with a brush and with the dental floss in proximal areas.

The onlay is secured in position and light-cured for one minute under different angles.

After polymerization, small excesses can be eliminated with a blade and with metal strips for the gingival margins. For larger excesses, multifluted carbide burs or fine-grain diamond burs are used.

Once restorations have been cleaned and occlusion has been checked, there is one important step before final polishing, namely sealing the margins and surface of the restorations. For that purpose, all accessible limits are etched for 10 seconds, rinsed, dried, impregnated with a liquid resin (Fortify, Bisco), and light-cured for 20 seconds.

Blocking tubules with a protective hybrid layer and sealing the margins and the surfaces are two very important steps for achieving excellent bonding.

The inlay/onlay is finally polished with several silicone cusps, disks, points and wheels, and lustered with a diamond paste (Truluster, Brasseler-Komet) on a Prophy cup.

Critical factors and failure rate

Over a 10-year period (1984–1994) we have used several ceramic materials and have met with a few failures, which have enabled us to assess our clinical results (Table 11.1) and seek answers to the following questions:

- Are ceramic inlays and onlays useful as long-term restorations?
- What are the most frequent causes of failure?
- Are onlays safer than inlays?
- What is the mean failure rate?

Table 11.1 provides a breakdown of the failure rate for a total of 1214 inlays/onlays (974 inlays and 240 onlays) over the 10-year period. It seems that deterioration of margins and proximal fractures are the failures most often encountered, accounting for more than half the total number of failures. It may be concluded that there is no significant difference between inlays and onlays in terms of failure rate (Roulet and Losche, 1996).

Laboratory considerations

The simplest technique for production of inlays/onlays relies on refractory investments for firing feldspathic or

Table 11.1 *Analysis of inlays/onlays during the period 1984–94 (1214 cases; 974 inlays and 240 onlays)*

	Number of failures	
	Inlays	Onlays
Defective margin	24	8
Recurrence of caries	4	1
Splitting of ceramic	4	3
Proximal fracture	14	5
Fracture of isthmus	3	—
Deterioration of base	3	1
Debonding	1	1
Fracture during try-in	3	—
Total	**56**	**19**
Total		
Inlays	5.7%	
Onlays	7.9%	
Average failure rate over 10 years	6.2%	

Layering

Layering of inlays/onlays makes it possible to regulate setting shrinkage satisfactorily and achieve a highly natural esthetic effect, restricting the response of the dentin and enamel to light. The ceramist should always be shown any sites of discoloration, such as patches of sclerotic dentin, in order to make the best use of opacious dentin to camouflage these unsightly areas.

These layered inlays, unlike surface-colored heat-pressed or castable glass ceramics such as Dicor or Empress, can subsequently be corrected for occlusal adjustment without altering the esthetic effect (Figures 11.63 and 11.64). Highly successful esthetic integration can be achieved without any visible line between tooth and ceramic by using a semitranslucent ceramic enamel. This approach of using the natural tooth color as 'underlay' to maximize camouflaging effects illustrates our present views on esthetic considerations: we endeavor to re-establish light transmission resembling that of natural tooth in all our bonded ceramic prostheses (Figures 11.65–11.67).

Laboratory-fabricated composite inlays/onlays

Although this book is principally concerned with current prospects for ceramics, mention should also be made of the decisive advances made with second-generation laboratory composite resins. These appear to offer great prospects for use in inlays/onlays with good esthetic properties.

The limitations of the first generation of microfilled laboratory composite resins, such as Dentacolor (Kulzer), Isosit N (Ivoclar) and Visiogem (ESPE), which were developed in the 1980s, soon became evident (Miara, 1988). This was especially the case for inlays – and even more for onlays. These disadvantages included (Figure 11.68):

- partial or complete fracturing
- lack of stiffness
- opening of margins
- risk of deformation under high stress levels
- heavy abrasion
- fairly rapid staining.

These first-generation laboratory composite resins were gradually phased out in favor of ceramic

glass ceramics. These investments have now made great advances, and have reached a highly satisfactory level of clinical accuracy. Their application does not require any special equipment, and all porcelain manufacturers now offer an investment suited to their ceramic (Cosmotech-G, Cera; Optec, PVS, Mirage, and others). After fabrication of the laboratory model, a duplicate is made using addition silicone and the double-mix technique. Dies will already have been coated with spacer varnish before duplication, to preserve the space allocated for the resin cement.

Duplicating material, as its name implies, must lend itself to reproducing the preparation faithfully in all its detail. Hence the grain of the refractory raw material (pure quartz) must be of a suitable shape and grain size distribution to allow optimum surface conditions (maximum density and minimum space between grains). Condensing build-up also contributes to higher mechanical and heat resistance, possibly at the expense of porosity, but this is not of major concern because the amount of refractory material applied is of limited volume relative to a tooth.

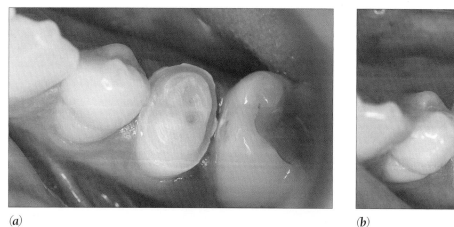

(a)

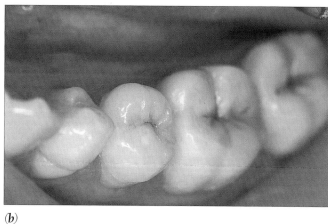

(b)

Figure 11.63 Empress onlay (layering technique). (**a**) Tooth preparation. (**b**) Surface and occlusal corrections can be achieved after bonding, without affecting the esthetic outcome.

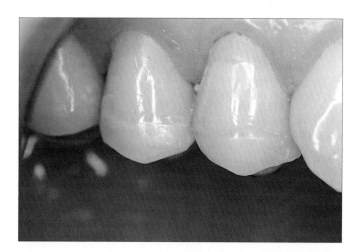

Figure 11.64 When Dicor onlays are trimmed and polished, the surface color layer is removed, resulting in an unesthetic appearance.

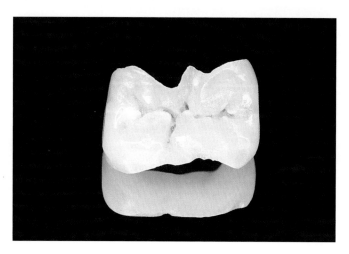

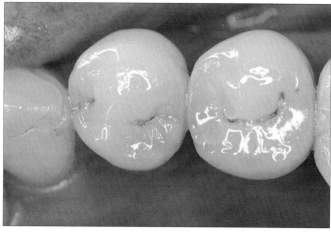

Figure 11.65 DO inlay in the first premolar and MOD inlay in the second premolar: 5 years postoperatively after repolishing.

Figure 11.66 MOD ceramic inlay (IPS Classic, Ivoclar). (Ceramist: Gérald Ubassy.)

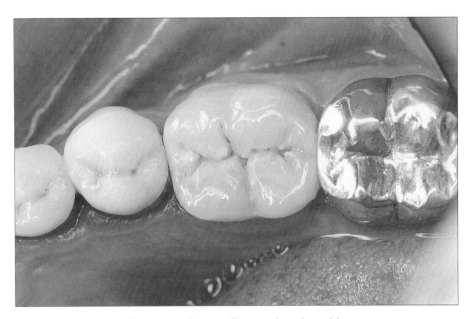

Figure 11.67 *An excellent camouflaging effect can be achieved by incorporating variations in hue and chroma inside the onlay.*

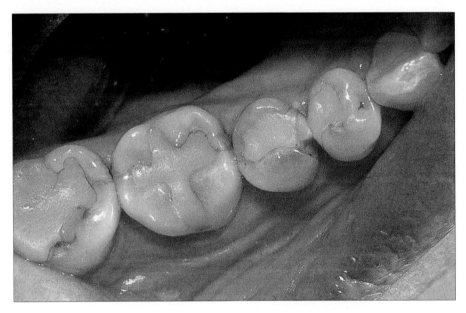

Figure 11.68 *First-generation laboratory composite resins are subject to fairly rapid degradation, with fracturing and different degrees of opening of margins.*

inlays/onlays in the mid-1980s. However, since then, there has been a revival of interest in a second-generation of composite resins, which, in terms of their mechanical properties, are closer to mineral than to organic substances.

The advances involved in the development of these new polymers have been made principally in three areas, namely their structure and composition, their degree of polymerization, and their reinforcement with fibers.

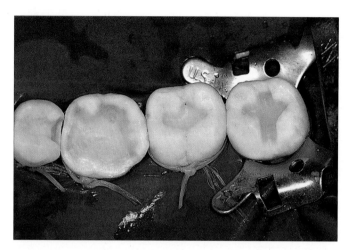

Figure 11.69 *Example of preparation for a composite resin inlay/onlay. This differs very little from the preparations described for ceramic inlays/onlays.*

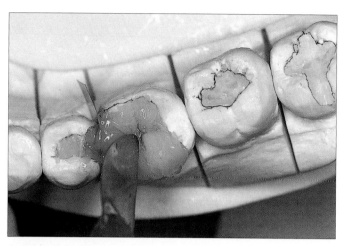

Figure 11.70 *The composite resin is built up by progressive layering. (Technician: JP Levot.)*

Structure and composition

The structure and composition of the second-generation laboratory resins is of a type known as 'micro-hybrid', very similar to those used for direct application in the clinic. This indicates the inclusion of small-sized mineral fillers measuring between 0.05 and 1.0 μm with a high percentage by volume (66%) and by weight (80%). The shape, size, distribution and proportion of filler vary from one composite resin to another, but in second-generation resins the proportions by volume are two-thirds mineral filler and one-third resin matrix. It should be borne in mind that first-generation composite resins had a so-called 'micro-filled' structure, with the reverse proportion, i.e. one-third mineral filler and two-thirds resin.

This major increase in filler associated with particle size and arrangement has a direct bearing on mechanical properties. Moreover, the reduced proportion of resin also has a major influence on contraction during polymerization and on degradability (Touati, 1996; Touati and Aidan, 1997).

Polymerization

Owing to the hardening of the resin matrix, polymerization brings about a more or less successful 'fixing' of the filler, and, together with composition and structure, represents one key aspect of composite strength and durability. The higher the degree of the polymerization, the better will be the properties of the composite.

It should be noted that a monomer cannot be completely transformed into a polymer by photopolymerization alone – however powerful the light source used, or however long its duration. In order to increase the final degree of polymerization, it is necessary to apply a thermal treatment, either under low pressure, or, better still, in the complete absence of oxygen (atmospheric oxygen interferes with both surface and deeper-lying polymerization of the resin matrix, inhibiting carbon–carbon bonding).

The use of furnaces with temperatures of 140°C under a nitrogen atmosphere, associated with heat-cured composite resins, would appear to be the solution most conducive to a high degree of polymerization (98.5%) for the HP enamels of Belle Glass HO (Belle de St Claire).

Reinforcement by addition of fibers

In a number of industrial applications, fibers have long been incorporated in resin matrices, to enhance mechanical properties in particular. Some manufacturers now intend to reinforce second-generation laboratory composite resins by the addition of fibers that have previously undergone special surface treatment,

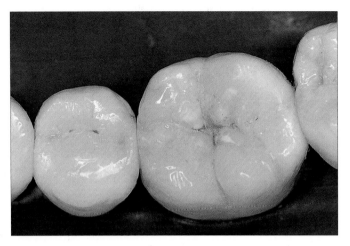 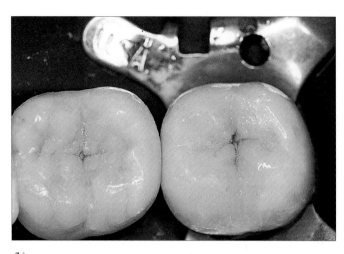

(a)   (b)

Figure 11.71 (a,b) Excellent simulation of tooth structure by second-generation laboratory composite.

enabling them to bind perfectly to the resin matrix (Dickerson and Rinaldi, 1996). This is the case with the Targis Vectris system (Ivoclar), involving silanization followed by polymer coating, the Fiberkor process (Conquest) and Connect (Belle de St Claire).

We are unable to recommend one particular material at present because of a lack of clinical history, but our clinical experience of composite resins, especially with regard to inlays/onlays, has enabled us to draw up guidelines for selecting the most suitable system.

A laboratory composite resin for inlays/onlays must possess the following properties:

- It should have a micro-hybrid structure – above all, with a percentage of filler in excess of 55% by weight or 70% by volume. The ratio by volume between filler and resin is more indicative of the true nature of the composite resin than the ratio by weight, in view of the great differences in density between organic and mineral constituents.
- It should have an elastic modulus of over 8000 MPa – the greater this modulus, the more resistant to deformation will an inlay/onlay be.
- It should have a flexural strength of over 120 MPa – the greater this factor is, the more fracture-resistant will an inlay be.
- It should have a compressive strength of over 350 MPa – the greater this factor is, the more fracture-resistant will an inlay be. With the given elastic modulus and flexural strength requirements satisfied, the compressive strength is the parameter to be taken into account in the selection of a composite resin for restoration purposes.
- It should be subject to as little contraction upon polymerization as possible. Accuracy of inlays/onlays is closely connected with the final degree of polymerization, which remains low for most second-generation laboratory composite resins.
- A sufficiently wide range of color shades should be available.
- Effective polishing should be possible.
- A functioning polymerization system should be available.

Preference should be given to systems combining photopolymerization with thermal treatment under low pressure or, better still, in the complete absence of oxygen, with the air replaced by an inert gas such as nitrogen under pressure.

Other characteristics, such as water absorption, solubility, abrasion resistance and abrasiveness, also have an influence on the aging, brittleness and degradability of these materials.

There are currently several systems in existence that more or less fulfil these requirements, but treatment of the inner surfaces of inlays/onlays and the quality of composite bonding resins need to be optimized for these systems to succeed.

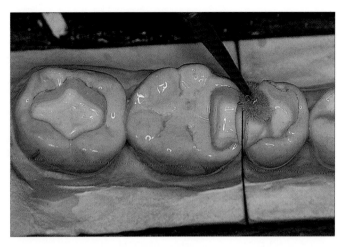

Figure 11.72 The master model: Belle Glass HP (Belle de St Claire) composite resin is being used here.

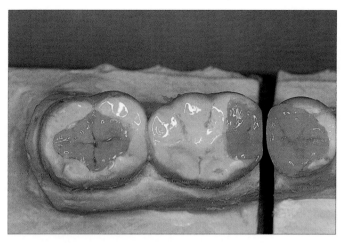

Figure 11.73 Inlays/onlays are built up in two stages: first, using dentin and light-cured incisal resins (different characterizations can be incorporated at this stage); these are then overlaid by heat-cured composite resins (HP enamels).

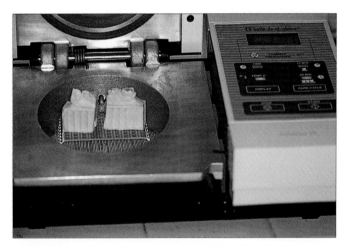

Figure 11.74 The advantage of this technique lies in the fact that heat-curing takes place in a furnace at 140°C under a pressure of 5.5 bars nitrogen.

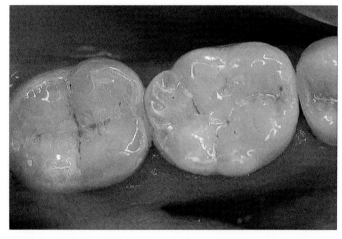

Figure 11.75 Composite resins with remarkable mechanical and esthetic qualities can be produced by heat curing under nitrogen pressure, since the degree of polymerization reaches 98.5% for surface enamels. This is considerably lower for dentins and subsurface enamels in order to promote good bonding with the composite resin adhesive.

We have insufficient clinical experience at present to claim that these composite substances will oust ceramics in the case of inlays/onlays, although their excellent mechanical properties, which closely resemble those of dental tissue, open up prospects that we cannot afford to ignore. The procedures involved in the preparation and insertion of composite inlays/onlays are shown in Figures 11.69–11.79.

Summary

- Ceramic inlays/onlays are contraindicated in the event of parafunctional activity.
- In the absence of parafunction, they are indicated for premolars, and may be used on first and second molars.

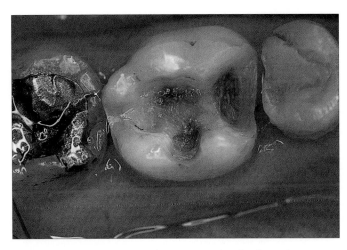

Figure 11.76 Preparation of a mesio-occlusal inlay/onlay on a lower first molar.

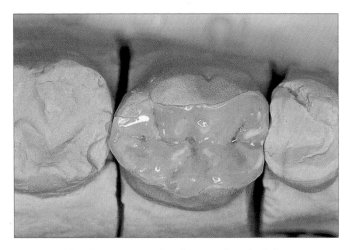

Figure 11.77 A composite inlay fabricated in the laboratory (Targis, Ivoclar).

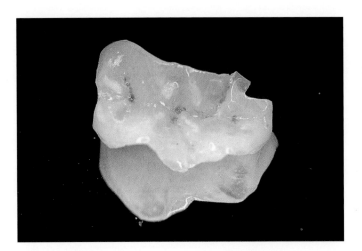

Figure 11.78 The inlay has good esthetic qualities, with a wide range of translucent and opaque materials being available, and different values, which give vitality.

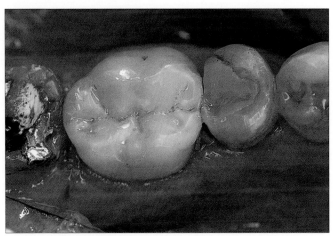

Figure 11.79 The final result after bonding with a fifth-generation adhesive and a dual-cure composite cement. The restorations on the premolar and second molar will be redone.

- Cavity design differs markedly from that required for gold inlays, but is very similar to that for ceramic inlays.
- Good case selection is a major factor determining the success of ceramic inlays and onlays.
- In small cavities, direct placement composite resin restorations prove satisfactory and cheaper alternatives (Figures 11.80–11.82).

- In large cavities, ceramic inlays are superior (see Figures 11.15–11.19).
- With attention to detail, the failure rate of ceramic inlays/onlays is low.
- In situations where one cannot provide enough compressive strength inside ceramic inlays and onlays, second-generation laboratory composites would be the preferred clinical choice.

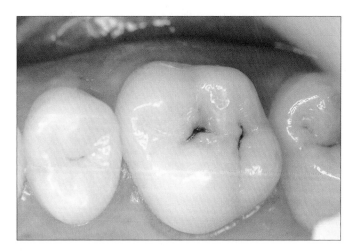

Figure 11.79 Occlusal caries in the first molar.

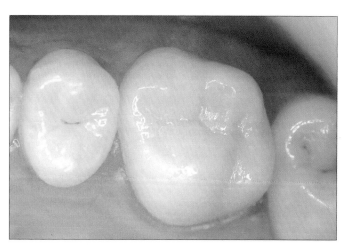

Figure 11.80 Direct freehand composite restoration (Herculite, Kerr). For small cavities, composite resins are considered the best clinical option.

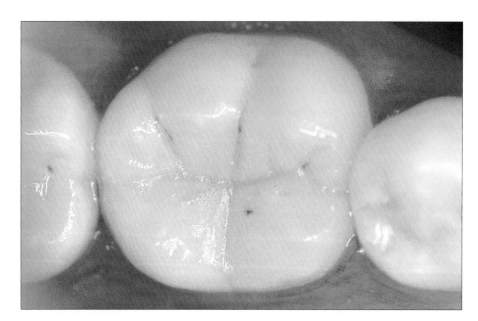

Figure 11.81 Direct freehand composite restoration (Herculite, Kerr) on the first lower molar: the esthetic outcome is excellent, and can compete with a ceramic restoration.

References

Degrange M, Charrier J-L, Attal JP et al, Bonding of luting materials for resin-bonded bridges: clinical relevance of in vitro tests. *J Dent* 1994a; **22(Suppl 1)**: S28–S32.

Degrange M, Attal JP, Theimer K, Aspects fondamentaux du collage appliqués à la dentisterie adhésive. *Réalités Cliniques* 1994b; **5**: 371–82.

Dickerson W, Rinaldi P, The fiber reinforced inlay supported indirect composite bridge. *Pract Periodont Aesthet Dent* 1996; **8**: 8–12.

Dietschi D, Spreafico R, *Adhesive Metal-Free Restorations*. Berlin: Quintessence, 1997.

Dietschi D, Spreafico R, Current clinical concepts of adhesive cementation of tooth-colored posterior restorations. *Pract Periodont Aesthet Dent* 1998; **10**: 47–54.

Magne P, Dietschi D, Holz J, Esthetic restorations for posterior teeth: Practical and clinical considerations. *Int J Periodont Rest Dent* 1996; **16**: 104–119.

Miara P, Nouveau composite de laboratoire pour inlays et onlays collés. *Rev Odontostomatol (Paris)* 1998; **17**: 9–27.

Mormann WH, Ameye C, Lutz F, Komposit Inlays: Marginale Adaptation, Randdichtigkeit, Porosität und okklusaler Verschleiss. *Dtsch Zahnärztl Z* 1982; **37**: 438–41.

Roulet JF, Losche GM, Tooth-colored inlays and inserts – long-term clinical results. *Acad Dental Mat, Transactions* 1996; **9**: 200–15.

Touati B, Une nouvelle application du collage en prothèse conjointe: inlays-onlays et couronnes jackets en résine composite. *Rev Odontostomatol (Paris)* 1984; **3**: 171–80.

Touati B, Pissis P, L'inlay collé en résine composite. *Cah Prothèse* 1984; **48**: 29–59.

Touati B, Pissis P, L'inlay-onlay compo-métal: Restauration unitaire et moyen d'encrage de bridge. *Actual Odontostomatol (Paris)* 1986; **155**: 453–84.

Toauti B, The evolution of aesthetic restorative materials for inlays and onlays. *Pract Periodont Aesthet Dent* 1996; **8**: 657–66.

Touati B, Aidan N, Second generation laboratory composite resins for indirect restorations. *J Esthet Dent* 1997; **9**: 108–18; 250–3.

CHAPTER 12

Dental Ceramics and Laboratory Procedures

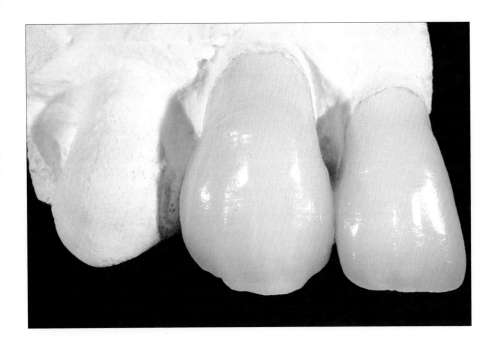

An esthetically successful dental prosthesis is the result of a number of decisions and actions. While the practitioner assesses the case, draws up a program of treatment, performs the preparation, produces the impression, and eventually fits the prosthesis, it is the ceramist who is responsible for recreating the appearance and function of natural teeth by an appropriate ceramic build-up.

The importance of communication between the practitioner and the ceramist has been pointed out repeatedly throughout various chapters. A common language must be adopted to set up this dialogue, which is one reason why every practitioner should get to know the basics of laboratory procedures. He or she should, for instance, become acquainted with the different materials required for producing ceramic prostheses so as to be aware of their potential, their constraints, and, above all, the fabrication procedures in the laboratory.

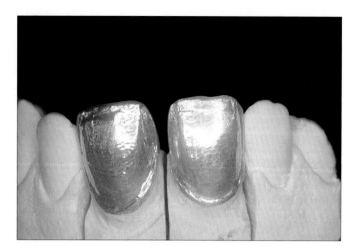

Figure 12.1 Platinum foil swaged onto the dies allows application, sculpting and firing of the feldspathic ceramic.

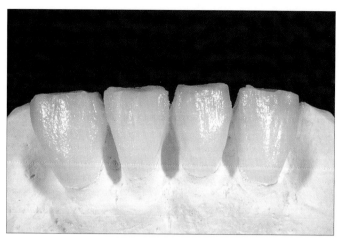

Figure 12.2 Ceramic restorations processed directly over refractory investment model. (Ceramist: Gérald Ubassy.)

This chapter provides the reader with a brief update on the major aspects of various modern techniques for producing all-ceramic restorations.

Laboratory prescription forms

It can sometimes be difficult to bring together the practitioner, patient and ceramist, which means that the practitioner has to communicate a body of information to the ceramist, using a language he or she can understand.

Besides impressions and interocclusal records, the laboratory prescription form constitutes the main connection between the patient, practitioner and ceramist. Ideally, it combines, as clearly and accurately as possible, information on the type of prosthesis to be constructed, including basic data on color, shape, different features or peculiarities, and brings together the observations, analyses and aims of the practitioner, patient and ceramist. It can also be complemented by other items, such as photographs, study models, diagnostic wax-ups, etc. The different options now available for data transmission have been amply described in Chapter 7, 'Transfer of Esthetic Information'.

The choice of support for ceramic powders

The build-up and firing of metal-free ceramic substructures requires a support. Two alternative types of support are suitable for conventional feldspathic ceramic: these are platinum foil (Figure 12.1) and refractory investment (Figure 12.2).

For firing of the latest ceramics, such as Duceram-LFC (Ducera), Empress (Ivoclar) and In-Ceram (Vita), the substructure is ceramic and the final stratification is made directly on a ceramic core. The production of this ceramic core will vary from one procedure to the next:

- with Duceram-LFC, the core is produced by conventional firing of a high-fusing feldspathic ceramic fabricated on a refractory investment die;
- in the Empress procedure, the core is produced from a pressed ceramic ingot;
- with the In-Ceram procedure, the core is produced by slip casting and sintering alumina on a special investment; the solid porous alumina core is then infiltrated with a high-fusing glass at a later stage.

Despite the indisputable virtues of these new procedures, traditional feldspathic ceramics still remain the most widely used, especially for fabricating laminate veneers and inlays/onlays.

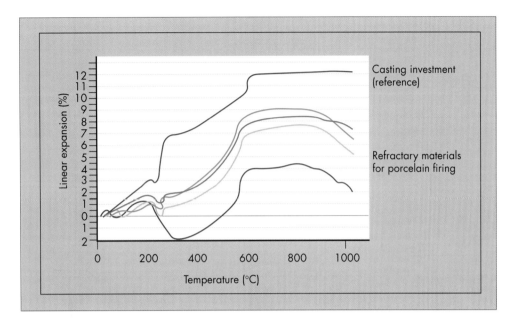

Figure 12.3 *Comparison between heat expansion of four materials for firing of ceramic and that of standard investment for casting alloys (Vestrafine). Note the absence of cristobalite at 250°C for the four materials intended for ceramic firing. Key: red, Vestrafine (Unitek); yellow, Symphyse (Symphyse Cie); blue, Cosmotech Vest (GC); pink, Mirage (Miron Laboratories); green, VHT (Whip Mix). (Courtesy of Dr JC Senoussi.)*

Platinum foil has long been used as substrate for fabricating porcelain jacket crowns and, more recently, ceramic laminate veneers. Although this technique still has certain applications and a number of advocates, especially for fabricating laminate veneers without incisal overlay, it is now simpler to use refractory dies. In the case of inlays and onlays, only the refractory investment is used.

The accuracy and quality of the latest refractory investments make it possible to produce all types of ceramic-based dental restorations whether laminate veneers, jacket crowns or inlays/onlays.

Duplicating material

Duplicating material, as its name implies, must lend itself to reproducing the preparation faithfully in all its detail. Hence the grain of the refractory raw material (pure quartz) must have a shape and grain size distribution to allow a compact build-up. This guarantees optimum surface conditions (maximum density and minimum space between grains). Compact build-up also contributes to higher mechanical and heat resistance – possibly at the expense of porosity, but this is not of major concern because the amount of refractory material applied is of limited volume relative to a tooth.

Support material

Support material for the ceramic paste must have excellent mechanical and heat resistance properties, since it undergoes repeated firings, and must expand and shrink exactly as does the ceramic, but must remain chemically non-reactive with the ceramic.

For a true understanding of how these substances behave during firing, it should be remembered that they both closely resemble and differ significantly from the phosphate-bonded investment material currently used in precision casting (Figure 12.3). The main difference is the almost total absence of cristobalite in the powder of refractory materials for ceramics, in favor of quartz, which accounts for the majority of the refractory filling. When cristobalite passes from a low to high temperature, its crystalline structure undergoes reversible transformation from the alpha to the beta form at around 250°C, with isothermal expansion in the neighborhood of 1%. This is a highly advantageous property in precision casting, compensating as it does for the shrinkage during casting, but is obviously incompatible with the almost linear expansion of the ceramic in the solid phase. The refractory material must therefore satisfy the essential condition of matching this expansion in order

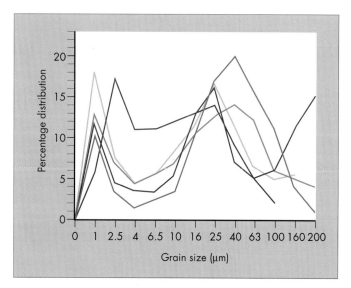

Figure 12.4 *Comparison between granular distribution of four materials for ceramic firing, and that of type 1 investment for casting alloys (Vestrafine). Key: red, Vestrafine (Unitek); yellow, Symphyse (Symphyse Cie); blue, Cosmotech Vest (GC); pink, Mirage (Miron Laboratories); green, VHT (Whip Mix). (Courtesy of Dr JC Senoussi.)*

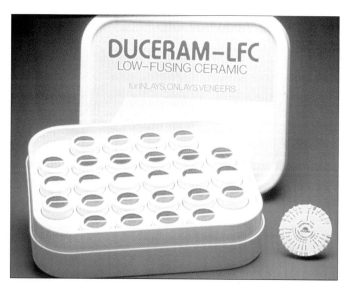

Figure 12.5 *Duceram-LFC ceramic kit (Ducera).*

to serve as a reliable support for the ceramic component during firing (Figure 12.4). Quartz meets these requirements most satisfactorily. Despite its isothermal transformation, which appears detrimental to a good match with ceramic expansion, the temperature of this process, at 575°C, is 50°C above that of the initial softening of the ceramic during glass transition, this glass transition temperature being around 520°C–524°C, depending on the ceramic concerned.

The abrupt expansion of quartz occurring at 575°C has no notable effect on the ceramic, which, being at the doughy stage at that temperature, 'accommodates' the variations in the volume of the support. Nevertheless, variations in the volume of the ceramic and refractory material will only coincide if one follows a strict procedure of slow heating and equally gradual cooling, taking proper account of all thermal parameters (such as expansion, contraction, constraints, and inertia) as well as the set or doughy phase of the ceramic.

Low-fusing ceramics (Duceram-LFC)

The development of very low-fusing ceramics (fusing temperature 660°C) meant that a simple and accurate technique for building up and firing all-ceramic prostheses could be adopted (Figure 12.5).

A fine layer of conventional ceramic (Duceram) is fired on a refractory die (Ducera-lay); the ceramic core is then separated from the refractory by sand blasting (50 µm of aluminum) and replaced on the plaster die of the master cast. This combination will provide the support for building up and firing low-fusing powders without deformation.

The difference of 260°C between the firing temperature of conventional and low-fusing ceramics (920°C and 660°C respectively) allows repeated firing to be carried out without the risk of distortion of the margins.

Advantages

The advantages of the low-fusing system include (Figures 12.6–12.15):

- excellent marginal adaptation;
- use of a plaster master cast;
- no special equipment required;
- allows for modification by repeat firings;
- abrasion rate closely resembling that of natural teeth;
- reduced abrasion of opposing teeth;
- excellent visual qualities, including best reproduction of opalescence of natural teeth.

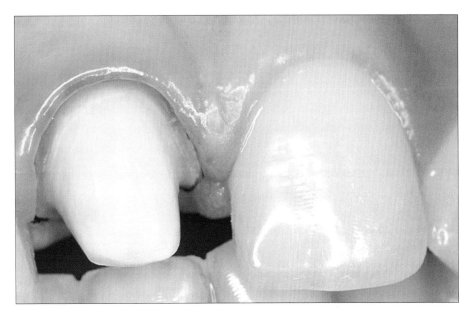

Figure 12.6 *Preparation for a ceramic jacket crown with a peripheral shoulder.*

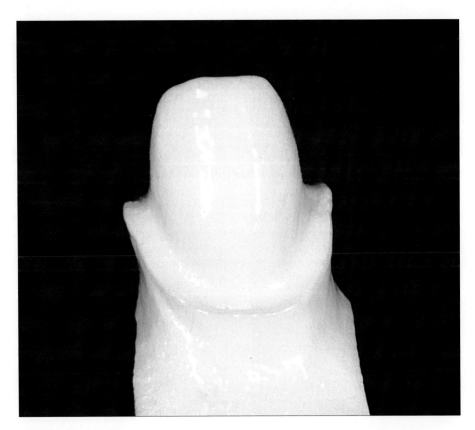

Figure 12.7 *A fine layer of initial ceramic (connector) over a Ducera-lay die in refractory investment is fired at 980°C. This connector layer should be bright and even.*

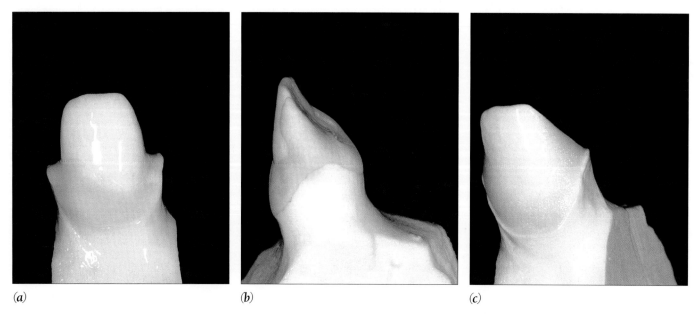

(a)   (b)   (c)

Figure 12.8 (*a–c*) *Lamination in traditional Duceram ceramic directly on the refractory die to produce a ceramic coping 0.3 mm thick.*

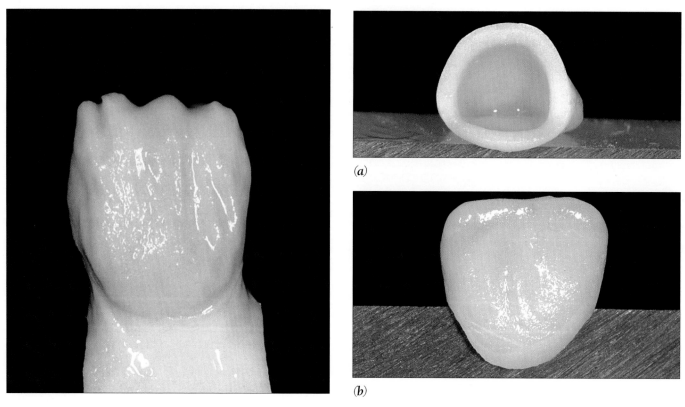

(a)

(b)

Figure 12.9 *Firing of coping at 940°C. Various shades can be introduced at this stage.*

Figure 12.10 (*a,b*) *The ceramic coping after gently sand-blasting off the refractory material.*

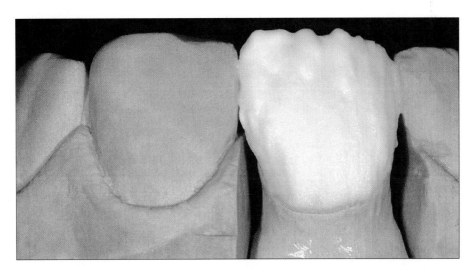

Figure 12.11 *The coping is replaced on the plaster cast. Lamination can then be completed using a low-fusing ceramic, which will be fired at 660°C in a vacuum.*

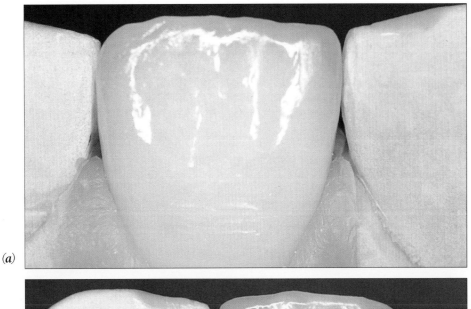

(a)

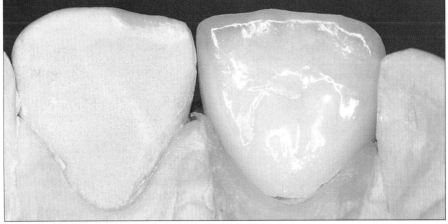

(b)

Figure 12.12 *Completed ceramic crown:* (a) *facial view;* (b) *lingual view. (Courtesy of Marc Cristou.)*

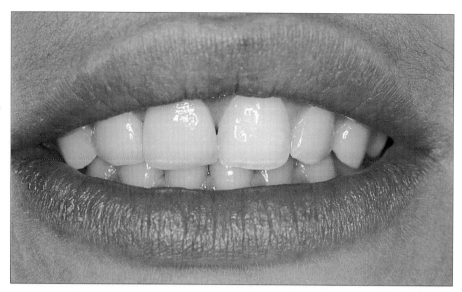

Figure 12.13 *The opalescence of the natural tooth can be reproduced using this type of ceramic crown.*

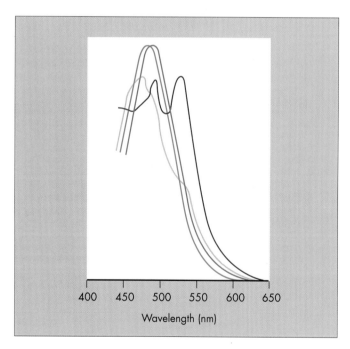

Figure 12.14 *Comparison of fluorescence of natural teeth (green), Duceram-LFC (blue) and two traditional ceramics (yellow and red). (Courtesy of Ducera.)*

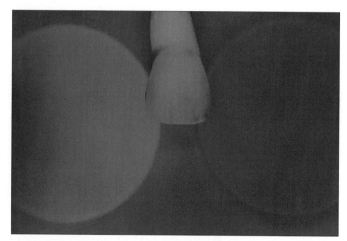

Figure 12.15 *It can be seen that fluorescence of LFC (see circle on left) is very close to natural tooth, whereas traditional ceramic material (circle on right) is devoid of fluorescence. (Courtesy of Ducera.)*

- requirement for high-transparency ceramic;
- requirement for pronounced opalescence (more suitable than Empress or In-Ceram in this respect).

Applications for low-fusing ceramics:

- laminate veneers, jackets/crowns, inlays and onlays;

Low-fusing ceramics are contraindicated for masking grossly discolored teeth and, in particular, when aiming for high fracture resistance.

Feldspathic ceramics

Feldspathic ceramics allowed the development of bonded ceramics (Figure 12.16). Their original application and the subsequent surge in their use stems from the development of accurate phosphate investment, enabling ceramic powders to be built up and fired.

They are widely used for fabricating laminate veneers and inlays/onlays (Figures 12.17–12.34). However, their mechanical properties appear inadequate for fabricating ceramic jacket crowns.

Advantages

The advantages of feldspathic ceramics are:

- excellent visual qualities due to the wide selection of ceramic powders;
- no special equipment is required;
- can be built up in fine layers.

Feldspathic ceramics are recommended for laminate veneers when the underlying tooth is not grossly discolored, and especially when tooth reduction is minimal. Feldspathic ceramics are also recommended for inlay/onlay techniques where esthetics are paramount.

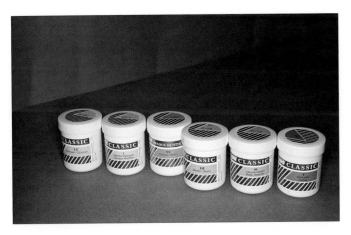

Figure 12.16 IPS Classic feldspathic ceramic powder (Ivoclar).

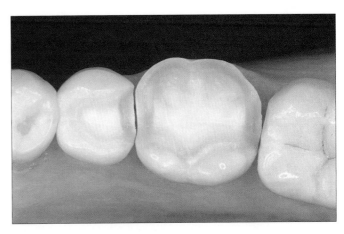

Figure 12.17 Preparations for ceramic inlay and onlay on model teeth.

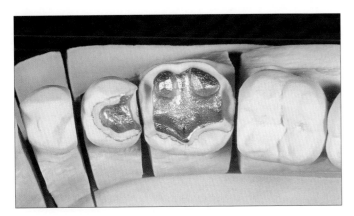

Figure 12.18 Master model with preparations for a ceramic inlay (premolar) and a ceramic onlay (molar), showing layer of spacer applied away from margins.

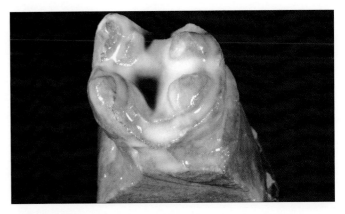

Figure 12.19 Application of first layer of ceramic powder and liquid over refractory die, extending beyond the margins of the preparation.

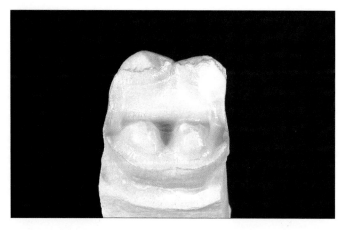

Figure 12.20 *First layer of porcelain after firing: this fine transparent layer must not display cracking or debonding.*

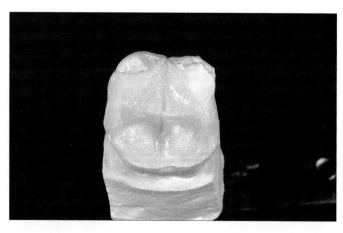

Figure 12.21 *The second firing creates a deep layer of high-chroma porcelain, simulating dentin.*

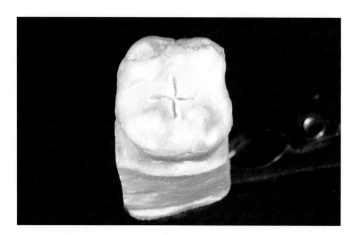

Figure 12.22 *Transparent porcelain is applied to margins of the preparation.*

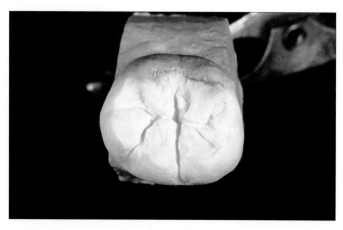

Figure 12.23 *The complete porcelain build-up is slightly oversized in order to compensate for shrinkage during firing.*

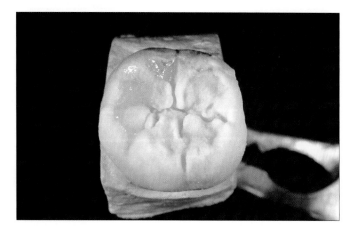

Figure 12.24 *Final firing of porcelain onlay.*

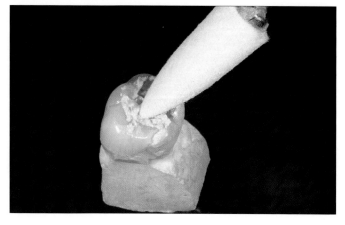

Figure 12.25 *A natural sheen is obtained using a felt tip and diamond paste. (Ceramist: Gérald Ubassy.)*

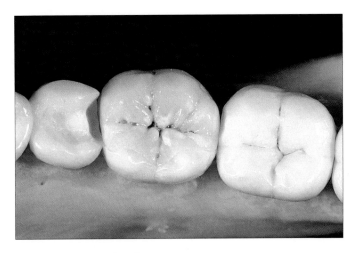

Figure 12.26   *Onlay during try-in.*

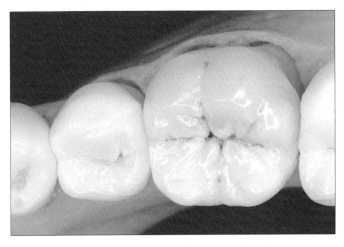

Figure 12.27   *The ceramic inlay and onlay after cementation.*

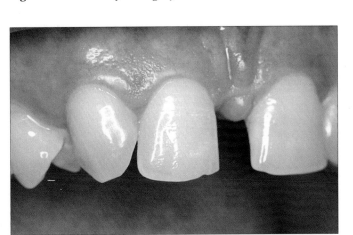

Figure 12.28   *This female patient wishes to convert a canine into a lateral tooth. A laminate feldspathic ceramic veneer (Shofu) will be produced, with extensive incisal overlap.*

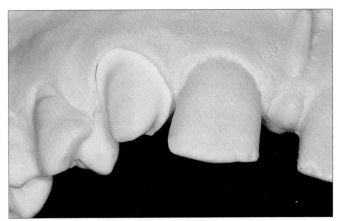

Figure 12.29   *Master casts with a special die: the gingival contour in plastic will be kept throughout the fashioning of the veneer.*

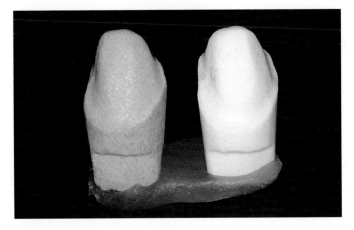

Figure 12.30   *A die in refractory investment is produced from the plaster die (Lamina Vest, Shofu).*

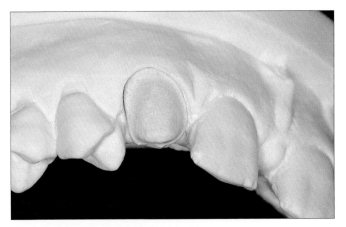

Figure 12.31   *View of refractory die after firing of connector layer.*

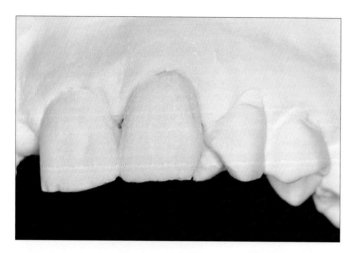

Figure 12.32 *Build-up of ceramics.*

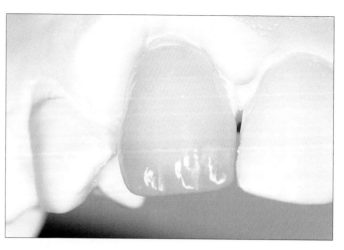

Figure 12.33 *Completed laminate veneer. (Ceramist: Jean-Pierre Levot.)*

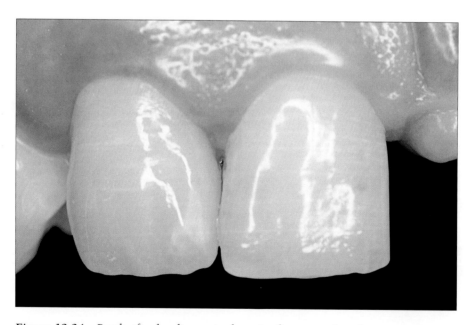

Figure 12.34 *Result after bonding: note character features and surface appearance.*

IPS Empress

IPS Empress is a leucite-reinforced feldspathic ceramic with good mechanical and visual properties. IPS Empress employs wax models that are invested with subsequent heat pressing of glass–ceramic; this makes it possible to produce particularly accurate ceramic restorations.

This is a highly versatile technique that can be used for laminate veneers, jacket crowns, inlays and onlays, whether by surface staining or conventional build-up layering or lateral segmentation over glass–ceramic cores (Figures 12.35–12.52).

Advantages

The advantages of IPS Empress are:

- allows for any kind of build-up;
- excellent mechanical properties;
- excellent optical properties;
- excellent marginal fit.

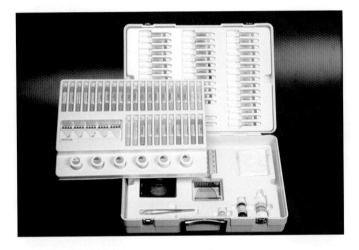

Figure 12.35 *IPS Empress ceramic kit.*

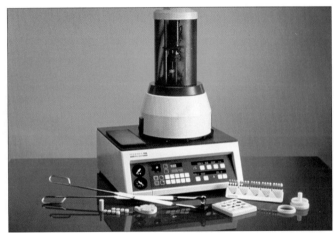

Figure 12.36 *Furnace used for injection molding of IPS Empress restorations.*

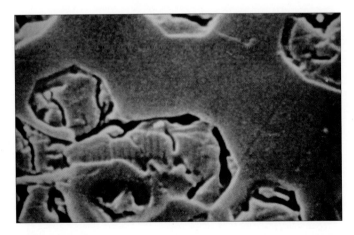

Figure 12.37 *SEM view of the microstructure peculiar to IPS Empress after pressing. (Courtesy of Ivoclar.)*

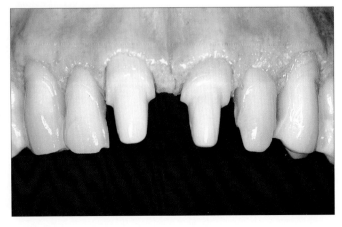

Figure 12.38 *Model teeth prepared for all-ceramic restorations. Centrals are prepared for IPS Empress crowns; laterals and canines are prepared for feldspathic porcelain veneers.*

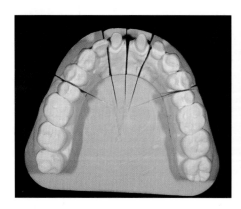

Figure 12.39 *Master cast obtained from a silicone impression.*

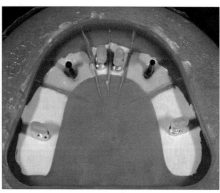

Figure 12.40 *Preparations for veneers are cast in investment. The other parts of the cast are in a silicone impression (Zermack).*

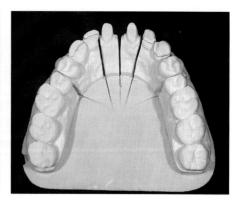

Figure 12.41 *Working model where the dies have been trimmed.*

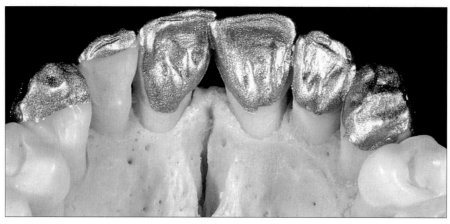

(a)

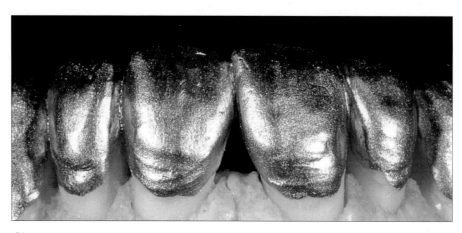

(b)

Figure 12.42 *Wax-up of restorations on model. Gold varnish is applied to the surface to help visualize the texture and microgeometry of future restorations. (**a**) Facial view; (**b**) lingual view. (Ceramist: Gérald Ubassy.)*

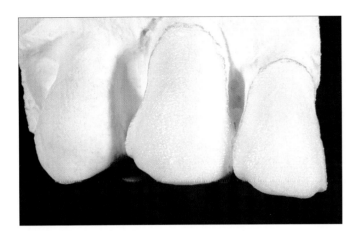

Figure 12.43 *First firing of connector ceramic over investment for build-up of veneers.*

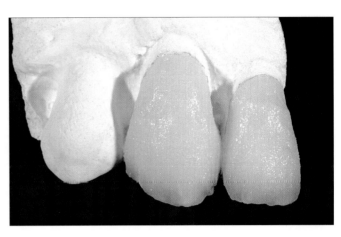

Figure 12.44 *Second firing of dentin porcelain with internal effects.*

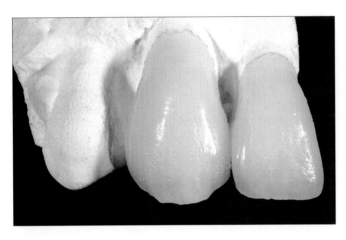

Figure 12.45 *Third firing, adding translucent and transparent effects.*

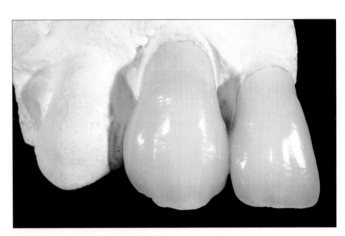

Figure 12.46 *Result after polishing.*

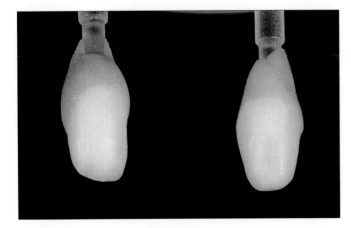

Figure 12.47 *Once the IPS Empress ceramic copings are completed, they are inserted over dies made of light-cured resin of the same color as the abutment teeth. The dies are utilized to check the shade.*

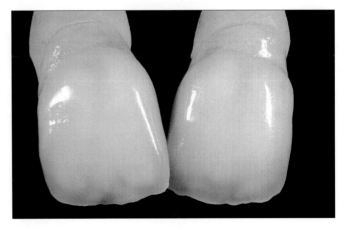

Figure 12.48 *Finished IPS Empress crowns.*

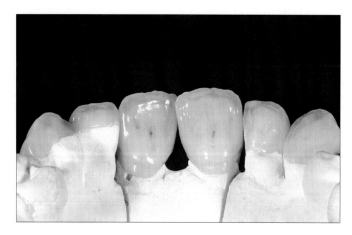

Figure 12.49 Lingual view of all restorations positioned on refractory model.

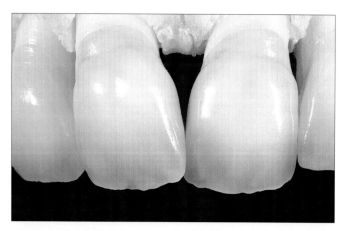

Figure 12.50 IPS Empress crowns placed on model teeth.

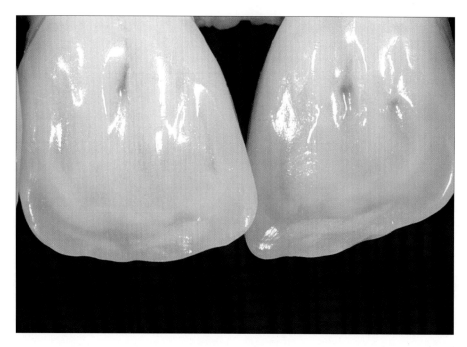

Figure 12.51 Close-up view of lingual aspects of IPS Empress crowns, showing detail of incisal edges.

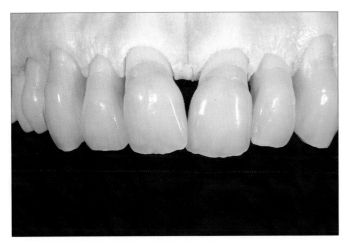

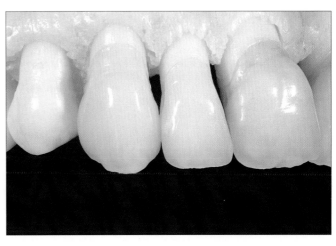

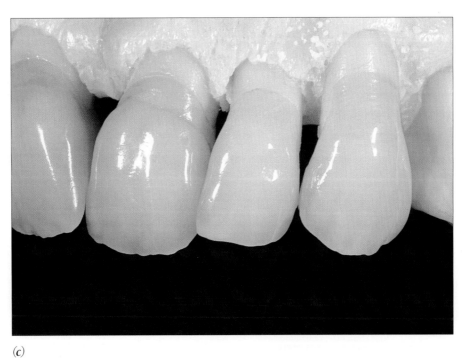

(c)

Figure 12.52 (a) *Finished restorations placed on model showing a good color match and harmony between feldspathic porcelain veneers and IPS Empress injection molded crowns. Close-up views of the restorations are shown:* (b) *right side;* (c) *left side. (Ceramist: Gérald Ubassy.)*

In-Ceram

Since the time of Pierre Fauchard (1747), all dental ceramics have conformed to more of less the same vitreous structure. Additional components have been added to produce variations in color, opacity, mechanical resistance or coefficient of thermal expansion.

In the case of In-Ceram, however, the structure of the basic material is a matrix of crystals joined to each other and subsequently infiltrated with colored glass. This particular structure allows for a considerable improve-ment in the mechanical properties of the material, reaching a flexural strength of 600 MPa, which is higher than that of any other dental ceramic and 3.5 times that of glass–ceramics.

The extraordinary mechanical advantages and dimensional accuracy of the In-Ceram system have made it a favorite material for the manufacture of ceramic copings and infrastructures for crowns and short-span bridges (Figures 12.53–12.65).

In-Ceram was invented by Dr Mickaël Sadoun, and was marketed in 1989 by Vita.

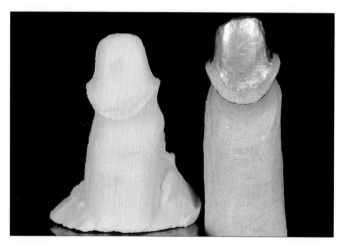

Figure 12.53 *Die for In-Ceram crown (with spacer) and duplicate die in special plaster.*

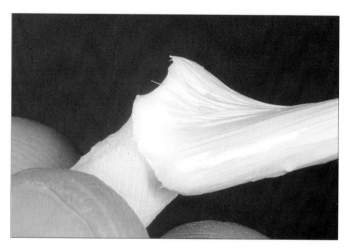

Figure 12.54 *Painting of alumina solution ('slip') onto plaster die.*

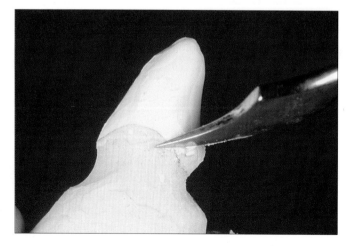

Figure 12.55 *Margins of alumina core are finished using a blade. (Ceramist: H Levy.)*

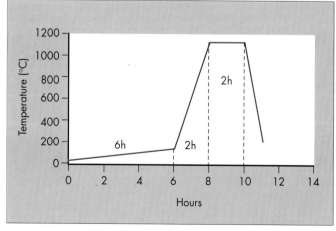

Figure 12.56 *Sintering program for In-Ceram alumina core.*

Application

To produce In-Ceram copings the dies are first separated and duplicated using a special plaster with a predetermined expansion rate. The ceramist will build up the coping on this duplicate die by brushing on a paste made up of very fine alumina crystals (measuring approximately 3 μm) in an aqueous suspension. On coming into contact with the plaster duplicate, the moisture from the paste is absorbed and the granules compact onto the die. Contour and margins are shaped by scalpel. The copings are then fired in a special furnace that reaches a temperature of 1120°C within 7.5 hours. They remain at a steady state for 2 hours, allowing the plaster of the duplicate to contract, thus releasing the copings. At the same time, the aluminum oxide crystals fuse to form a continuous, porous polycrystalline matrix.

Following initial firing, the copings are checked and coated with glass powder of a chosen shade. They again undergo firing, during which the molten glass is absorbed by capillarity and infiltrates the porous matrix. This infil-

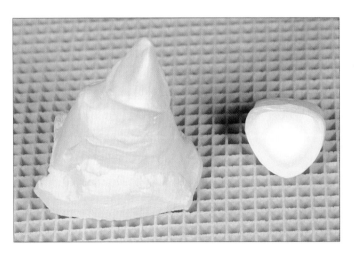

Figure 12.57 *The In-Ceram alumina core is released by removal of the plaster.*

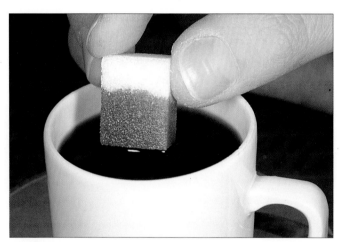

Figure 12.58 *Glass infiltration of the alumina coping is similar to coffee spreading through a sugar cube.*

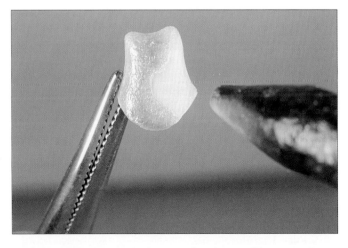

Figure 12.59 *Removal of excess glass by sandblasting with alumina particles.*

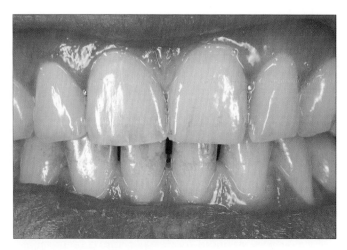

Figure 12.60 *Cemented In-Ceram crown on maxillay right central incisor. (Courtesy of Dr Eskenazi; Ceramist: H Levy.)*

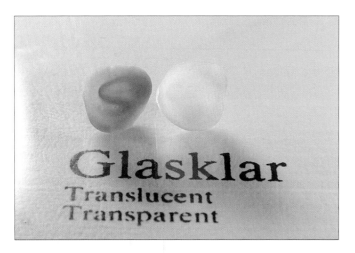

Figure 12.61 *A new material: framework of spinel (right) and alumina (left).*

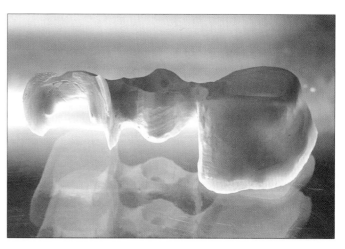

Figure 12.62 *Framework of a posterior bridge in zirconium with cervical margins of alumina.*

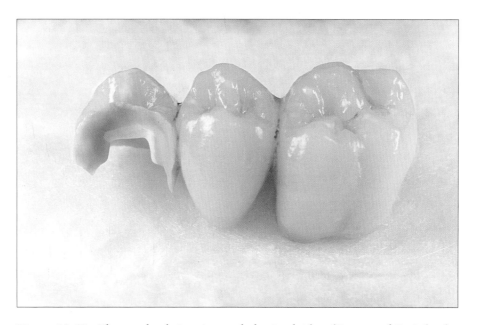

Figure 12.63 *The completed zirconium and alumina bridge. (Courtesy of Dr Laborde; Ceramist: H Levy.)*

tration makes the coping translucent and strong. After this second firing, excess glass is eliminated by sandblasting.

Vitadur Alpha ceramic is used on this alumina coping – it is the only porcelain compatible with alumina under thermal expansion.

This product has good esthetic properties because, unlike powders intended for metal–ceramic techniques, it does not contain leucite. The accuracy of margins obtained at the initial firing will not alter further, despite repeated firings, owing to the fact that these are fired at a lower temperature (lower by 200°C). The mechanical properties of the In-Ceram core allow crowns and bridges to be cemented without reinforcement by adhesion to dental structures, as is necessary with any other all-ceramic procedure at present.

A choice therefore exists between conventional luting (zinc phosphate, glass ionomer) and bonding with composite or even 4-meta-based (Superbond) resin.

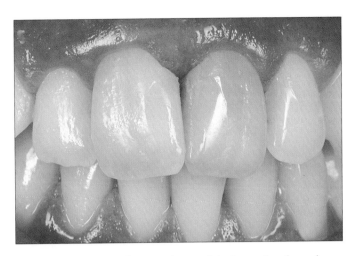

Figure 12.64 Heavily stained central incisors: the planned restoration includes the use of two In-Ceram crowns.

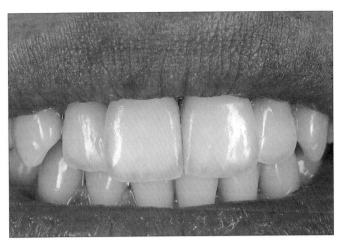

Figure 12.65 Finished restoration. (Courtesy of Dr J Pimenta; Ceramist: H Levy.)

Indications

The basic substance for the In-Ceram technique is aluminum oxide. Its dentin shade, accuracy and ease of use make it the preferred material for ceramic crowns and short-span bridges.

A second, more translucent, material based on the spinel of magnesium and aluminum oxides has been on the market since 1993 (see Figure 12.61). It has better esthetic properties but a 30% reduction in strength, and is more specifically suited to inlays, laminate veneers and crowns for vital teeth.

A third formulation containing 33% zirconium oxide is now undergoing trials, and should soon be available to complete the range (see Figures 12.62 and 12.63). It has poorer esthetic properties but is far tougher, and is intended for posterior bridges and splints.

Eventually, three different formulations will be available for fabrication of copings. As all three could be juxtaposed on the same coping, zirconium–aluminum oxide or spinel combinations might well be envisaged in order to take advantage of all the benefits offered.

This procedure is particularly recommended for the production of ceramics in the following cases:

- where great mechanical strength is required;
- if, for special reasons, bonding is preferable;
- where underlying teeth are stained;
- for producing short bridges or splints with no metal substructure.

Selected Reading

Current ceramic systems

Campbell SD, Kelly JR, The influence of surface preparation on the strength and surface microstructure of a cast dental ceramic. *Int J Prosthodont* 1989; **2**:459–66.

Giordano RA, Dental ceramic restorative systems. *Compendium* 1996; **17**:779–94.

Kelly J, Nishimura I, Campbell S, Ceramics in dentistry: historical roots and current perspectives. *J Prosthet Dent* 1996; **75**:18–32.

Lange FF, The interaction of a crack front with a second phase dispersion. *J Philos Mag* 1970; **22**:983–92.

Sadoun M, Bridges tout céramique avec la technique du "slip-casting". 7ème Symposium International de Céramique, Paris, Septembre 1988.

Sadoun M, Asmussen F, Bonding of resin cements to an aluminous ceramic: a new surface treatment. *Dent Mater* 1994; **10**:185–9.

Senoussi J-C, Les revêtements compensateurs a liant de phosphate en prothèse conjointe. Theses 3ème cycle en sciences ondontologiques, Académie de Paris, Juillet 1997.

Color and Light Transmission

Allen E, Metamerism – A study of dimension. *Color Eng* 1968; **6**:38–43.

Allen E, Some new advances in the study of metamerism. *Color Eng* 1969; **7**:35–40.

Bourrelly G, La vitalité en céramo-métallique. *Prothèse Dent* 1991; **56–57**:9–17.

Byou A, Kaoun K, Laâlou Y, Mariani P, Enquête épidermiologiques sur la vision des couleurs. *Cah Prothèse* 1997; Juin, no. 98.

Clark EB, The Clark Tooth Color System, Parts I & II. *Dent Mag Oral Top* 1933; **50**:139–52; 249–58.

Davis BK, Aquilino SA, Lund PS et al, Colorimetric evaluation of the effect of porcelain opacity on the resultant color of porcelain veneers. *Int J Prosthodont* 1992; **5**:130–6.

Duret F, Communication sur la spectrocolorimétrie. 7ème Symposium International de Céramique, Paris, Septembre 1988.

Hegenbarth EA, *The Creative Color System*. Chicago, IL: Quintessence, 1989.

Iranside JC, Light transmission of ceramic core material used in fixed prosthodontics. *Quintessence Dent Technol* 1993; **16**:103–6.

Jinoian V, Importance of proper light source in metal ceramics. In: Preston JD (ed) *Perspectives in Dental Ceramics. Proceedings of the Fourth International Symposium on Ceramics.* Chicago, IL: Quintessence, 1988: 229.

Jorgenson MW, Goodking RJ, Spectrophotometric study of five porcelain shades relative to the dimension of color, porcelain thickness and repeated firings. *J Prosthet Dent* 1979; **42**:96.

Kato T, Kuwata M, Tamura K, Yamamoto M, The current state of porcelain shade guides: A discussion. *Quintessence Dent Technol* 1984; **8**:559.

Lanthony P, Pathologie de la vision des couleurs, EMC. *Ophtalmologie* 1987; **1**:210–30.

Lemire PA, Burk BB, *Color in Dentistry*. Bloomfield, CT: Ney, 1975.

Levy H, Technique rationnelle de prise de teinte en prothèse dentaire. *Prothèse Dent* 1988; **6**:5–10.

Lombardi RE, The principles of visual perception and their clinical application to denture esthetics. *J Prosthet Dent* 1973; **29**:358.

Miller L, Organizing color in dentistry: esthetic dentistry. *J Am Dent Assoc* 1987; **26** (special issue):E-40.

Muia P, *The Four Dimensional Tooth Color System*. Chicago, IL: Quintessence, 1982.

Panier C, Approche de la spectrocolorimétrie dentaire. *Prothèse Dent* 1992; **67**:33–43.

Paul S, Pliska P, Pietrobon N, Schärer P, Transmission de la lumière par les composites de scellement. *Paradontie Dent Rest* 1996; **19**:165–73.

Pincus CL, Color and esthetics. In: *Dental Porcelain: The State of the Art*. Los Angeles: University of Southern California, School of Dentistry, 1977: 303.

Preston J, Etat actuel du choix de la teinte et de l'harmonisation des couleurs. *Odontologia* 1985; **2**:77–88.

Seghi RR, Johnson WM, O'Brien WJ, Spectrophotometric analysis of color differences between porcelain systems. *J Prosthet Dent* 1986; **56**:35.

Sieber C, Illumination in anterior teeth. *Quintessence Dent Technol* 1992; **15**:81–8.

Sieber C, A key to enhancing natural esthetics in anterior restorations: The light optical behavior of spinell luminaries. *J Esthet Dent* 1996; **8**:101–6.

Wright WD, *The Measurement of Colour, 3rd edn*. London: Hilgar & Watts, 1964: 185.

Yamamoto M, *Metal Ceramics*. Chicago, IL: Quintessence, 1985.

Yamamoto M, Une nouvelle évolution: la céramique OPALE, 1ère partie. *ATD* 1990; **1**:7–16.

Yamamoto M, Une nouvelle évolution: la céramique OPALE, 2è partie. *ATD* 1990; **1**:81–91.

Color of Natural Teeth

Atkinson D, Tetracycline and its effect on teeth. *Dent Assist* 1978; **47**:36–40.

Bailey RW, Christen AG, Bleaching of vital teeth stained with endemic fluorosis. *Oral Surg* 1968; **26**:871.

Baker KL, The fluorescent, microradiographic, microhardness and specific gravity properties of tetracycline-affected human enamel and dentin. *Arch Oral Biol* 1972; **17**:525–36.

Berman LH, Intrinsic staining and hypoplastic enamel: Etiology and treatment alternatives. *Gen Dent* 1980; **30**:484–8.

Bhasker SN (ed) *Orban's Oral Histology and Embryology, 11th ed*. St Louis, MO: Mosby, 1991.

Christensen GJ, Bleaching vital tetracycline stained teeth. *Quintessence Int* 1977; **8**:33–9.

Dzierzak J, Factors which cause tooth color changes: Protocol for in-office 'power' bleaching. *Pract Periodont Aesthet Dent* 1991; **3**:15–20.

Goldberg RA, Fortier JP, Garber DA, *Bleaching Teeth*. Chicago, IL: Quintessence, 1987.

Goldstein RE, *Change Your Smile*. Chicago, IL: Quintessence, 1984.

Hefferen JJ, Hefferen SM, Hoerman KC, Balekjian AY, Phosphorescence of enamel treated with stannous salts. *J Dent Res* 1967; **46**:196.

McDevitt CA, Armstrong WG, Investigation into the nature of the fluorescent material in calcified tissues. *J Dent Res* 1969, **48**:1108.

Horsley HJ, Isolation of fluorescent materials present in calcified tissue. *J Dent Res* 1967; **46**:106.

Nutting EB, Poe GS, A new combination for bleaching teeth. *Dent Clin North Am* 1967: 655-62.

Nyborg H, Bränström M, Pulp reaction to heat. *J Prosthet Dent* 1968; **19**:605–12.

Seale NS, McIntosh JE, Taylor AN, Pulpal reaction to bleaching of teeth in dogs. *J Dent Res* 1981; **60**:948–53.

Sieber C, *Voyage: Visions in Color and Form*. Chicago, IL: Quintessence, 1994.

Walton E, Eisenmann DR, Ultrastructural examination of various stages of amelogenesis in the rat following parenteral fluoride administration. *Arch Oral Biol* 1974; **19**:171–82.

Yamamoto M, *Metal Ceramics*. Chicago, IL: Quintessence, 1985.

Zaragoza VMT, Bleaching of vital teeth: technique. *Esto Modeo* 1984; **9**:7–30.

Treatment of Tooth Discoloration

Albers HF, Home bleaching. *Adept Report* 1991; **2**:9–17.

Aldana L, Wagner M, Frysh H, Baker F, Inactivation of tooth whitener peroxide by oral fluids. *J Dent Res* 1991; **70** (special issue): 424 (abstract 1266).

Bailey RW, Christen AG, Bleaching of vital teeth stained with endemic dental fluorosis. *J Dent Res* 1970; **49**:168–70.

Belkhir MS, Douki N, A new concept for removal of dental fluorosis stains. *J Endodont* 1991; **17**:288–92.

Bowles W, Lancaster LS, Wagner MJ, Reflectance and texture changes in bleached composite resin surfaces. *J Esthet Dent* 1996; **8**:229–33.

Bowles WH, Bokmeyer TJ, Staining of adult teeth by minocycline: Binding of minocycline by specific proteins. *J Esthet Dent* 1997; **9**:30–34.

Brighton DM, Harrington GW, Nicholls JI, Intracanal isolating barriers as they relate to bleaching. *J Endodont* 1994; **20**:228–32.

Brown G, Factors influencing successful bleaching of the discolored root-filled tooth. *Oral Surg* 1965; **20**:238–44.

Colon PG, Removing fluorosis stain for teeth. *Quintessence Int* 1971; **2**:89–93.

Costas FI, Wong M, Intracoronal isolating barriers: Effect of location on root leakage and effectiveness of bleaching agents. *J Endodont* 1991; **17**:365–8.

Croll TP, Enamel microabrasion followed by dental bleaching: Case reports. *Quintessence Int* 1992; **23**:317–21.

Croll TP, Segura A, Donly KJ, Enamel microabrasion: New considerations in 1993. *Pract Periodont Aesthet Dent* 1993; **5**:19–29.

Dishman MV, Corvey DA, Baughan LW, The effects of peroxide bleaching on composite to enamel bond strength. *Dent Mater* 1994; **10**:33–6.

Feinman RA, Bleaching vital teeth. *Curr Opin Cosmet Dent* 1994; 23–9.

Garcia-Godoy F, Dodge WW, Donohue M, Composite resin bond strength after enamel bleaching. *Oper Dent* 1993; **18**:144–7.

Goldberg M, Fortier JP, Guillot J, Lys Masanes J, Colorations de l'émail dentaire. *Actual Odontostomatol (Paris)* 1987; **157**:99–118.

Goldstein RE, *Esthetics in Dentistry*. Philadelphia, PA: Lippincott, 1976.

Goldstein RE, Garber DA, *Complete Dental Bleaching*. Chicago, IL: Quintessence, 1995.

Harrington GW, Natkin E, External resorption associated with bleaching of pulpless teeth. *J Endodont* 1979; **5**:344–8.

Haywood VB, Leech T, Haymann HO et al, Nightguard vital bleaching: Effects on enamel surface texture and diffusion. *Quintessence Int* 1990; **21**:801–6.

Haywood VB, Houck V, Heymann HO, Nightguard vital bleaching: Effects of varying pH solutions on enamel surface texture and color change. *Quintessence Int* 1991; **22**:775–82.

Haywood VB, History, safety and effectiveness of current bleaching techniques and applications of the nightguard vital bleaching technique. *Quintessence Int* 1992; **23**:471–88.

Haywood VB, Bleaching of vital and nonvital teeth. *Curr Opin Dent* 1992; **2**:142–9.

Haywood VB, Leonard RH, Nelson CF, Brunson WD, Effectiveness, side effects and long term status of nightguard vital bleaching. *J Am Dent Assoc* 1994; **125**:1219–26.

Haywood VB, Achieving, maintaining and recovering successful tooth bleaching. *J Esthet Dent* 1996; **8**:31–8.

Haywood VB, Leonard RH, Dickinson LG, Efficacy of six months of nightguard vital bleaching of tetracycline-stained teeth. *J Esthet Dent* 1997; **9**:13–19.

Heithersay GS, Dahlstrom SW, Marin PD, Incidence of invasive cervical resorption in bleached root-filled teeth. *Aust Dent J* 1994; **39**:82–7.

Holmstrup G, Palm AM, Lambjerg-Hansen H, Bleaching of discolored root-filled teeth. *Endodont Dent Traumatol* 1988; **4**:197–201.

Howell RA, The prognosis of bleached root filled teeth. *Int Endodont J* 1981; **14**:22–6.

Kehoe JC, pH reversal following in vitro bleaching of pulpess teeth. *J Endodont* 1987; **13**:344–8.

Kendell RL, Hydrochloric acid removal of brown fluorosis stains: clinical and scanning electron micrographic observations. *Quintessence Int* 1989; **20**:837–9.

Killian CM, Croll TP, Enamel microabrasion to improve enamel surface texture. *J Esthet Dent* 1990; **2**:125–8.

Lado FA, Stanley HR, Weisman MI, Cervical resorption in bleached teeth. *Oral Surg* 1983; **55**:78–80.

Leonard RH, Phillips C, Haywood VB, Predictors for sensitivity and irritation in nightguard trays. *J Dent Res* 1996; **75**:286.

Love MR, Effects of dental trauma on the pulp. *Pract Periodont Aesthet Dent* 1997; **9**:427–36.

McEvoy SA, Chemical agents for removing intrinsic stains for vital teeth: I Technique development. *Quintessence Int* 1989; **20**:323–8.

McEvoy SA, Chemical agents for removing intrinsic stains for vital teeth: II. Current techniques and their clinical application. *Quintessence Int* 1989; **20**:379–83.

MacIsaac AM, Hoen CM, Intracoronal bleaching: Concerns and considerations. *J Canad Dent Assoc* 1994; **60**:57–64.

Madison S, Walton RE, Cervical resorption following bleaching of endodontically treated teeth. *J Endodont* 1990; **16**:570–4.

Magne P, Megabrasion: a conservative strategy for the anterior dentition. *Pract Periodont Aesthet Dent* 1997; **9**:389–95.

Meyenberg KH, Luthy H, Schärer P, Zirconia post: A new all-ceramic concept for non-vital abutment teeth. *J Esthet Dent* 1995; **7**:73–80.

Miara P, Aesthetic treatment of discoloration of non-vital teeth. *Pract Periodont Aesthet Dent* 1995; **7**:79–84.

Nathoo SA, Richter R, Smith SF, Zhang YP, Kinetics of carbamide peroxide degradation in bleaching trays. *J Dent Res* 1996; **75**:286.

Rivera ME, Vargas M, Ricks-Williamson L, Considerations for the aesthetic restoration of endodontically treated anterior teeth following intracoronal bleaching. *Pract Periodont Aesthet Dent* 1997; **9**:117–28.

Rotstein I, Zalkind M, Mor C et al, In vitro efficacy of sodium perborate preparations used for intracoronal bleaching of discolored non-vital teeth. *Endodont Dent Traumatol* 1991; **7**:177–80.

Rotstein I, Friedman S, pH variation among materials used for intracoronal bleaching. *J Endodont* 1991; **17**:376–9.

Rotstein I, Friedman S, Mor C et al, Histological characterisation of bleaching – induced external root resorption in dogs. *J Endodont* 1991; **17**:436–41.

Rotstein I, Zyskind D, Lewinstein I, Bamberger N, Effect of different protective base materials on hydrogen peroxide leakage during intracoronal bleaching in vitro. *J Endodont* 1992; **18**:114–7.

Rotstein I, Lehr Z, Gedalia I, Effect of bleaching agents in inorganic components of human dentin and cementum. *J Endodont* 1992; **18**:290–3.

Rotstein I, Mor C, Friedman S, Prognosis of intracoronal bleaching with sodium perborate preparation in vitro: 1-year study. *J Endodont* 1993; **19**:10–12.

Rotstein I, Role of catalase in the elimination of residual hydrogen peroxide following tooth bleaching. *J Endodont* 1993; **19**:567–9.

Seale NS, McIntosh JE, Taylor AN, Pulpal reaction to bleaching of teeth in dogs. *J Dent Res* 1981; **60**:948–53.

Sommer R, *Clinical Endodontics*. Philadelphia, PA: W.B. Saunders, 1956: 456–9.

Steiner DR, West JD, A method to determine the location and shape of an intracoronal bleach barrier. *J Endodont* 1994; **20**:304–6.

Steiner DR, West JD, Bleaching pulpless teeth. In: Goldstein RE, Garber DA (ed) *Complete Dental Bleaching*. Carol Stream, IL: Quintessence, 1995: 101–36.

West JD, The aesthetic and endodontic dilemmas of calcific metamorphosis. *Pract Periodont Aesthet Dent* 1997; **9**:289–93.

Zach L, Cohen G, Pulp response to externally applied heat. *Oral Surg* 1965; **19**:515–30.

Zaragoza VMT, Bleaching vital teeth. *Bulletin d'Information Dentaire* 1983; 325.

Zaragoza VMT, Bleaching vital teeth: technique. *Esto Modeo* 1984; **9**; 7–30.

Transmission of Esthetic Information

Bengel W, The ideal dental photographic system? *Quintessence Int* 1993; **24**:251–6.

Chiche G, Pinault A, *Esthetics of Anterior Fixed Prosthodontics*. Chicago, IL: Quintessence, 1994.

Durand A, *La Pratique de la Macrophotographie, 2ème Edition*. Paris: Montel Editions, 1987.

Freehe C, Clinical dental photography. *Clinic Dent* 1976; **50**:1.

Ganz CH, Brisman SA, Tauro V, Computer video imaging: computerization, communication and creation. *QDT Yearbook* 1989; **13**:64.

Golub-Evans J, Unity and variety: essential ingredients of a smile design. *Curr Opin Cosmet Dent* 1994; 1–5.

Hornbrook DS, Porcelain jacket crowns: diagnostic try – ins for optimal aesthetics. *Pract Periodont Aesthet Dent* 1995; **7**:23–37.

Levine JB, Esthetic diagnosis. *Curr Opin Cosmet Dent* 1995; 9–17.

Magne P, Magne M, Belser UC, Natural and restorative oral aesthetics. Part 1: Rationale and basic strategies for successful aesthetic rehabilitations. *J Esthet Dent* 1993; **5**:161–73.

Magne P, Magne M, Belser UC, Natural and restorative oral aesthetics. Part 2: Aesthetic treatment modalities. *J Esthet Dent* 1993; **5**:239–46.

Magne P, Magne M, Belser UC, Natural and restorative oral aesthetics. Part 3: Fixed partial dentures. *J Esthet Dent* 1994; **6**:15–22.

Magne P, Magne M, Belser UC, The diagnostic template: key element of comprehensive aesthetic treatment concept. *Int J Periodont Rest Dent* 1996; **16**:561–9.

Mousques T, Benque G, La macrophotographie: la photographie argentine, 1ère partie. *Clin Odontologia* 1990; **2**:45–51.

Mousques T, Benque G, La macrophotographie: la photographie magnétique, 2ème partie. *Clin Odontologia* 1990; **2**:135–41.

Nathanson D, Current developments in aesthetic dentistry. *Curr Opin Dent* 1991; **1**:206–11.

Preston JD, Bergen SF, *Color Science and Dental Art: A Self-Teaching Program*. St Louis, MO: Mosby, 1980.

Qualtrough AJ, Burk FJT, A look at dental aesthetics. *Quintessence Int* 1994; **25**:7–14.

Rifkin L, Materdomini D, Facial lip reproduction system for anterior restorations. *J Esthet Dent* 1993; **5**:126–31.

Roach RR, Muia PJ, Communication between dentist and technician: An aesthetic checklist. In: Preston JD (ed) *Perspectives in Dental Ceramics: Proceedings of the Fourth International Symposium on Ceramics*. Chicago, IL: Quintessence, 1988: 445.

Rogé M, Preston JD, Color, light and the perception of form. *Quintessence Int* 1987; **18**:391.

Rufenacht C, *Fundamentals of Esthetics*. Chicago, IL: Quintessence, 1990.

Schärer P, Rinn LA, Kopp FR, Aesthetic guidelines for restorative dentistry. *Quintessence Int* 1982; **9**:179–86.

Shavell HM, Dentist–laboratory relationships in fixed prosthodontics. In: Preston JD (ed) *Perspectives in Dental*

Ceramics: Proceedings of the Fourth International Symposium on Ceramics. Chicago, IL: Quintessence, 1988: 429.

Stein RS, Kuwata M, A dentist and a dental technologist analyze current ceramo-metal procedures. *Dent Clin North Am* 1977; **21**:729.

Tjan AHL, Miller GD, The JGP: Some aesthetic factors in the smile. *J Prosthet Dent* 1984; **51**:24–8.

Tripodakis AP, Dental aesthetics, "oral personality" and visual perception. *Quintessence Int* 1987; **18**:405–18.

Ubassy G, *Shape and Color: The Key to Successful Ceramic Restorations.* Berlin: Quintessence, 1993: 31–9.

Yamamoto M, Bases fondamentales de l'esthétique (4 parties). *ATD* 1991, 1992; Vols 2 and 3.

Shape and Position of Teeth

Albino JE, Cunnat JJ, Fox RN et al, Variable discriminating individuals who seek orthodontic treatment. *J Dent Res* 1981; **60**:1661.

Ballard ML, Asymmetry in tooth size: A factor in the etiology, diagnosis and treatment of malocclusion. *Angle Orthodont* 1994; **14**:67.

Brigante RF, Patient-assisted esthetics. *J Prosthet Dent* 1981; **46**:18.

Dietschi D, Free-hand bonding in the esthetic treatment of anterior teeth: creating the illusion. *J Esthet Dent* 1997; **9**:156–64.

Fillion D, *The Resurgence of Lingual Orthodontics: Clinical Impressions, Vol 7.* Ormco Corporation, 1997.

Fillion D, Improving patient comfort with lingual brackets. *J Clin Orthodont* 1997; **31**:689–94.

Garn SM, Lewis AB, Walenga AJ, Maximum-confidence value for the human mesiodistal crown dimension of human teeth. *Arch Oral Biol* 1968; **13**:841.

Kokich VK, Aesthetics and anterior tooth position: An orthodontic perspective. Part III: Mediolateral relationship. *J Esthet Dent* 1993; **5**:11.

Lavelle CLB, The relationship between stature, skull, dental arch and tooth dimensions in different racial groups. *Orthodontist* 1971; Spring: 7.

Lombardi RE, The principles of visual perception and their clinical application to denture aesthetics. *J Prosthet Dent* 1973; **29**:358.

Mankoo T, Functional, biologic and esthetic considerations in the contemporary management of posterior endentulous areas in extensive rehabilitation. *J Esthet Dent* 1997; **9**:137–45.

McArthur RD, Determining approximate size of maxillary artificial teeth when mandibular anterior teeth are present. Part 1: Size relationship. *J Prosthet Dent* 1973; **29**:358.

Pound E, Applying harmony in selecting and arranging teeth. *Dent Clin North Am* 1962; March: 241–58.

Ricketts RM, The biologic significance of the divine proportion and Fibonacci series. *Am J Orthodont* 1982; **81**:351–70.

Salama MA, Aesthetic considerations for the generalist in the pre-adolescent orthodontic patient. Part 1: Dental alignment and soft tissue concerns. *J Esthet Dent* 1994; **6**:10–14.

Touati B, Improving aesthetics of implant-supported restorations. *Pract Periodont Aesthet Dent* 1995; **7**:81–92.

Touati B, The double guidance concept. *Int J Dent Symp* 1997; **4**:4–9.

Touati B, Excellence with simplicity in aesthetic dentistry. *Pract Periodont Aesthet Dent* 1997; **9**:806–12.

Williams JL, A new classification of human tooth forms with a special reference to a new system of artificial teeth. *Dent Cosmos* 1914; **56**:627.

Ceramic Laminate Veneers

Albers HF, *Tooth Colored Restoratives, 7th edn.* Cotati, CA: Alto Books, 1985.

Albers HF, Porcelain veneers. *Adept Report* 1990; **1**:17–28.

Augereau D, Tirlet G, Pierrisnard L, Les facettes céramiques collées. *Le Chirurgien Dentiste de France* 1992; **626**:69–76.

Barghi N, Berry TG, Post-bonding crack formation in porcelain veneers. *J Esthet Dent* 1997; **9**:51–4.

Barkmeier W, Menis D, Barnes DM, Bond strength of a veneering porcelain using newer generation adhesive systems. *Pract Periodont Aesthet Dent* 1993; **5**:50–5.

Bichacho N, Porcelain laminate veneers. Part 1: Preparation techniques. *Isr J Dent Technol* 1994; **3**:59.

Bichacho N, Porcelain laminates: Integrated concepts in treating diverse aesthetic defects. *Pract Periodont Aesthet Dent* 1995; **7**:13–22.

Black JB, Esthetic restoration of tetracycline-stained teeth. *J Am Dent Assoc* 1982; **104**:846–52.

Bowen RL, Development of a silica-resin direct filling material. Report 6333. Washington: National Bureau of Standards, 1958.

Bowen RL, A method for bonding to dentin and enamel. *J Am Dent Assoc* 1983; **107**:734–6.

Cavanaugh RR, Croll TP, Bonded porcelain veneer masking of dark tetracycline dental stains. *Pract Periodont Aesthet Dent* 1994; **6**:71–9.

Chalifoux P, Darvish M, Porcelain veneers: Concept, preparation, temporization, laboratory and placement. *Pract Periodont Aesthet Dent* 1993; **5**:11–17.

Chalifoux PR, Porcelain veneers. *Curr Opin Cosmet Dent* 1994; 58–66.

Chpindel P, Cristou M, Tooth preparation and fabrication of porcelain veneers using a double-layer technique. *Pract Periodont Aesthet Dent* 1994; **6**:19–28.

Chpindel P, Cristou M, Facettes en céramiques montées en double structure. *Quintessence Int* 1996; **17**: 9–16.

Chpindel P, Cristou M, Facettes en céramiques montées en double structure. *Clinic* 1996; **17**:9–17.

Christensen GJ, Veneering of teeth: State of the art. *Dent Clin North Am* 1985; **29**:373–91.

Christensen GJ, Procelain veneer update '93. *Clin Res Assoc Newsltr* 1993; 17.

Christensen GJ, Christensen RP, Clinical observations of porcelain veneers: A three-year report. *J Esthet Dent* 1991; **3**:174–9.

Crispin BJ, Full veneers: the functional and esthetic application of bonded ceramics. *Compendium* 1994; **15**:284–8.

Cristou M, Mise en oeuvre et applications des céramiques basse fusion. *Réal Clin* 1991; **2**:491–8.

Davis BK, Aquilino SA, Lund PS et al, Subjective evaluation of the effect of porcelain opacity on the resultant color of porcelain veneers. *Int J Prosthodont* 1990; **3**:567–72.

Degrange M, Influence des traitements de surface et des promoteurs d'adhésion sur les mécanismes d'adhérence des biomatériaux aux tissus dentaires calcifiés. Thèse: Doctorat d'état en odontologie, Paris V, 1990.

Degrange M, Sadoun M, Heim N, Les céramiques dentaires. 2e partie: les nouvelles céramiques. *J Biomater Dent* 1987; **3**:61–9.

Dunne SM, Millar BJ, A longitudinal study of the clinical performance of porcelain veneers. *Br Dent J* 1993; **175**:317–21.

El Sherif M, Jacobi R, The ceramic reverse three-quarter crown for anterior teeth: preparation design. *J Prosthet Dent* 1989; **61**:4–6.

Fahl N, Predictable esthetic reconstruction of fractured anterior teeth with composite resins: A case report. *Pract Periodont Aesthet Dent* 1996; **8**:17–30.

Faunce FR, Myers DR, Laminate veneer restoration of permanent incisors. *J Am Dent Assoc* 1976; **93**:790–2.

Freedman GA, McLaughlin GL, *Color Atlas of Porcelain Laminate Veneers*. St Louis, MO: Ishiyaku Euroamerica, 1990.

Fradeani M, Baducci G, Versatility of IPS Empress restorations. Part II. Veneers, inlays and onlays. *J Esthet Dent* 1996; **8**:170–6.

Fuzzi M, Bouillaguet S, Holz J, Improved marginal adaptation of ceramic veneers: A new technique. *J Esthet Dent* 1996; **8**:84–90.

Garber D, Porcelain laminate veneers: ten years later. Part I: Tooth preparation. *J Esthet Dent* 1993; **5**:56–62.

Garber DA, Porcelain veneers: to prepare or not to prepare? That is the question. *Cont Esthet Dent* 1996; **2**:1–7.

Gilmour AS, Stonee DC, Porcelain laminate veneers: a clinical success? *Dent Update* 1993; **20**:167–9.

Goldstein RE, Diagnostic dilemma: to bond, laminate, or crown? *Int J Periodont Rest Dent* 1987; **5**:9–29.

Gribble AR, Multiple diastema management: An interdisciplinary approach. *J Esthet Dent* 1994; **6**:97–102.

Haller B, Klaiber B, Hofmann N, Bonded all-ceramic restorations with the IPS Empress System. *Pract Periodont Aesthet Dent* 1993; **5**:39–48.

Harris JH, Temporization of teeth prepared for porcelain veneers. *Gen Dent* 1991; **39**:84.

Hartster P, Martinez J, Lingual-reverted laminate veneers: Clinical procedure and case presentation. *Pract Periodont Aesthet Dent* 1993; **5**:57–64.

Hastings JH, Conservative restoration of function and aesthetics in a bulimic patient: A case report. *Pract Periodont Aesthet Dent* 1996; **8**:726–36.

Hobo S, Porcelain laminate veneers with three dimensional shade reproduction. *Int Dent J* 1992; **42**:189–98.

Hsu CS, Stangel I, Nathanson D, Shear bond strength of resin to etched porcelain. *J Dent Res* 1985; **64**:296 (abstract 1095).

Huseyin A, Crack propagation within dental ceramic materials. MS Thesis, Columbus, Ohio: The Ohio State University, 1993: 109.

Ibsen R, *The New Cosmetic Dentistry Syllabus*. Santa Maria, CA: Dent-Mat Corp, 1987.

Jenkins CBG, Aboush YEY, Clinical durability of porcelain laminates over 8 years. *J Dent Res* 1987; **60**:1081.

Jordan RE, Suzuki M, Gwinnett AJ, Conservative applications of acid etch-resin techniques. *Dent Clin North Am* 1981; **25**:307–36.

Kinderknecht KE, Kupp LI, Aesthetic solution for large maxillary anterior diastema and frenum attachment. *Pract Periodont Aesthet Dent* 1996; **8**:95–102.

King DG, Methods and materials for porcelain veneers. *Curr Opin Cosmet Dent* 1995; 45–50.

Knellesen C, Editorial spécial collages. *Cah Prothèse* 1985; **52**:31.

Knellesen C, Une nouvelle céramique dentaire: la céramique de verre coulé. *Cah Prothèse* 1985; **50**:129–40.

Knight LD, Use of porcelain for treating a maxillary central diastema. *Gen Dent* 1992; **40**:498–9.

Laswell HR, Welk DA, Regenos JW, Attachment of resin restorations to acid pretreated enamel. *J Am Dent Assoc* 1971; **82**:558–63.

Liger F, Perelmuter S, Facettes et céramique. *Inf Dent* 1990; **72**:1425–32.

Lim CC, Case selection for porcelain veneers. *Quintessence Int* 1995; **26**:311–5.

Livaditis GJ, Cast metal resin-bonded retainers for posterior teeth. *J Am Dent Assoc* 1980; **101**:926–9.

Magne P, Facettes en céramique. *Cah Prothèse* 1996; Décembre, no. 96.

Magne P, Holz J, Stratification of composite restorations: Systematic and durable replication of natural aesthetics. *Pract Periodont Aesthet Dent* 1996; **8**:61–8.

Malament KA, Grossman DG, The cast glass ceramic restoration. *J Prosthet Dent* 1987; **57**:674–83.

Manolakis K, Paul SJ, Schärer P, Schmeltzhaftung aus gewahlter adhasiver Zementsysteme. *Dtsch Zahnarztl Z* 1995; **50**:582–4.

Mayenberg KH, Modified porcelain fused-to-metal restorations and porcelain laminates for anterior aesthetics. *Pract Periodont Aesthet Dent* 1995; **7**:33–44.

McLaren EA, Luminescent veneers. *J Esthet Dent* 1997; **9**:3–12.

Miller LL, Les systèmes de céramique: clinique et esthétique. *Cah Prothèse* 1993; **83**:73–9.

Miller MB, Porcelain veneers. *Reality Inform Sources Esthet Dent* 1996; **10**:443.

Môrig G, Aesthetic all-ceramic restorations: a philosophic and clinical review. *Pract Periodont Aesthet Dent* 1996; **8**:741 9.

Nakabayashi N, Kojima K, Masuhara E, The promotion of adhesion by the infiltration of monomers into tooth substrates. *J Biomed Mater Res* 1982; **16**:265–73.

Nakabayashi N, Identification of a resin-dentin hybrid layer in vital human dentin created in vivo: durable bonding to vital dentin. *Quintessence Int* 1992; **23**:135–41.

Nash RW, Closing a large central diastema. *Dent Econ* 1992; **10**:80–1.

Nash R, Indirect composite resin restorations: esthetic and function without wear of opposing natural teeth. *Compendium* 1997; **18**:838–42.

Nathanson D, Etched porcelain restorations for improved esthetics: 1. Anterior veneers. *Compend Contin Educ Dent* 1986; **7**:706–11.

Nixon RL, *The Chairside Manual for Porcelain Bonding*. Wilmington, DE: BA Videographics, 1987.

Nixon RL, Mandibular ceramic veneers: An examination of diverse cases integrating form, function and aesthetics. *Pract Periodont Aesthet Dent* 1995; **7**:17–26.

Nixon RL, Mandibular ceramic veneers: An examination of complex cases. *Pract Periodont Aesthet Dent* 1995; **7**:17–28.

Nixon RL, Masking severely tetracycline-stained teeth with ceramic laminate veneers. *Pract Periodont Aesthet Dent* 1996; **8**:227–35.

Nixon RL, Provisionalization for ceramic laminate veneer restorations: A clinical update. *Pract Periodont Aesthet Dent* 1997; **9**:17–27.

Nordbo H, Rygh-Thoresen N, Henaug T, Clinical performance of porcelain laminate veneers without incisal overlapping: 3 years' results. *J Dent* 1994; **22**:342–5.

Paul SJ, Schärer P, Effect of provisional cements on the bond strength of various adhesive bonding systems on dentin. *J Oral Rehab* 1997; **24**:8–14.

Paul SJ, Pliska P, Pietrobon N, Schärer P, Light transmission of composite luting resins. *Int J Periodont Rest Dent* 1996; **16**:164–73.

Pensler AV, Multiple-diastema porcelain laminate veneers: A case study. *Compend Contin Educ Dent* 1993; **14**:1470–8.

Perelmuter S, Launois C, Facettes de céramique collées. *Inf Dent* 1987:no. 1.

Perelmuter S, *L'Esthétique en Odontologie*. Paris: SNPMD Editeur, 1992.

Phillips RW, *Science of Dental Materials, 8th edn*. Philadelphia, PA: WB Saunders, 1982: 510.

Pinhas A, Avoiding patient disappointment with trial veneer utilization. *J Esthet Dent* 1997; **6**:277–84.

Portalier L, Diagnostic use of composite in anterior aesthetics. *Pract Periodont Aesthet Dent* 1996; **8**:643–52.

Rada RE, Jankowski JB, Porcelain laminate veneer provisionalization using light-curing acrylic resin. *Quintessence Int* 1991; **22**:291–4.

Radiguet J, Genini P, Les facettes de céramique collées. *Actual Odontostomatol (Paris)* 1988; **164**:781–90.

Retief D, Austin J, Fatt L, Pulpal response to phosphoric acid. *J Oral Pathol* 1974; **3**:114–22.

Robbins JW, Color characterization of porcelain veneers. *Quintessence Int* 1994; **22**:853–6.

Robbins JW, Porcelain veneers. In (ed R Schwartz et al): *Fundamentals of Operative Dentistry: Contemporary Concepts*. London: Quintessence, 1996; 349–71.

Rochette AL, Les onlays moyen d'ancrage en prothèse fixée – 14 ans de recal. St Paul, MN: 3M Company, 1975.

Rochette AL, A ceramic bonded by etched enamel and resin for fractured incisors. *J Prosthet Dent* 1975; **33**:287–93.

Rosenthal L, Diastema closure utilizing porcelain veneers – simple and advanced. *Dent Econ* 1994; **84**:63–4.

Rouse JS, Full veneer versus traditional veneer preparation: discussion of interproximal extension. *J Prosthet Dent* 1997; **6**:545–9.

Seghi RR, Dery IL, Rosenstiel SF, Relative fracture toughness and hardness of new dental ceramics. *J Prosthet Dent* 1995; **74**:145–50.

Senoussi JC, Les revêtements compensateurs à liant de phosphate en prothèse conjointe. Thèse pour le doctorat en sciences odontologiques, Paris, 1977.

Sheets CG, Taniguehi T, Advantages and limitations in the use of porcelain veneer restorations. *J Prosthet Dent* 1990; **64**:406.

Silverstone LM, Dogon IL, *Proceedings of an International Symposium on the Acid Etch Technique.* St Paul, MN: North Central Publishing, 1975.

Simonsen RJ, Thompson VP, Barrack G, *Etched Cast Restorations: Clinical and Laboratory Techniques.* Chicago, IL: Quintessence, 1983.

Sorensen JA, Strutz JM, Avera D, Materdomini D, Marginal fidelity and microleakage of porcelain veneers made by two techniques. *J Prosthet Dent* 1992; **67**:16.

Touati B, Pissis P, Miara P, Restaurations unitaires collées et concept des préparations pelliculaires. *Cah Prothèse* 1985; **13**:95–130.

Touati B, Aesthetic dentistry: not just "icing on the cake". *Pract Periodont Aesthet Dent* 1993; **5**:10–11.

Touati B, Miara P, Light transmission in bonded ceramic restorations. *J Esthet Dent* 1993; **5**:11–18.

Touati B, Bonded ceramic restorations: achieving predictability. *Pract Periodont Aesthet Dent* 1995; **7**:33–7.

Touati B, Préparation modifiée du bord incisif pour facettes de céramique. *Inf Dent* 1997; **21**:1396–9.

Trushkowsky RD, Masking tetracycline staining with porcelain veneers. *Dent Econ* 1994; **84**:64–5.

Ubassy G, *Formes de Contours.* Paris: Quintessence, CDP Ed, 1992.

Williamson RT, Techniques for aesthetic enhancement of porcelain laminate veneer restorations: A case report. *Pract Periodont Aesthet Dent* 1994; **6**:73–80.

Wohlwend A, Schärer P, The Empress technique: a new technique for the fabrication of full ceramic crowns, inlays, and veneers (in German). *Quitessenz Zahntech* 1990; **16**:966–78 (English reprints, 1991).

Wohlwend A, Schärer P, Céramique sans métal pour couronnes, inlays et facettes. *Art et Technique Dentaire* 1992: vol. 3, no. 1, Février.

Winter R, Visualizing the natural dentition. *J Esthet Dent* 1993; **5**:102–16.

Zappala C, Bichacho N, Prosper L, Options in aesthetic restorations: Discolorations and malformations – problems and solutions. *Pract Periodont Aesthet Dent* 1994; **6**:43–52.

Zyman P, Traitement de bords incisifs fracturés à l'aide de facettes céramique. *Inf Dent* 1997; **21**:23–9.

Ceramic and Modified Metal–Ceramic Crowns

Altglas SL, Conservation de l'esthétique du secteur incisivo-canin: apport de l'éruption forcée. *Actual Odontostomatol (Paris)* 1988; **42**:767–79.

Altglas A, Intérêt du lambeau esthétique pré-prothétique dans la réhabilitation du secteur antérieur. *Inf Dent* 1997, **21**:1149–54.

Boghosian A, Sunrise: A new and versatile ceramic system. *Pract Periodont Aesthet Dent* 1990; **3**:21–4.

Chalifoux P, Aesthetics of the single anterior temporary crown. *Pract Periodont Aesthet Dent* 1991; **3**:15–18.

Chiche G, Aoshima H, Functional versus aesthetic articulation of maxillary anterior restorations. *Pract Periodont Aesthet Dent* 1997; **9**:335–42.

De Rouffignac M, De Cooman J, Aesthetic, all-porcelain anterior restorations. *Pract Periodont Aesthet Dent* 1992; **4**:9–13.

El Mowafy OM, Fenton AH, Forrester N, Milenkovic M, Retention of metal–ceramic crowns cemented with resin cements: Effects of preparation taper and height. *J Prosthet Dent* 1996; **76**:524–9.

Ferrari M, Dalloca L, Kugel G, Bertelli E, An evaluation of the effect of the adhesive luting on microleakage for the IPS Empress crowns. *Pract Periodont Aesthet Dent* 1994; **6**:15–23.

Ferrari M, Tissue management and retraction technique combined with all-ceramic crowns: A case report. *Pract Periodont Aesthet Dent* 1995; **7**:87–94.

Ferrari M, All-ceramic fixed restorations: A preliminary clinical evaluation. *Pract Periodont Aesthet Dent* 1996; **8**:73–80.

Ferrari M, Cagidiaco MC, Kugel G, All ceramic fixed

restorations: a preliminary clinical evaluation. *Pract Periodont Aesthet Dent* 1996; **8**:73–80.

Fradeani M, Anterior maxillary aesthetic utilizing all–ceramic restorations. *Pract Periodont Aesthet Dent* 1995; **7**:53–66.

Haller B, Klaiber B, Hofmann N, Bonded all-ceramic restorations with the IPS Empress system. *Pract Periodont Aesthet Dent* 1993; **5**:39–48.

Holloway JA, Miller B, The effect of core translucency on the aesthetics of all-ceramic restorations. *Pract Periodont Aesthet Dent* 1997; **9**:567–74.

Hornbrook DS, Repair of class IV fractures utilizing resin and porcelain. *Pract Periodont Aesthet Dent* 1993; **5**:55–64.

Hornbrook DS, Porcelain jacket crowns: Diagnostic try-ins for optimal aesthetics. *Pract Periodont Aesthet Dent* 1995; **7**:29–37.

Howard NY, Optimizing anterior esthetics: Combining porcelain and periodontal considerations in single-tooth replacement. A case report. *J Esthet Dent* 1997; **9**:295–305.

Kern M, Thompson VP, Bonding to glass-infiltrated alumina ceramic: Adhesive methods and their durability. *J Prosthet Dent* 1995; **73**:240–9.

Lehner CR, Männchen R, Schärer P, Variable reduced metal support for collarless metal–ceramic crowns: A new model for strength evaluation. *Int J Prosthodont* 1995; **8**:337–45.

Leibenberg W, Achieving interdental integrity in resin-bonded posterior ceramic restorations. *Pract Periodont Aesthet Dent* 1994; **6**:43–51.

Levartovsky S, Golstein GR, Georgescu M, Shear bond strength of several new core materials. *J Prosthet Dent* 1996; **75**:154–8.

Magne P, Dietschi D, Holz J, Esthetic restorations for posterior teeth: practical and clinical considerations. *Int J Periodont Rest Dent* 1996; **16**:104–19.

McComb D, Adhesive luting cements – classes, criteria, and usage. *Compendium* 1996; **17**:759–73.

Meyenberg KH, Modified porcelain fused to metal restorations and porcelain laminates for anterior aesthetics. *Pract Periodont Aesthet Dent* 1995; **7**:33–44.

Meyenberg KH, Lüthy H, Schärer P, Zirconia posts: A new all-ceramic concept for nonvital abutment teeth. *J Esthet Dent* 1995; **7**:73–80.

Miller MB, Aesthetic anterior reconstruction using a combined periodontal/restorative approach. *Pract Periodont Aesthet Dent* 1993; **5**:33–40.

Mörig G, Aesthetic all-ceramic restorations: A philosophic and clinical review. *Pract Periodont Aesthet Dent* 1995; **8**:741–9.

Nixon RL, Masking severely tetracycline-stained teeth with ceramic laminate. *Pract Periodont Aesthet Dent* 1996; **8**:227–35.

Paul S, Schärer P, Post and core reconstruction for fixed prosthodontic restoration. *Pract Periodont Aesthet Dent* 1997; **9**:513–20.

Pietrobon N, Paul S, All-ceramic restorations: A challenge for anterior aesthetics. *J Esthet Dent* 1997; **9**:179–86.

Ross W, The all-porcelain bonded crown. *Pract Periodont Aesthet Dent* 1990; **2**:21–4.

Seymour K, Zou L, Samarawickrama DYD, Lynch E, Assessment of shoulder dimensions and angles of porcelain bonded to metal crown preparations. *J Prosthet Dent* 1996; **75**:406–11.

Wiskott HWA, Nicholls JL, Belser US, The relationship between abutment taper and resistance of cemented crowns to dynamic loading. *Int J Prosthodont* 1996; **9**:117–30.

Ceramic Inlays and Onlays

Bourrelly G, Comprendre les composites de laboratoire. *Prothèse Dent* 1996; Novembre, no. 121: 29–31.

Bourrelly G, Layet G, Clavel B, Polycarbonate micro chargé, applications en implantologie. *Prothèse Dent* 1997; Septembre, no. 130:12–21.

Christensen GJ, Acceptability of alternatives for conservative restoration of posterior teeth. *J Esthet Dent* 1995; **7**:228–32.

Dalloca LL, Brambilla R, Indirect ceramic system for posterior esthetics. *J Esthet Dent* 1997; **9**:119–23.

Ferrari M, Davidson CL, In vivo resin-dentin interdiffusion and tag formation with lateral branches of two adhesive systems. *J Prosthet Dent* 1996; **75**:250–3.

Finger WJ, Fritz U, Laboratory evaluation of one-component enamel dentin bonding agents. *Am J Dent* 1996; **9**:206–10.

Fuhrer N, Restoring posterior teeth with a novel indirect composite resin system. *J Esthet Dent* 1997; **9**: 125–30.

Fuhrer N, Helft E, A combined porcelain onlay/amalgam restoration for an endodontically treated posterior tooth. *Pract Periodont Aesthet Dent* 1995; **7**:13–20.

Jackson R, An aesthetic, bonded inlay–onlay technique using "total etch". *Pract Periodont Aesthet Dent* 1990; **2**:26–31.

Jackson R, Aesthetic inlays and onlays: A clinical technique update. *Pract Periodont Aesthet Dent* 1993; **5**:18–26.

Jackson R, Esthetic inlays and onlays. *Curr Opin Cosmet Dent* 1994; 30–9.

Koczarski M, Utilization of Ceromer inlays/onlays for replacement of amalgam restorations. *Pract Periodont Aesthet Dent* 1998; **10**:405–12.

Lutz F, Krejci I, Besek M, Operative dentistry: The missing clinical standards. *Pract Periodont Aesthet Dent* 1997; **9**:541–8.

Miara P, Semi-indirect technique for a composite onlay. *Fenestra* 1997; no. 8:5–9.

Miara P, Aesthetic guidelines for second-generation indirect inlay and onlay composite restorations. *Pract Periodont Aesthet Dent* 1998; **10**:423–31.

Nash R, Leinfelder K, Radz G, An improved onlay system. *Compendium* 1997; **18**:98–104.

Perdigao J, Lambrechts P, Van Meerbeek B et al, The interaction of adhesive systems with human dentin. *Am J Dent* 1996; **9**:167–73.

Rifkin RL, Maxillary reconstruction utilizing a second generation glass reinforced resin material. *Pract Periodont Aesthet Dent* 1998; **10** (March suppl):2–7.

Tay FR, Gwinnett AJ, Wei Shy, Micromorphological spectrum from overdrying to overwetting acid-conditioned dentin in water-free, acetone-based, single-bottle primer/adhesives. *Dent Mater* 1996; **12**:236–44.

Terata R, Characterization of enamel and dentin surfaces after removal of temporary cement: Study on removal of temporary cement. *Dent Mater* 1993; **12**:18–28.

Terata R, Nakashima K, Obara M, Kubota M, Characterization of enamel and dentin surfaces after removal of temporary cement: Effect of temporary cement on tensile bond strength of resin luting cement. *Dent Mater* 1994; **13**:148–54.

Tirlet G, Vers une prothèse moins mutilante, bridge d'inlay onlay en fibres de verre et Ceromer collé. *Inf Dent* 1998; 15 janvier, 73–82.

Trushkowsky RD, Ceramic optimized polymer: the next generation of esthetic restorations: Part 1. *Compend Contin Educ Dent* 1997; **18**:1101–10.

Tyas MJ, Clinical evaluation of five adhesive systems: Three-year results. *Int Dent J* 1996; **46**:10–14.

Van Meerbeek B, Conn LJ Jr, Duke ES, et al, Correlative transmission electron microscopy examination of nondemineralized and demineralized resin–dentin interfaces formed by two dentin adhesive systems. *J Dent Res* 1996; **75**:879–88.

Weaver WS, Blank LW, Pelleu GB, A visible light - activated resin cured through tooth structure. *Gen Dent* 1988; **36**:236–7.

Index

Page numbers in *italic* refer to illustrations and tables.